The Body Almanac

Also by Neil McAleer

EARTHLOVE: A SPACE FANTASY
THE COSMIC MIND-BOGGLING BOOK

THE
BODY
ALMANAC

Mind-Boggling Facts About
Today's Human Body
and High-Tech Medicine

NEIL McALEER

Doubleday & Company, Inc., Garden City, New York 1985

Library of Congress Cataloging in Publication Data

McAleer, Neil, 1942–
   The body almanac.

   Bibliography: p. 350.
   Includes index.
   1. Body, Human—Miscellanea.   2. Medical technology—
Miscellanea.   I. Title.
QP38.M38   1984   612   82-45298
ISBN 0-385-17982-0
ISBN 0-385-17983-9 (pbk.)
Copyright © 1985 by Neil McAleer

TO
Anna Hollek Strauss
Sophia Strauss Green
Constance Green-McAleer

Contents

Foreword

Doctors and demographers disagree with one another as to the exact date when medicine began to make a substantial contribution to human welfare. Even today there are those who insist that improvements in diet and in public hygiene outweigh the contributions of technical medicine. Certainly, if one looks back over the last two hundred years one can see improvements in life expectancy which were underway long before it was possible to identify any particular advance in scientific medicine; and most of these favorable changes can be explained in terms of social policy as opposed to drugs or surgery. Nevertheless, the comfort and safety which we've come to regard as part of our birthright in the Western world are increasingly dependent upon the technical services which the medical profession can now offer; and although it would be foolish to deny how much we owe to clean cities and rational nutrition, it would be just as rash to overlook the safety net which medical science extends beneath us. Unfortunately this safety net is usually represented in terms of miracle drugs and heroic operations, whereas the efficiency of modern medicine is largely due to the fact that we now have an accurate working model of the human body which allows us to make interventions whose outcome can be predicted with increasing certainty.

To a large extent this is the result of our having mechanized the picture of biological function and this in turn is the consequence of mechanizing our picture of the natural world—a development which became irreversibly established after the scientific revolutions of the seventeenth century. Naturally the discovery of new drugs and the invention of surgical techniques have given doctors a power which their ancient predecessors would have envied. In fact it's hard to imagine what it must have been like to practice medicine without antibiotics or anesthetics. I suspect however that none of these would make a noticeable difference without the scientific knowledge which guides their administration.

Without our having to deny whatever it is that makes our humanity such a distinctive feature of the natural world, we have come to accept the fact that the best way of describing our biological functions is in terms which resemble the ones which explain the action of machines and chemical systems. Far from dehumanizing us, this has given us a better opportunity of enjoying our humanity in safety. And in Neil McAleer's splendidly illustrated book you can see just how far we've come from the days when William Harvey turned the medical world upside down.

JONATHAN MILLER
Camden Town
London, England

Preface

The largest medical library in the world, the National Library of Medicine near Washington, D.C., contains over 3.1 million items of medical information in its collection. This international resource is an ideal example of the information explosion that has overwhelmed all of us in the latter half of the twentieth century.

This book intends, in an entertaining way, to shrink this "information overwhelm" and focus on today's human body as well as on the high-tech medical technology that helps to keep it healthy. No claim of completeness is made for obvious reasons. All medical specialties are going through constant and rapid transformation. There is no way to freeze this change, capture a topic thoroughly, and keep it completely up-to-date.

Some 24,000 medical periodicals from around the world are subscribed to by the National Library of Medicine each year; and tens of thousands of new books and other printed matter are added to the collection annually, bringing in about 18 million new pages of material. This does not include the dozens of computer data bases that provide easy access to some 5 million references, nor does it include thousands of audiovisual resources.

The total holdings of the National Library of Medicine amount to more than 1 billion pages of medical information. If they were laid end to end, these pages could encircle the planet earth at the equator about 7 times. No single human being, indeed no large professional group of scientists and doctors could possibly comprehend, retain, or fully utilize this vast depository of information. Certainly no one book or multivolume set of books can do more than scratch the surface. R. R. Bowker's *Medical Books and Serials in Print, 1984* lists some 70,000 books and periodicals in its pages—just a healthy *selection* of the total in-print literature. If the amount of medical literature astounds us, it is nothing compared to how the human body itself can boggle our minds. Just as the quasar—that bewildering, superpowerful, billions-of-light-years-distant cosmic object—is at the edge of human comprehension, so too is the human body with its microcosmic mysteries and its 100 trillion cells.

For example, the genetic stuff of life, the molecules of DNA, bend and twist 1 billion times every second. If all *your* body's tightly coiled DNA material in its trillions of cells could be unraveled, it would stretch from the earth to the sun and back 1,000 times!

The human brain, with its 10 billion nerve cells packed more densely than any other tissue in the body, has the ability to record over 86 million bits of information each day of our lives. Memory, it has been estimated, can hold some 100 trillion bits of information in a lifetime. The brain's electrical circuitry alone, discounting its extremely complex chemistry, is some 1,400 times more complex than today's global telephone network. Each and every second, your brain forms at least 100,000 different chemical reactions which in turn create thoughts, emotions, and actions.

The senses provide a constant flow of information to the brain, but 99 percent is screened out as irrelevant. The human eyes provide 80 percent of the raw sensory data that does reach the brain—the same sensory data that is used as the basis for all our knowledge. Our marvelous eyes are so sensitive that, under ideal conditions from a mountaintop at night, they can detect a match flame some 50 miles (80 kilometers) away.

While our eyes look outward to the world, medical technology has created high-tech eyes that peer into the living body and its organs. Where once the scalpel cut into flesh and muscle to uncover a medical problem, today safe, computerized scanning devices allow doctors to see inside the patient—a blocked coronary artery, perhaps, or the living brain processes of an epileptic patient. The Dynamic Spatial Reconstructor is a state-of-the-art example of this imaging equipment. It can generate 75,000 cross sections of the body in 5 seconds, the same time it took an earlier-generation CAT scanner to produce just one.

Technology is not just "seeing" inside the body as never before, re-creating microcosmic structures for the first time ever; it is also replacing portions of broken or diseased bodies with used donor parts or man-made parts—from an ever-increasing inventory which includes arms, eyes, and hearts, and even sexual organs. In a 5-year period, some 4 million people—more than the population of Chicago, Madrid, or Manchester, England—have had replacement body parts implanted. At the same time, the uses of medical lasers as a surgical tool are growing and hold great promise for the twenty-first century. Even today laser microbeams can scour coronary arteries of plaque or repair the aging, deteriorating eye and restore sight.

It is, however, medical technology's successes with the life process itself—gene manipulation, in vitro fertilization, embryo transfers, surgery in the womb—that have profound implications for human life. While some of these breakthroughs can give the joy of children to childless couples, they also present unsettling moral dilemmas and potential for abuse that disturb many people. Some of us ask: Will a brave new world of assembly-line reproduction and programmed lives become a reality?

Then there is the fun of sex. All of us spend much more time thinking about sex than actually having it. An average sex life of 50 years—between the ages of 20 and 70—amounts to only about 600 hours of actual intercourse, which averages out to an unimpressive 2 minutes each day. In actual time, it's mental sex that dominates our lives. However, during a sexually active lifetime of 50 years, a couple releases enough energy to equal that of 1 ton of TNT or one great and spectacular fireworks display. Just 10 minutes of sexual pleasure generates enough energy to run all household appliances—including a bedroom air conditioner—for those 10 minutes.

On a larger scale, humanity's total sexual energy, including every person who has ever lived, would equal about 25,000 megatons of TNT. If such energy were released all at once, it would render planet earth uninhabitable. As it happens, the billions of little sexual explosions that constantly occur on planet earth give us sexual pleasure, satisfied bodies, and sometimes offspring.

Today's human body and high-tech medicine are without question the stuff of information overwhelm. *The Body Almanac* breaks up this overwhelm into accessible nuggets of entertaining facts. So enjoy, learn, marvel . . . let your body boggle your mind.

Acknowledgments

Two Doubleday editors deserve my special gratitude: Betty Heller, who gave me encouragement and fresh-eyed editorial advice throughout the project; and Jim Menick, my sponsoring editor, who thought well of the book proposal and took it to the editorial board.

My wife Connie helped me with some of the research, sorting through subjects within the "information overwhelm," as did Timothy M. Erdman and Mary Jane Francis Smith.

For information and photographs, I especially thank Dale Blumenthal of the Audio-Visual Branch of the National Institutes of Health. I also thank the following people at the various institutes of NIH for their generous help: Dr. Jeffery Barker, Larry Blaser, Don Bradley, Marsha Corbett, Dr. Monique Dubois-Dalcq, Richard J. Feldmann, Susan Johnson, Arlene Soodak, and Lynn Trible.

In addition, for helping to obtain hard-to-find or one-of-a-kind micrographs and photographs, I wish to thank: Deborah Clayton and Betty Partin at the Centers for Disease Control; Janet Deg and Edward Y. Zavala of Sharp Cabrillo Hospital; Ronald G. Cohn of Syntex Research; Barbara Clark, Collagen Corporation; Al Hicks and Dr. Arnold Scheibel, UCLA School of Medicine; Dr. Karen Holbrook, University of Washington; John M. Basgen, University of Minnesota; Stacie W. Newman, Stanford University Medical Center; Rosemary Klein, Mayo Clinic; Sharon Herczog, Medical Engineering Corporation; Harold May, Dow-Corning Wright; Corinna Kaarlela, University of California at San Francisco; Dr. Lourens J. D. Zaneveld, University of Illinois; Dr. E. S. E. Hafez, Wayne State University School of Medicine; Dr. Frederick D. Curcio III, Sherman Associates; Deborah A. Pitzrick, Dacomed Corporation; and Mary P. Grein, Eli Lilly and Company.

The Body Almanac

Chapter One

Room at the Top:
The Human Brain

Brain Ahoy!

The brain is a soft lump of tissue, weighing about 3 pounds in the average adult. It is so full of water that it would slump like Jell-O if taken out of the skull and placed on a flat surface. The brain's outer portions are 85 percent water, which makes it one of the most watery solid tissues in the body. It also floats in liquid—the cerebrospinal fluid —which is derived from blood, itself composed of 80 percent water. Our thoughts are therefore anchored in a portable ocean.

Brain Spurts

There are 2 important growth spurts in the human brain after conception. The first takes place 8 to 13 weeks into pregnancy, when billions of cells called neuroblasts are formed. These eventually develop into the all-important nerve cells (neurons). Prenatal nutrition at this time is known to affect the number of neurons in the embryo's brain.

The second brain spurt begins some 2½ months before birth and continues until about the age of 2. Rapid growth of the interconnections between neurons takes place during this period. The degree to which the neurons are wired up and connected is a more important factor in intelligence than the number of neurons.

On the average, over 30,000 neurons are formed each minute from the time of conception to the baby's birth.

The General Store

How much information can the human brain store? During a lifetime of 70 years, a person's memory holds at least 100 trillion (100,000,000,000,000) bits of information. The entire *Encyclopaedia Britannica* is only 200 million bits. One hundred trillion is 10,000 times the number of neurons (nerve cells) in the brain, which would give each cell 10,000 bits of information. For a transistorized computer to have the same potential as the brain, it would have to be larger than Carnegie Hall. An advanced computer with microelectronic "chip" innards would still weigh more than 20,000 pounds (9,072 kilograms).

Chasing Evolution

A very simple worm has about 23 neurons in its nervous system; an ant has about 250, a bee about 900. The entire human brain has about 10 billion neurons.

A team of researchers analyzed and mapped nerve-cell connections of the simple worm; it took them 3 years with the help of a computer to do the job. If the same rate of progress were made with a bee, it would take the team 117 years. For a human brain, it would take more than 1.3 billion years. If human evolution continues, the cerebral cartographers would never catch up with the brain's growth.

Brains on Brains

Many human brains are concentrating on human brains—inside-the-head research. These scientists produce more than 500,000 research papers every year.

Brain in the Eye

A Stockholm researcher has found an unusual place to study brain tissue and its development. Nerve tissue from various regions of the brain such as the cerebellum, hippocampus, and cerebral cortex have

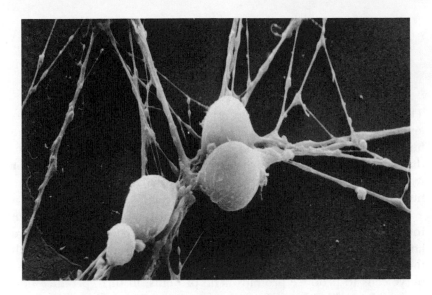

The human brain contains some 10 billion nerve (neuron) cells. On the average, over 30,000 neurons are formed each minute from the time of conception to the baby's birth. Magnification: 2,400X. Courtesy Monique Dubois-Dalcq, M.D., Steve Waisbren, and the National Institutes of Health.

usually been placed into a laboratory culture dish for study. The unique, new method transplants the brain tissue (about 1/12 of an inch, 2 millimeters in size) into the living eyes of laboratory animals by inserting it through an incision in the cornea. The slit heals quickly, and the graft, on the outer surface of the iris, is fed by the animal's blood supply.

The brain-in-the-eye technique enables researchers to record the tissue's electrical activity and to actually see it develop by looking deep into a mouse's or a rat's eye!

Needling the Brain

Modern research has developed an electrode that can painlessly penetrate a single brain cell and record its activity. The electrode, made of extremely fine glass, is invisible to the human eye—only 1 millionth of an inch (2.5 millionths of a centimeter) in diameter. This is over 6,000 times finer than a human hair.

Sexual Brains

The brains of women and men are different—that is the consensus emerging from several specialized disciplines of brain research. The final conclusions are not yet in, but there is enough data to indicate that the sexual hormones—testosterone for men and estrogen for women—affect structures such as the hypothalamus deep within the human brain.

The primitive hypothalamus at the base of the brain stem has been found to contain specific areas where hormones accumulate. These are known as receptor sites. When either of the 2 hormones match up with the specific receptors, they shape the brain's structure by directing the nerve cells to produce proteins. The proteins, in turn, produce new nerve cells early in life which may create permanent brain structures that differ in men and women.

Some researchers have also found evidence that the cerebral cortex is different in men and women. The right eye and ear (controlled by

The gray and furrowed cerebral cortex is more densely packed with cells than any other part of the human body.

The hippocampus, part of the primitive limbic system deep inside the brain, plays an important role in short-term memory and learning. Courtesy National Institutes of Health.

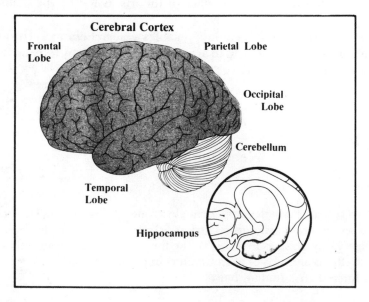

Cerebral Cortex

Frontal Lobe

Parietal Lobe

Occipital Lobe

Cerebellum

Temporal Lobe

Hippocampus

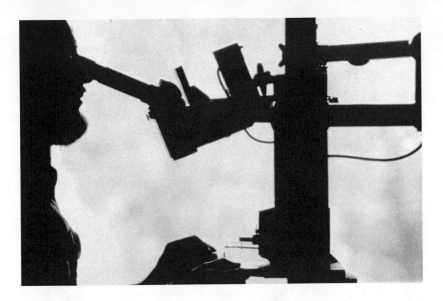

A researcher uses apparatus that enables microelectrodes to penetrate a single brain nerve cell. Made of extremely fine glass, the microelectrodes are only 1 millionth of an inch (2.5 millionths of a centimeter) in diameter. Courtesy National Institutes of Health.

the left brain hemisphere) are more sensitive in women, while the opposite is generally true for men. Men are usually better at spatial (right-hemisphere-controlled) tasks, women at verbal (left-hemisphere-controlled) ones. This further supports the view that the right hemisphere dominates the brains of men, the left hemisphere the brains of women.

This research is controversial and will no doubt be misinterpreted by many. But it has great potential value. Every woman and man may someday have his or her own personal brain profile, detailing the strengths and weaknesses of each individual's cerebral matter and allowing each person to make more intelligent decisions about his or her life's work and style. But domestic chores will conveniently fall in the space between the left and right hemispheres for both sexes and will no doubt still be negotiated.

Between the Hemispheres

A dense bundle of nerves, about 4 inches (10 centimeters) long, connects the left and right cerebral hemispheres in the human brain. This bridge, the corpus callosum, has steadily thickened and increased in size during the course of human evolution. Only in the last few decades has its main function been discovered: It is the link between 2 brains, the left and right hemispheres, that are specialized and serve different functions. This bundle of 200 million nerve fibers unifies awareness and allows our left and right brains to share their unique memories and learning.

Each of the 200 million nerve fibers in the corpus callosum fires a nerve impulse on the average of 20 times a second, which means that each second—right now, in fact—there are 4 billion nerve impulses firing back and forth *between* your left and right hemispheres.

Deceptive Symmetry

The apparent physical symmetry of the brain's 2 hemispheres is deceptive. Even though it has been known for some time that the right half of the brain controls vision, movement, and sensation for the left side of the body, and that the left half does the same for the right side of the body, the last 3 decades of brain research have discovered much about the left and right specializations in the human brain. Among other discoveries has been the detection of physiological differences in the

A bridge of brain tissue—the corpus callosum—connects the left and right hemispheres, and each second 4 billion nerve impulses fire back and forth between the 2 hemispheres. Courtesy National Institutes of Health.

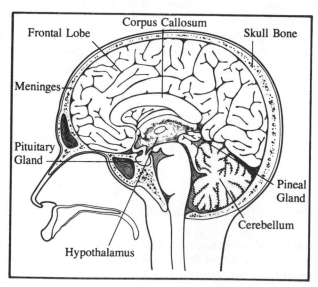

relative sizes of specific areas. This active area of research will no doubt yield many fruitful discoveries in the next few decades.

The left hemisphere has been labeled "the talking hemisphere." It almost always dominates in speech, reading, writing, and logical thinking. This side specializes in analytical and verbal skills and excels in processing information in a serial, linear fashion, bit by bit. Some scientists refer to the functioning of the brain's left side as the active mode.

The right side of the brain is adept at space and pattern perception. While the right is nonverbal and cannot express speech, it dominates in visual imagery (color patterns, face recognition) and spatial relations (math, perception of depth, and music). When you see an image in your "mind's eye" or in a dream, it comes from the right side of your brain. This hemisphere processes information differently than the left; it synthesizes, putting ideas together in a holistic fashion, and grasps relationships.

These are strong brain-side preferences, but they are rarely cut and dried—nature has provided a good degree of redundancy for survival. Both left and right hemispheres have decision-making ability, and it is probable that the logical and long-term storage processes (subverbal) occur on both sides. Even though the right side cannot produce speech, it still can comprehend it.

The discoveries of right and left brain specialization should not blind us to the fact that the 2 hemispheres interact and cooperate in an integrated way—they do, in a variety of ways, many of which are not now understood.

All in all, the 2 hemispheres are fairly similar at this point of human evolution, with some functional specialization. Possibly these specializations have evolved in relatively recent human history. The hemispheres in the brains of early Homo sapiens may well have been wholly redundant as survival backups for one another (considering all the skull smashing that went on back then).

The future of the human brain may be further differentiation. Specialization of the hemispheres may be the first step in the long-term process of cerebral evolution. In the distant future, our right and left brains may no longer be symmetrical and may appear physically different. They may even comprehend and communicate in entirely different languages. This will happen on an evolutionary time scale if it happens at all—a gradual process over thousands, perhaps millions, of years.

Sex Life of the Hypothalamus

The limbic system is a primitive region of the human brain that evolved millions of years ago. It is made up of several structures and is located around the brain stem (reptilian brain), the most primitive area that regulates vital organs such as heart and lungs. Because the limbic system evolved before the cerebrum, which houses our higher thought processes, it has been called the "old mammalian brain." Another nickname, the "nose brain," came about because it contains so many connective nerves involved with our sense of smell.

The hypothalamus, a cluster of nerve cells at the center of the limbic system, controls our basic drives and emotions—hunger, thirst, aggression, rage, pleasure, sex. Electrical stimulation of this region has provoked all the basic emotional responses, including sexual arousal. The hypothalamus interacts with the pituitary gland to control sexual behavior by releasing hormones into the bloodstream, and if certain areas of the hypothalamus are injured, the sex urge disappears completely.

The continued sex life of the hypothalamus, however, seems assured for most of us because it is so well protected by its location in the middle of the limbic system, which is in the middle of the brain. This physical protection helps to ensure the continuation of our species.

More than Ma Bell

The brain's neuron circuitry, only partly mapped by neurologists after hundreds of years, is just one dimension of the human mind. These signal pathways interact with the intricate molecular chemistry that does everything from rejuvenating neuron cells to creating long-term memories. Considered alone for comparison, our head's circuitry is still impressive: It is 1,400 times more complex than today's global telephone network.

Going to Great Lengths

If all the nerve-cell connections—the axons and dendrites—from a human brain could be placed end to end to form a living wire, it would

---

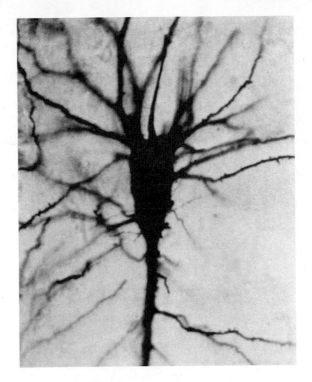

If all the brain's nerve-cell connections were stretched out end to end, they would encircle the earth many times. Our brain's circuitry, not including its chemistry, is 1,400 times more complex than today's global telephone network. Courtesy Arnold Scheibel, M.D., UCLA School of Medicine.

be long enough to encircle the earth many times. The dendrites alone could stretch an estimated 100,000 miles (160,000 kilometers).

The Microelectric Brain

The amount of electricity involved in sending brain signals along nerve fibers is infinitesimal when compared to the amount used by common household appliances.

The difference in electrical potential between the outside and inside of a nerve-cell membrane is usually between 1/20 and 1/10 of a volt, and it is this difference (constantly maintained by the inside-outside sodium and potassium ionic balance) that propagates the nerve impulse along the axon.

This microelectricity is equal to about 1/40 the amount it takes to light up a standard 2-battery flashlight, and $1/1,600$ the amount used to heat up a toaster.

Global Brain Power

If the brain's metabolism were converted into energy, it would equal that of a 20-watt light bulb. All the energy of the 4.6 billion brains of planet earth would add up to 90 billion watts—enough energy to keep 15 New York Cities well lit and humming, and equal to one fourth of the present energy capacity of the United States.

Raceways of the Mind

The fastest nerve impulses travel from neuron to neuron in the brain at about 250 miles (402 kilometers) per hour. These record in-skull speeds occur in the long nerve fibers—the longer the fiber, the faster the electrical impulse. The insulation in the membranes of these nerve fibers cannot compete with well-insulated, man-made copper wire—a million times more energy leaks out. But because these signals are chemically amplified at each neuron, this energy loss does not hinder their transmission. The brain can easily generate 100 impulses every second along the nerve fibers. This amounts to more than 225 billion in an average lifetime—as many as there are stars in the Milky Way Galaxy. But the speed of the brain's impulses is slow by cosmic standards. At their top speed of 250 miles an hour, it would take them an average human lifetime to reach the planet Mars. The *Viking 1* spacecraft reached the planet in 11 months.

Rapid Fire

Most brain nerve cells have the ability to rapid-fire repeatedly—200 times per second is not uncommon. Some specialized neurons—for example, the Renshaw cells in the spinal cord that act as a negative feedback control of motor neurons—can fire up to 1,600 times a second. The fastest turnaround time for a cell to fire its signal again is about $1/500$ of a second, about the same time it takes a balloon to pop (not the noise of course, which is longer).

Make no mistake; this is fast by human standards. We can take no voluntary action in this time span. But this microspeed pales when compared to computers that have switching speeds of a billion times each second. The human mind has created something many times faster than itself—well over a half a million times faster.

Axon Relay

Each neuron has a major fiber extension called an axon, which conducts impulses away from the nerve-cell body toward the synapse (the gap between 2 adjacent nerve cells), and a number of fibrous branches called dendrites, which receive the incoming signals. Axons are much longer than dendrites, up to several feet in some parts of the body, and end with microscopic branches that have "terminal buttons" at their ends. These send signals to receiving dendrites of another cell.

The axons of most large neuron cells are covered by myelin, a fatlike substance that insulates and accelerates the electrical impulse as it travels to the terminal buttons. Along this myelin sheath are the nodes of Ranvier, small gaps which allow the extracellular fluid to directly contact the cell membrane. These are the sites of electric excitation of the nerve impulse, which is reinforced at each gap. Ranvier's nodes are about 1 micron* (1/25,000 of an inch) in width, and there is one node about every 1,000 microns (1/25 of an inch).

This means that there could be more than 1,000 Ranvier's nodes in the body's longest axons—those of the motor neurons to the lower limbs, which can be over 40 inches (1 meter) in length. Who would have thought that 1,000 microamplifiers are needed to send a 1/10 of a volt signal such a short distance?

Molecules Galore

The transmitter molecules that translate the electrical impulses of the brain into chemical ones before they are squirted across the synaptic gap can be produced in microtime—over 1,500 each second. Before their journey they are stored in tiny pockets called synaptic vesicles, and a single axon terminal may have thousands of these. Each of these pockets contains between 10,000 and 100,000 molecules, and so 100 million (50,000 molecules times 2,000 pockets) transmitting molecules at the terminal of an axon would be a good average. Multiply this

---

* The *micron*, 1 millionth of a meter (1/25,000 of an inch) in length, is usually referred to as the "micrometer" in today's usage. For space considerations, this book uses the shortened form, "micron."

number by 100 trillion (the number of synapses) and you have a total number that would take 300-plus generations over 10,000 years to count.

The Axon Express

Each neuron has a complex two-way transportation system, and it all takes place within nerve-cell dimensions that range in size from $1/2,500$ of an inch (10 microns) to $1/250$ of an inch (100 microns). In the 1960s, scientists learned that the entire contents of a brain cell's axon move toward its terminal buttons and the synaptic gap.

The cell's nucleus synthesizes enzymes and other complex molecules to constantly renew the neuron—the only body cell that cannot reproduce itself. The transport system is needed to move proteins and other molecules from the cell body down the length of the axon to the transmitting terminals and back again. There is a one-way flow from the cell body to the axon terminals that is important for regeneration. This is the slow traffic, which moves about $1/25$ of an inch (1 millimeter)

Neurons are the only body cells that cannot reproduce themselves, and each one contains a complex two-way circulation system to rejuvenate the cell and replenish the chemical transmitters at the end of the axons. This all takes place in cells as small as $1/2,500$ of an inch (10 microns) in diameter. Courtesy Dr. Jeffery Barker, National Institutes of Health.

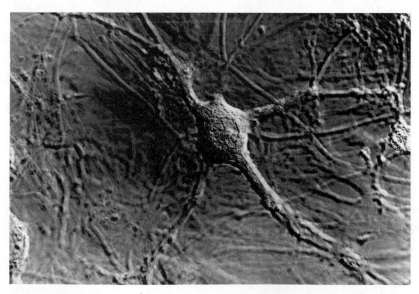

each day. The other system has two-way traffic and is a superhighway. These fast lanes move more specialized cellular components, such as some of the enzymes that help to produce the chemical transmitters, at speeds of between 4 and 8 inches (10 and 20 centimeters) a day. These are long distances, relatively speaking, representing a distance that is 20,000 times the length of a small neuron cell. It is analogous to the extinct Brachiosaurus dinosaur, about 100 feet (30 meters) in length, walking 380 miles (608 kilometers) in 1 day.

The Dendrite Nexus

The receiving dendrites of the brain's neurons display a myriad variety of branching patterns. Tens and often hundreds of them branch out like a tree from a single cell, each one again branching into smaller twigs that finally become tiny terminal "spines." These spines, small bumps that can number in the thousands, are where the nerve impulses are received from other cells.

The spines are the finest dendritic branches in the human brain and can be as small as 1 millionth of an inch (1/40 of a micron) wide, and an average of 1/12,500 of an inch (2 microns) in length. Divide a fine human hair about 7,000 times and you have the width.

The output neuron of the brain's cortex (pyramidal neuron) has some 4,000 spines to receive impulses; they are able to receive nerve information from upward of 100,000 other fibers.

Microgaps by the Trillions

The microscopic gap between 2 neurons (from the terminal buttons of an axon to the tiny spines of a dendrite) is called the "synapse," which is from the Greek word *synaptein,* meaning to clasp tightly. These sites are where the neurons communicate to one another through a complex electrochemical process whereby the cell's electrical pulse is converted into a chemical squirt that travels to receptors on the dendrite of the next cell and is, most of the time, again converted to an electrical pulse that travels onward.

Each synaptic gap is less than 1 millionth of an inch (2.5 millionths of a centimeter) wide. It has been estimated that the number of synapses in the human brain may be as many as 100 trillion (10^{14})—at least 500 times the number of stars in our Milky Way Galaxy.

The Head's Glue

The cells that support, protect, and nourish the neuron cells in the human brain and central nervous system are called glia cells *(glia means glue in Greek)*. They are 10 times more numerous than neurons —the average human brain has about 100 billion glia, which make up about half its mass.

Brain researchers generally agree that these cells do more than protect and nourish neurons, but all their functions are not yet clearly understood. Some researchers believe that glia play a vital role in the memory process, and there is some evidence that, like neurons, they form their own communicating network. They may have a more direct role in processing information than traditionally believed, perhaps by regulating the electric field around neurons. One theory states that glia cells absorb and store potassium released by neuronal activity. This would make neurons directly dependent on glia for their activity.

Glia, like all other body cells except neurons (whose numbers are more or less fixed at birth), retain the ability to reproduce themselves throughout a person's lifetime. Recent animal research indicates that the brain's cortex can increase in size at any age. This is contrary to the

Glia cells nourish and support the brain's nerve (neuron) cells. The human brain contains about 100 billion glia cells, which make up half its mass. Courtesy National Institutes of Health.

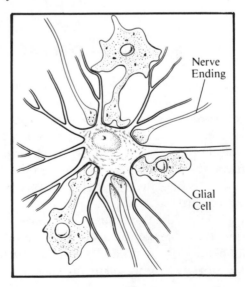

traditional belief that intelligence inevitably declines with age. How can this happen if the number of neurons cannot increase? The answer: The number of glia increases around the neurons and the cell bodies of the neurons increase in size. But the environment must be rich in stimuli for this to happen. It won't happen to older people who sit in easy chairs all day.

The Brain's Barricades

Brain neurons are extremely specialized cells, and they pay the price by being extremely sensitive to toxic substances and small molecules such as amino acids that are in the bloodstream. Because of this sensitivity, a protective mechanism has evolved for nerve cells—a selective filtration system known as the blood-brain barrier which, in effect, isolates the brain from the body's general circulation system. The brain is thereby protected from surges in the levels of blood sugar, amino acids, and toxic substances that come from everyday eating and drinking. If a person's diet is drastically altered and harmful to health, the brain is the most protected organ in the human body.

How are these toxic substances kept away from the brain? The blood vessels have a tight sheath of glia cells (the supporting brain cells), and this makes them impermeable to all but the smallest molecules such as those of life-giving oxygen. Even glucose, the blood sugar that along with oxygen allows the brain to stay alive, must be taken into the inner sanctum by special transport mechanisms.

The blood-brain barrier is therefore an important consideration in the research and development of drugs that act directly on the brain. To be effective, the drug's molecules must be either very small or soluble in the membrane fat of the glia cells. If not, they are denied entry by the protective sheaths. These microbarricades, at their thickest, are 60 times thinner than a human hair.

Rewiring the Brain

The future looks bright for correcting central nervous disorders caused by brain damage, stroke, senility, and Parkinson's disease. Recent animal research has shown that severed central nerves regenerate themselves in a useful way, and that implanted young nerve cells grow well and help to correct damaged areas of the brain. Researchers have observed the implanted nerves hooking up to blood vessels in the animal brains, suggesting that the conducting axons of the grafted nerve cells grow functional connections.

The nerves to be transplanted may be hard to come by, however. The use of nerves taken from aborted or miscarried human fetuses will no doubt be ethically controversial. A more likely source may be nerves taken from the patient's own body. For example, nerve tissue from the adrenal gland could be transplanted into the brain's damaged area.

The distant future promises to reverse brain damage—no matter what the cause.

Patched-Up Brains

The brain is a privileged site for tissue transplants because, unlike other parts of the body, it does not reject them with immune defenses.

Probably one of the first disorders that will be successfully treated with brain tissue transplants is Parkinson's disease, which is caused by

In the future, tissue transplants from the adrenal glands to the substantia nigra area of the brain may cure Parkinson's disease. Courtesy National Institutes of Health.

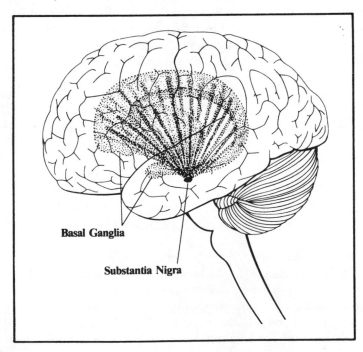

Basal Ganglia

Substantia Nigra

the degeneration of nerve cells deep within the brain. These specialized neurons produce dopamine, a substance important to the control of body movements. The tremors and other symptoms of Parkinson's disease are caused when these cells degenerate and fail to secrete dopamine.

Encouraged by laboratory successes, surgeons believe they can transplant healthy cell tissue from the adrenal glands into the brain. The new tissue will produce dopamine and normal body movement will be restored.

The same methods may eventually be applied to other brain disorders such as replacing damaged tissue caused by strokes. Candace Pert, a neurologist at the National Institute of Mental Health, good-humoredly speculates that in the far future "kindness" neurons could be transplanted from the brains of women to the brains of men.

Renewed Brains

All the molecules of the human body are constantly being broken down and rejuvenated. The smallest molecules in the human brain may live for just a few minutes. Ninety percent of all protein molecules in the brain are broken down and replaced in no more than 2 weeks. This fact should give rise to great optimism during our duller moments.

Future Brains

The size of the human brain has not changed much in the last 50,000 years, but size is not everything. Cooperation among many human brains, unified in their goals, means collective brainpower that transcends any individual, even a genius. The footprints on the moon are tangible evidence of this enhanced power of the collective brain.

In the last 3 decades, brainpower has left the confines of the human skull and is making explosive advances in computer technology. It has been predicted that the storage capacity of computers will equal that of the human brain by the end of this century—some 10 billion facts in a brain-sized space, running on about 20 watts of power. After that, watch out! Once computers have reached the general intelligence of a human being and are able to educate themselves, their powers will increase exponentially and their capacity will be incalculable.

There will therefore be 2 types of brains in the future—our inside-

.the-skull brains and our outside-the-skull brainchildren, the computers and their artificial intelligence.

Our in-skull brains will be enhanced or treated with novel products coming from brain chemistry research. Our mental powers will probably be retained throughout our lives, without the usual deterioration of memory and other faculties. Some mental powers such as learning and memory will be enhanced as well as prolonged. Brain pacemakers, groups of targeted electrodes, will help control the pain and destructiveness of severely neurotic and schizophrenic patients. Damaged brains will be repaired with tissue transplants and regenerated tissues.

Some scientists believe that our outside-the-skull brainchildren—the computers—will be the future direction of our evolution. But there is no reason why humankind and computers cannot work in cooperation with one another. They could, in fact, be electronically linked as some scientists have suggested. Tiny bionic computer terminals could be surgically implanted in the skull or any fleshy part of the body, or for that matter carried in a pocket or built into eyeglasses. These "biocomps" would have radio contact with the large computers, which would assist the human brain in calculations, handling information, and so forth. These bionic computer terminals would wed the human brain and its own original creation, the computer, and they would be very small—about the size of a postage stamp and less than 1/12 of an inch thick. In this way, human brains grow into the future.

The Head's Pharmacy

Brain chemistry research has exploded in recent years, leading to the general view that the neurons' complex circuitry and currents are anchored in an ocean of chemicals and chemical reactions. Much of this research is focusing on the brain's tiny peptides (short chains of amino acids) that are believed to carry signals between the nerve cells and produce countless effects on behavior and emotion.

In the mid-1970s, a group of tiny peptides named enkephalens was found whose members acted as natural painkillers of the brain. A few years later, the peptide dynorphin (from the Greek word *dynamikos*) was identified as an extremely powerful analgesic—200 times greater than morphine. Spin-off research is soon expected to develop a potent and nonaddictive painkiller. Drug companies, in fact, are already hard at work.

The number of chemical reactions in the human brain is enough to intimidate the most dedicated specialist. Each second—right now—some 100,000 different chemical reactions are occurring in your brain, forming your thoughts, emotions, and actions.

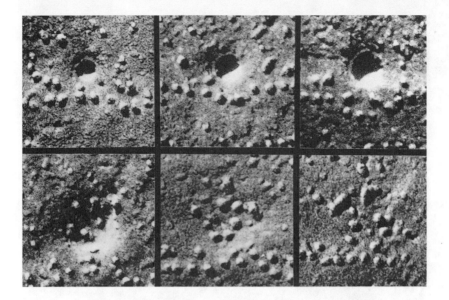

The release of neurotransmitters, magnified 500,000 times. This 6-step sequence occurred in about 1/4 of a second. Some 1,500 transmitting molecules squirt across the synaptic gap between 2 brain cells each second, activating the neuronal network that gives us thought, memory, and dreams. Courtesy National Institutes of Health.

Chemical Communicators

More than 30 different chemical transmitters (neurotransmitters) have been discovered in the human brain, each one of which has a unique molecular structure, which can be "recognized" and "judged" by a specialized receptor on the next cell's dendrites across the synaptic gap. Each of these chemical transmitters is found in specific populations of neurons that serve specialized functions in the brain. They are chemically coded messengers that communicate throughout the brain and activate the neuron network. Because of this complex chemistry, each receptor site "knows" the source of the signal and can accept or reject it.

Acetylcholine, the first neurotransmitter identified and the most common one found in the human brain, is a simple organic molecule (acetic acid and choline). In animal research, administration of acetylcholine to different sites of a cat brain caused strikingly different kinds of behavior. Injection in one area caused circling movements; in an-

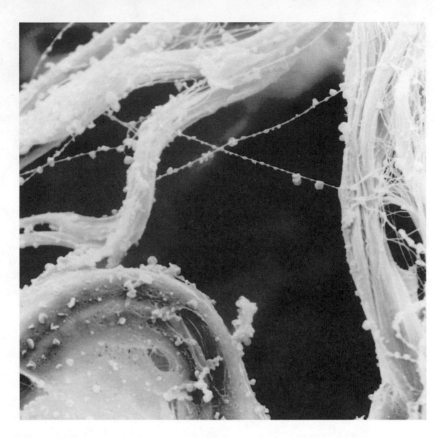

Brain tissue, frozen in time by a scanning electron microscope and magnified 4,000 times. The beaded strands are believed to be nerve networks along which packets of neurotransmitter molecules move toward the synapse. Courtesy Arnold Scheibel, M.D., Linda Paul, Itzhak Fried, and the UCLA School of Medicine.

other, a catatonic-like response; in another, rage and attack; and in still another, peaceful purring.

Immediately after acetylcholine is transmitted across the nerve synapse, it is broken down into acetic acid and choline again. If this did not happen, the molecule would accumulate in the human brain, the nervous system would be overstimulated, and the muscular control of breathing would eventually fail, causing paralysis and death. This important communicating chemical for the brain is actually very toxic. In fact, the lethal effects of nerve gas and some insecticides are caused by the toxic accumulation of acetylcholine. The human brain, luckily, knows when to use it, when to get rid of it, and when to create more of it. For us, it is a messenger of life, not of death.

ROOM AT THE TOP:

Memory Mysteries

On what physiological base does memory exist? Cells, molecules, circuits of cells? Final solutions to the mysteries of memory are decades away, but scientists have narrowed their area of search in the last few years. Memory is somehow created in the microscopic electro-chemical labyrinth of the human brain. Specific memories are not to be found in specific synapses or pathways of synapses as once believed; rather they are thought to be a pattern of chemical changes over the entire brain that involve synapses in some way.

The molecular key to learning behavior (as distinct from memory) appears to be in the protein synthesis of ribonucleic acid (RNA) which is found in all cells. Components of these proteins, peptides (small chains of molecules), have been linked to learned behavior in laboratory studies where rats were conditioned to stay in light areas and avoid dark areas, which they normally do not do. A brain extract from these trained rats was then injected into untrained rats and they then also avoided the dark! Next the extract was analyzed and chemically synthesized. This peptide was named scotophobin ("fear of darkness" in Greek), and was made up of 15 amino acids. Even more amazing is that the synthetic scotophobin also produced dark avoidance in goldfish.

This research, done in the 1970s by George Ungar and his associates at the Baylor University School of Medicine in Houston, was continued, and another specific protein called anelatin was found to be responsible for rats responding to an electric bell. What this research implies is that every learned skill (and think of the millions upon millions in contemporary society) has its own specific chemical!

The Memory Labyrinth

All the memories of a human brain are probably not encoded the way conditioned learning is—it would be mathematically impossible for each fact and concept in our memory bank to have a specific protein, even though encoding does work mathematically for learned behaviors. One theory proposes that memory is embedded in a particular nerve network by chemical changes. This is where synapses come into play. If a repeated flow of nerve impulses over a specific pathway could alter the existing synaptic connections and cause new ones to grow, this would result in a neuron network that holds a specific memory.

The synapse changes would be caused by proteins synthesized in the nerve cell's body, proteins that affect the rate at which transmitter substances are released in the synaptic gap. The difference between short- and long-term memory may be the difference between short-term electrical activity and long-term chemical imprinting at synapses over a neural circuit.

Another theory proposes that permanent traces of specific memories are distributed throughout the entire brain. This concept was made credible in the laboratory by neurologist Karl Lashley. After training rats to run mazes, he removed small parts of their brains, then larger portions, but the behavior memory remained, even though it became impaired as more tissue was removed. From this work evolved the theory of "equipotentiability," which states that memory is evenly distributed throughout the brain. If this theory proves correct, the human brain would be like a hologram, in which every single chip of the whole plate contains the complete image and can reproduce it, although not as sharply.

Whichever theory of memory eventually becomes fact, it cannot be a simple one—not when you know that our brains have the ability to record over 86 million bits of information each day of our lives.

Memory Pills?

Vasopressin, one of the brain's peptides (short chains of amino acids), has been found to improve memory and learning in laboratory tests in both animal and human subjects.

The human subjects were tested each day for memory and learning responses over a period of 2 and 3 weeks, sometimes being given a synthetic analogue of vasopressin and sometimes a placebo. The subjects consisted of 3 groups: healthy, depressed, and senile. All 3 groups showed improved memory and learning responses when they were given the synthetic vasopressin as compared to when they were given the placebo. The researchers do not yet know by which means vasopressin accelerates memory and learning, and so it may be several years before we can take memory pills.

Behavior's Building Blocks

If every possible learned behavior has its own unique protein chain, then the potential number of substances that can be coded to elicit specific behaviors is practically infinite. This is because each of these proteins is made up of amino acids, and 20 principal amino acids can be found in any position along the chain. Just a 2-amino-acid chain has 400 possible combinations.

The potential number of combinations in a chain of 15 amino acids (the same number that scotophobin, the fear-of-darkness peptide, has) is about 36.5 quintillion—36,500,000,000,000,000,000.

Nothing New

The hippocampus is a U-shaped structure at the base of the forebrain and is important in transferring information from short-term to long-term memory. This is also probably true for other structures on the inner surface of the temporal lobes. This specific memory function was discovered in the 1950s, when a patient with a brain disorder had much of his hippocampus and other temporal lobe structures removed. After the operation it was discovered that he could not learn new information and store it in the long-term memory. Even though this person's knowledge and skills up to the time of the operation were intact, new information could only be retained for a few minutes with the aid of verbal rehearsal and with no distractions. It never got transferred to long-term memory. For this man, nothing new could ever become something old. He lived moment by moment, never knowing where he kept his toothbrush or his dinner plates.

Face to Face

Faces. Who hasn't spent some leisure cafe time just watching the faces of people that pass? Who hasn't been jolted by the sudden recognition of a face from the past? None of us. It is therefore not surprising to learn that the human brain has a specialized neural network which exists just to recognize faces.

The brain receives the visual image of a human face in a few hundredths of a second, analyzes its many details in about a quarter of a second, and then totally synthesizes the face in less than a second. That's to say we recognize a face immediately, even if it sometimes takes considerably longer to "place" the face. Researchers have also learned that memory for photographs of faces previously unseen is best 1.5 minutes after they are seen, suggesting that optimal short-term memory can be formed in about 90 seconds.

A brain disorder, prosopagnosia, destroys a person's ability to recognize faces. It is a very specific limitation because the patient can read and name objects correctly; what he cannot do is form a connection between a person's face and that person's identity. A few words allow the patient to immediately identify the individual by voice, but he could never know a person by face recognition alone—not even when he faces his own face in the morning mirror!

The Night Jerk

All of us have experienced the sudden spasm that causes our entire body to jerk while falling asleep. It's as if our bodies have been zapped with an electric shock.

This spasm, referred to as a myoclonic jerk or nocturnal jerk, is a natural occurrence during light sleep and is believed to result from a release of muscle tension, brought about by a neural burst of activity in the cerebral cortex of the brain.

This night jerk is gone in a fraction of a second and deep nondreaming sleep usually follows. If your bed partner is close to you and also drifting off, your jerk may cause him or her to jerk in response. A few soothing words, however, should quickly bring on sleep.

Tossing and Turning by the Millions

Last night as many as 50 million Americans slept badly, and about half the population tossed and turned at least once last week.

There are hundreds of nondrug remedies for occasional insomnia, but the best by far—one that usually works and is preferred by most of us—is good sex.

A No-Sleep Death

A person will die from total lack of sleep sooner than from starvation. Death will occur after about 10 days without sleep, while starvation takes a few weeks. A no-sleep death is no gradual fadeaway affair—it is preceded by insanity.

Sleep Motions

During an average night's sleep, we move 40 to 70 times. These shifts help prevent the pooling of blood, maintain some muscle tone, and help keep the proper balance of oxygen and carbon dioxide.

These motions rarely have anything to do with the activities of our dreams—running, swimming, loving, even flying. What, then, causes the muscles to remain dormant during these often intense dream activities? Why aren't we enacting our dreams and sleeprunning, sleepswimming, sleeploving, and trying to play Peter Pan by attempting to fly out the bedroom window?

Recent research has shown that the motor neurons, which usually cause muscles to contract, are subjected to a chemical that inhibits them from responding during the dream state. If this dream chemical does not fire properly, the so-called paralysis mechanism does not function, and there is a sleep disorder.

Sleepwalking is a deep-sleep disorder rather than a REM-dream-period one. The chemical inhibitor obviously doesn't do its job, and the muscles work when they shouldn't. While there have been many humorous scenes and jokes about sleepwalking, the problem is no laughing matter. Sleepwalkers have killed their own family members by accident or have tried to elope with boyfriends on imaginary ladders.

Sleep Senses

Your brain can still register sounds when asleep, even distinguish between different noises and words, and no matter how deeply you're sleeping, you'll usually react to someone calling your name. The touch sense, too, remains alert during sleep, and you'll react when touched. How you respond (by movement or verbal response and to what degree) depends on whether you "know" the person's touch.

Sleeptalking

Talking aloud during sleep usually relates to a dream. Sleeptalkers can also hear someone talking to them and can often incorporate a question into the dream and answer the person. On waking, however, they don't remember talking.

Deep sleeptalking is more fragmented than shallow (rapid-eye-movement or REM) sleeptalking, and so an awake bed partner has a good idea of the sleeper's level of sleep.

Sleep's Thermometer

How many hours you sleep does not depend, as might be expected, on how many hours you've been awake. Instead, it is body temperature rhythms that determine the duration of sleep. If body temperature is low when you go to sleep, you'll probably sleep your normal number of hours. If you fall asleep when your temperature is high and do not have an alarm clock or other external stimuli, you'll likely sleep much longer.

Dream time is also affected by body heat—you'll have more dreams if sleep begins during a low-temperature cycle.

Sleep and LSD

Specialized neurons found in the brain stem secrete a transmitter substance called serotonin, which is believed to be one of the major substances involved in producing sleep. A drug, p chlorophenylalanine, has been found to inhibit the production of serotonin, and injections of it have caused prolonged wakefulness in laboratory animals. Some researchers believe that serotonin and less well-known sleep substances accumulate in the brain stem or the cerebrospinal fluid and eventually bring on sleep.

The drug LSD (lysergic acid diethylamide) resembles serotonin in chemical structure and counteracts some of its chemical actions by occupying the neuron receptor sites that usually receive serotonin. With both substances, the neural network that processes sensory data from the outside world is disrupted—that much sleep and LSD have in common.

Right-Side Dreams

Our dreams originate in the right hemisphere of our brain, which is known to be nonverbal, emotional, and laden with images. Case histories of patients with right-brain damage support this view; they stop dreaming and are no longer able to have internal visual images even while awake. The same holds true for split-brain patients who have had the bridge (corpus callosum) severed between their left and right hemispheres. They may have vividly recalled many dreams before the operation, but none afterward. Even though they still may be dreaming in their right hemisphere, there is no way their verbal-oriented left brain can know or recall the dreams.

While the right-brain hemisphere clearly dominates in the dream and REM state, the left hemisphere probably asserts itself gradually as sleep progresses. This would explain why verbal activity in dreams is reported most often just before waking and rarely earlier in the sleep cycle. Dream recall also increases dramatically toward morning, which may also be explained by the increasing influence of the left hemisphere.

Researchers know that everyone has several periods of REM each night, and so the people who say they do not dream really do. They just don't remember their dreams. They are unable to transfer the right-brain images to their verbal left brain, and this ability varies to a great extent among individuals. It may be that women remember dreams better than men because their hemispheres are more integrated and less specialized.

The imagery of right-brain dreams is not just with us during sleep. Studies have shown that most people daydream about one third of their waking hours, and some researchers believe that the daydream state may be the more natural, normal mode of the human mind, while action-oriented and problem-solving mental states require a willed effort that must be conditioned and learned. Right-side dreams are therefore always ready to appear—night or day, asleep or awake—and they affect what we actually do and achieve in complex ways we never fully understand.

Dreams and Drunks

If you like to dream, take it easy on the booze. Alcohol suppresses the periods of rapid eye movements when dreams occur, and overindulgence has also been shown to disrupt the second half of the sleep period. Suppression of REM sleep is dangerous. In the case of people with alcohol and other drug addictions, it can cause hallucinations and psychotic symptoms. Dreamlike images are forced from normal sleep by these addictions and erupt into the waking state. Such displaced images follow the same basic occurrence pattern as REM periods.

So if you drink heavily, perhaps in response to fading "dreams," just remember that you run the risk of real nightmares.

Sound Dreams

People born blind do not have dream images—no rapid eye movements during sleep. They do dream, but their dreams are sound tracks without pictures.

Dream Erections

Most men have erections every hour to hour and a half during sleep, and this frequency is equal to the number of dream (REM) periods each night. Involuntary sexual response during sleep also happens to women, who develop vaginal lubrications at about the same time intervals.

It is now known that almost all of a man's REM periods during sleep are preceded by an erection which may last for an entire REM period— be it the first short one (about 10 minutes) or the longest one (about an hour) that occurs just before waking. Even if the REM periods are prevented in the sleep laboratory, erections occur during other phases of sleep about the time the REM period would have occurred.

This rhythm of nightly erections is not fully explained, but it appears to be set by some internal clock rather than being a response to erotic dream images. Probably the hypothalamus, a primitive region of the brain that is known to exert control over our sexual behavior, is activated as a result of the electrical and chemical processes that occur during the REM sleep periods. Laboratory studies indicate that this archaic brain structure becomes active during REM.

Whatever the reason for nocturnal tumescences, it's too bad loving couples cannot take better advantage of them. Just as it is possible to develop better dream recall, it may also be possible to sacrifice a REM period to enjoy these nighttime male and female sexual responses. Some of our dreams would literally come true and the afterglow would make for happy mornings.

Wet Dreams

All men have experienced wet dreams or so-called nocturnal emissions during sleep. These ejaculations occur most often to young men in their teens and early twenties when they are at their "sexual peak"— their hormonal peak, at least. The number of wet dreams varies considerably—from 12 a week to 1 a month—and the frequency does not necessarily have a connection to the number of sexual encounters while awake.

Dreams Revisited

Most dreams are forgotten, but thanks to sleep researchers and their laboratories, verbal recall of dream experiences is now routinely recorded, analyzed, and compared. There is a growing dream library with branches all over the world that hold tens of thousands of recalled dreams. Studies have shown the differences between the dreams of women and men, children and adults. Generally, women dream more about family, men about money and jobs. While women dream about men and women, men tend to dream about other men. Women dream more often about indoor settings, men about outdoor ones. Young children have snapshot dreams without a story line, but these frame-by-frame dreams become movies with a plot after the age of 8 or 9.

For those of us who are unable to recall most of our dreams, there are some simple techniques that can improve recall without a visit to a sleep laboratory. During the workweek, set the alarm back 30 to 45 minutes. Chances are that you'll wake up during a dream period. On weekends, sleep late and don't set an alarm; wake up naturally. A tape recorder or pencil and notepad should be within easy reach.

Since about one fourth of our sleep time is spent dreaming, revisiting dreams can teach us much about ourselves.

> "We are such stuff
> As dreams are made on. . . ."

wrote Shakespeare in *The Tempest*.

Chapter Two

Filling Up the Furrows: The Senses

EYES AND SIGHT

The New Eye

A new, revised human eye has been created by advanced medical skills and technology over the last 3 decades, and the explosive pace of progress will continue to produce other marvelous medical feats that will save or improve our vision in the decades to come.

If the eye's cornea becomes scarred by injury or disease—and there are tens of millions of such cases worldwide each year—surgeons can remove the damaged cornea and transplant a healthy one from a donor, with a 75 percent chance of success. This operation has been performed for decades, and it will continue to be the main treatment for corneal replacement. Recently, however, success has been found using artificial cornea implants made of a semirigid synthetic called polysulphone.

Man-made plastic lenses now replace those all-but-useless lenses destroyed by cataracts and thereby restore vision. A recent alternative method brings forth the same results by taking a donated cornea, tailor-cutting it to the shape of a lens on a computerized lathe, and implanting it in the corneal layers, where it acts as a replacement lens for the extracted, diseased one.

Even diseased vitreous fluid, the gelatinous substance that fills most of the eyeball, has yielded to the new medical technology. If the vitreous becomes clouded because of hemorrhaging or disease, doctors can further liquify it with a microrotary blade, draw it out, and fill the eyeball with a clear fluid that once again allows unadulterated light to strike the retina. An amazing surgical instrument, the Vitreous Infusion Suction Cutter (VISC), performs all 3 tasks, and it is only 1/15 of an inch (1.7 millimeters) in diameter. The VISC is what makes the operation possible—that and the great skill and patience of the surgeon. Such an operation can take up to 7 hours to perform.

Not too many years ago, the back-of-the-eye retina, home of the light sensors for vision, was inaccessible to medical treatment, but today that is no longer true. If a torn retina is detached from its wall, threatening blindness, surgeons can—through a complex and intricate pro-

If the clear gel, the vitreous, that fills the eyeball becomes clouded because of hemorrhaging or disease, doctors can remove it and fill the eyeball with a clear fluid to restore vision. The surgical instrument used is a VISC (Vitreous Infusion Suction Cutter), and the operation can take up to 7 hours. Courtesy National Institutes of Health.

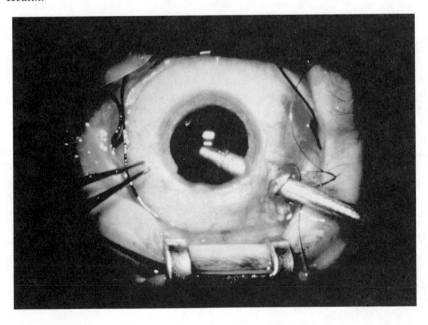

cedure—anchor the retina back in position with a microsurgical, burn-and-freeze, welding technique.

A new surgical treatment is also available today for extreme near-sightedness that is not correctable through optical means. Known as myopic keratomileusis (MKM for short), the procedure involves removing a portion of the cornea, freezing it, cutting and reshaping it with a computer-assisted scalpel, and then stitching it back in position. The newly shaped cornea properly focuses the incoming light, allowing it to fall onto, rather than in front of, the retina, and improved vision results.

The ultimate breakthrough, probably decades away, will be the completely artificial eye. Research for such a man-made eye has already begun at the Institute of Artificial Organs in New York, where 64 electrodes have been implanted in the visual brain areas of volunteers. Signals from a computerized stimulator travel through the electrodes and into the brain, where they are perceived as dots of light that form a pattern. This same basic reception method, once sophisticated with the help of high-tech microelectronics, eventually will be built into an artificial eyeball and connected to the visual cortex of the brain. Some people who were born blind will see the outside world for the first time in their lives. Think of the impact of seeing the people you love for the first time in your life!

The Active Iris

The iris, named for the Greek goddess of the rainbow, is the colored part of the eye, a circular membrane suspended between the cornea and the lens. It is composed of 2 types of involuntary muscle fibers (circular and radial) that, by contracting and dilating the pupil, control the amount of light entering the eye and striking the retina.

When the iris contracts, it protects the ultrasensitive retina from too bright light, and this is its most important reflex function. The circular muscles of the iris also contract and make the pupil smaller when the eyes focus on close-up objects or when a person is asleep. When the iris's radial muscles dilate the pupil, it is most often in response to dim light. However, a pinch on your neck will enlarge your pupils, and so will certain emotions—anxiety, fear, pain, and excitement, for example.

A high interest in subject matter or problem-solving will also dilate the pupils. One researcher slipped a photo of a nude female in with several landscape photos. Sure enough—when the male subjects came across the nude photograph, their irises dilated. In other words, their eyes popped out of their heads.

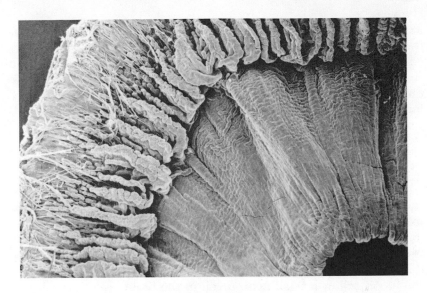

The iris, a circular, colored membrane of muscle fibers suspended between the cornea and the lens, contracts and dilates, thereby controlling the amount of light entering the eye. The iris also dilates during emotional states such as anxiety, fright, and sexual excitement. Courtesy Edward Y. Zavala, Sharp Cabrillo Hospital.

Colors Galore

Directly opposite the center of the pupil and lens is a small area of the retina known as the fovea, the point on the retina where the image is concentrated and focused. It is about the size of a pinhead, 1/40 of an inch (.625 millimeter) in diameter, and consists almost entirely of cones—photoreceptor cells that absorb light and encode it for color. Partly overlapping and surrounding the fovea is the macula ("yellow spot"), a pigmented central area of the retina, about 1/10 of an inch (2.5 millimeters) in diameter, that contains no blood vessels and is responsible for fine vision.

Within the pinhead-sized area of the fovea there are densely packed 1 million of the eye's 7 million cones, each with its own individual nerve fiber in the optic nerve. Each cone contains one of 3 pigments that is sensitive to different wavelength ranges of light—red, green, or blue. These cones transform the energy of light into electrical impulses through chemical changes in their pigment's protein molecules. These red, green, and blue cones provide the brain with the impulses that can mix any color. Because the red, green, and blue color cones have a degree of overlap in the wavelengths to which they respond, there will always be a dominant cone sending the electrical color-coded impulse to the brain, but the other 2 color cones will also be stimulated to some degree, even if it is a faint spark. This creates the rainbow of vision that healthy human eyes can paint—a palette of 7 million different shades of color!

The Eye's Image

Imagine a large beachball, about 3 1/4 feet (1 meter) in diameter, seen from a distance of 56 feet (17 meters). This sight would produce a tiny image on the retina that was 1/25 of an inch (1 millimeter) in size.

A point of light seen from afar would produce an image on the retina that was 1/9,000 of an inch (11 microns) in size—about the same size as a red blood cell or a small neuron cell in the brain.

Daily Fine Tuning, 2 x 10^5

Our ever-watchful eyes move constantly as we interact with the outside world, and the fine tuning needed depends on a harmonic complex of nerve and muscle fibers. In other parts of the body, the ratio of nerve to muscle is about 1 to 200, but in the human eye it is almost 1 to 2, which gives the superb control necessary for our busy vision. The muscles in both our eyes move some 200,000 times every day.

40 Minutes of Darkness

The human eye can adapt to a vast range of light intensity. After exposure to total darkness, the eye immediately begins to increase its sensitivity to light, but the fact that the pupil dilates to a maximum diameter of 1/3 of an inch (8 millimeters) from a minimum of 1/16 of an inch (1.5 millimeters), increasing its area about 16 times and letting up to 40 times more light in, is only a small part of the process.

It is the straight, thin rod cells—all 100 million of them in the light-sensitive retina at the back of the eyeball—that are responsible for dark adaptation and night vision. The rods contain the light-sensitive pigment rhodopsin (also called visual purple because of its hue) that bleaches in the light through a chemical process and regenerates in the dark. When the eye is completely dark-adapted, there are an estimated

10 million rhodopsin molecules in *each* of the retina's 100 million rods —a grand total of 1 trillion rhodopsin molecules in the onionskin-thin retina tissue.

After 1 minute of darkness, the eye's sensitivity to light increases 10 times; after 20 minutes, it increases 6,000 times; and after 40 minutes of complete darkness, the human eye reaches its limit of sensitivity to light—about 25,000 times more sensitive than before exposure to darkness.

The same sensitivity range is easily found in the world of light. Bright sunlight is about 30,000 times brighter than the light from the full moon, and the marvelous human eye automatically adjusts.

The Browns and the Blues

Research in the 1970s discovered an unexpected correlation between eye color and activity. Athletes with darker eyes did better in sports that required split-second timing (hitting a baseball, for example), whereas athletes with lighter eyes did better in sports that required self-paced response (like golf). Although there was doubt about the validity of such a linkage, further studies were conducted on animals and the same conclusions were reached—dark-eyed animals exhibited more reactive behavior and light-eyed ones were generally self-paced. Follow-up studies confirmed that people with medium-brown irises react faster than those with lighter-colored eyes.

Why? Experts are not absolutely sure, but one reasonable theory is that the dense pigmentation of darker eyes speeds up the nerve impulses from the eye to the brain. This could explain why dark-eyed people generally have faster reaction times.

Additional research to clarify and expand our knowledge of this link between eye color and behavior could eventually lead to better ways of matching a person's abilities and his or her life's work—by looking into his eyes.

Reworking Raw Light

The cornea and the lens bend and focus the light before the image reaches the retina and complex electrical codes are sent to the brain. The cornea does most of the light-bending and the lens behind it does the fine focusing. Because they both must be transparent, they have no blood supply and are nourished by the clear fluid (aqueous humor) inside them.

The human lens constantly changes shape in order to fine-focus light. When viewing a distant object 20 or more feet away, the lens flattens, the pupil dilates, and more light enters. As you read these words, your lens becomes rounder, your pupil contracts, and less light is absorbed.

The lens is composed of flat layers of cells (fibers), precisely aligned in regular rows. Under the extreme magnification of an electron microscope, they look like neat layers of lasagna. These cells are held together by ball-and-socket-type connections. This microsymmetry allows the light to pass smoothly through the lens without scattering.

The small muscles surrounding the lens of an eye move some 100,000 times each day. For leg muscles to work as much, they would have to be put through a 50-mile (80-kilometer) hike.

Extending the Human Eye

Our eyes provide 80 percent of the raw sensory data that is the basis for all our knowledge. Each second our eyes are capable of creating 10 new images by absorbing and sending 1 billion bits of information to the brain over tens of millions of nerve connections. In the optic nerve alone, there are about 1 million nerve fibers that pick up impulses from

The human eyes provide 80 percent of the raw sensory data that is the basis for human knowledge, absorbing 1 billion bits of information each second. This PETT scan image shows increased glucose metabolism (arrow) after stimulation by light in the left visual field. Courtesy National Institutes of Health.

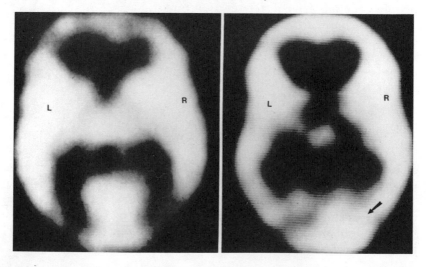

FILLING UP THE FURROWS:

the photosensitive retina and send the information to the visual cortex of the brain for processing.

The eyes are an extension of the human brain, and nowhere else on the human body is the central nervous system so directly exposed to the external world. But with the brain's power, humankind has mounted robot eyes on a spacecraft and sent them to the far reaches of our solar system. *Vikings 1* and *2* took more than 50,000 images of the Martian surface from 1976 to 1980. During their planetary encounters *Voyagers 1* and *2* transmitted about 70,000 images of Saturn and Jupiter back to earth. The four encounters took place over a period of about 2 years, even though the actual rendezvous times were measured in days. In all, the image data from both spacecraft were made up of 387 billion bits and took hundreds of hours to transmit. Our eyes can transmit the same amount of data to the brain in just 6¾ minutes.

Immediate Images

It takes 1/500 of a second for the brain to recognize an object after its light first enters the eyes.

The human eye can adapt to an immense range of light intensity. The retina's rod cells can sense some 10 million gradations of light. They can react to light as weak as 100 trillionths of a watt. Courtesy National Institutes of Health.

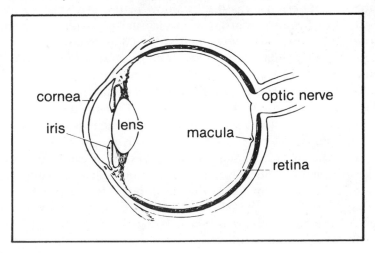

Light Sensitivity

The rod cells in the eye's retina—more than 100 million of them in each eye—register black and white only, whereas the retina's cone cells register color. The rod cells can sense some 10 million gradations of light, and they can react to light as weak as 100 trillionths of a watt. With this sensitivity, a person could see, on a clear, dark night, a "flick of a Bic" from some 50 miles (80 kilometers) away.

A Little Light for Human Sight

The amount of light energy required to stimulate the human optic nerve is infinitesimal—again, 100 trillionths of a watt. If the mechanical energy needed to lift a single small garden pea 1 inch (25 millimeters) above a dinner plate were converted to light energy, this energy would be more than enough to activate the optic nerves of every human being who has ever lived—an estimated 50 billion people.

The Vessel-less Cornea

The cornea covers the pupil and iris, and provides the outer protection for the eye. Referred to as the "window of the eye," the cornea is composed of 5 transparent layers, which make possible its primary focusing function. In fact, the cornea is about 3 times more powerful in its light-focusing ability than the lens behind it, and it does almost all the focusing of objects more than 20 feet (6 meters) away. (The lens handles the fine tuning of objects at closer distances.)

No blood vessels are in the cornea—one of the main reasons for its transparency. It must be fed by a watery fluid, the aqueous, that flows between it and the lens, as well as by local lymph circulation.

Because the cornea contains no blood vessels, it can withstand extremes of heat and cold. If healthy, it can function well in either polar or desert regions—from a teeth-chattering −100 degrees F to a scorching 140 degrees F (−148 degrees C to 60 degrees C)—which covers a temperature range of over 200 degrees, more than the range between ice and boiling water.

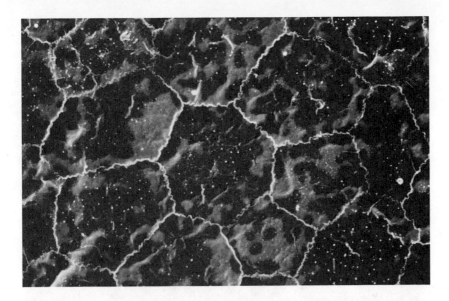

The eye's cornea, here magnified 1,400 times, focuses light before it reaches the lens for fine tuning. Like the lens behind it, the transparent cornea has no blood vessels and is fed by a clear fluid. Courtesy Edward Y. Zavala, Sharp Cabrillo Hospital.

Inner-Eye Sights

Afterimages. Normal light and dark adaptation of the eye can sometimes have a lasting effect. By steadily looking at a scene for several minutes, the microparts of the retina that receive the light from the brighter areas of the scene become less sensitive, and portions exposed to the darker areas become more sensitive. In other words, selective light and dark adaptations of specific parts of the retina have occurred because of the contrasting light and dark areas of the image.

Once the person moves his eyes away from the scene and stares at a bright white surface, he will see an afterimage of the same scene, but it will be a negative of what he actually saw—the light areas are dark and the dark areas are light. This is called a negative afterimage. Such an afterimage can be seen, under ideal conditions, for as long as an hour.

Flitting Flies. The largest part of the eye is the vitreous humor—a transparent, colorless mass of gelatinous tissue that fills the center of the eye behind the lens and keeps the eyeball under enough pressure to maintain its shape so that it can move smoothly. Sometimes dead red blood cells are released from the tiny capillaries in the retina and

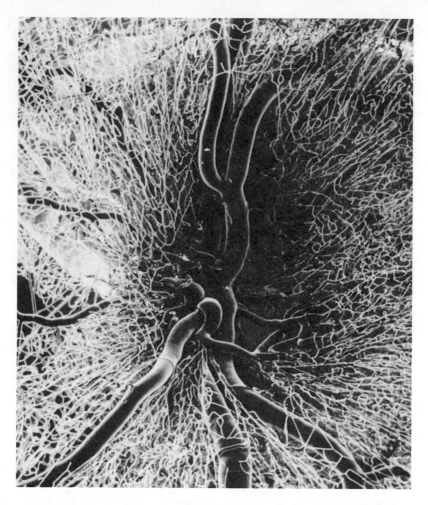

Sometimes tiny capillaries in the eye release dead blood cells into the jelly-like vitreous humor that fills the center of the eyeball. These trapped specks cast tiny shadows, causing us to see tiny spots when we stare at a neutral background. Courtesy University of Oregon Health Science Center.

work their way into the vitreous humor. These trapped specks of tissue debris cast minuscule shadows before our eyes, causing us to see tiny spots or filaments when we stare at a neutral background. These visual vagabonds are called *muscae volitantes,* Latin for "flying flies," and they float away when we try to focus on them directly.

The White Light. There is no single wavelength for white light because white is a combination of all wavelengths of the spectrum. If the 3 types (red, green, and blue) of the color-producing cones of the retina are all stimulated about equally, a person will only see a bright white light—a vision that over the centuries has been considered a mystical experience.

Computer Pink

If you're one of the millions of Americans who work at a computer video terminal for several hours each day, don't be surprised if you see some pink after staring at those green characters.

The visual pink is a harmless physiological afterimage that makes white things seem pink, and it's especially intense after several hours in front of the screen. Called the McCollough effect, this visual illusion was described in a letter to the *New England Journal of Medicine* in order to distinguish it from symptoms of neurological disease or hysteria.

After spending hours working before a video tube, look at a blank piece of white paper. It will probably appear pink.

The Eye's Rainbow

The color of the iris gives the human eye its color, and the amount of dark pigment, melanin, in the iris (genetically coded from one generation to the next) is what determines its color. Brown and other dark-colored eyes have the most pigment—the browner the iris, the more dense its melanin. Blue and light-colored eyes have the least amount. The eye's melanin is the same pigment that gives color to our skin and hair.

The fact that light-colored irises contain very little pigment causes the shorter wavelength colors—blue or green—entering the iris to be scattered within the top layer of nonpigmented fibers and bounced outward. The longer wavelength colors of yellow and red light, however, are absorbed at the back of the iris. Blue eyes are thus caused by the scattering of short wavelength light in the nonpigmented tissue, which is similar to why a blue sky appears blue—because the short wavelength light from sunlight is scattered by the air, moisture, and dust molecules in the atmosphere.

Newborns all have blue eyes because the pigment is concentrated in the folds of the iris. But when a baby is a few months old, the melanin moves to the surface of the iris and gives the baby his or her permanent eye color.

Experts believe that the evolution of blue and other light-colored eyes took place in the northern countries where sunlight is usually weak. But blue, green, or hazel eyes are in the minority. Most of the people on earth have brown eyes.

EARS AND HEARING

A Little Loud

Everyday sounds—those of passing cars, children's voices, singing birds, ringing telephones—represent extremely small amounts of energy compared to radiant energy sources such as a light bulb or a candle flame.

The acoustic power of a pneumatic drill breaking up cement (10,000 million times louder than the threshold of sound our ears can detect) or the even louder roar of a 747's engines is still negligible when put up against a radiant energy source. Such loud sounds put out less energy than a small flashlight!

Humanity in Unison

If all the people of the world were to speak at once—all 4.6 billion of us —the total acoustic energy would equal that produced by a small power plant (about 0.3 megawatt). If everyone in the world simultaneously shouted about 3 times louder than his or her normal speaking tone, and the volume were concentrated at a single point, then the level of sound would be equal to the power of a jet engine at full thrust.

Long-Distance Sound

Whatever the power of a sound source, our eardrum receives only a small fraction of the energy. Thinner than a page in this book and less than 1/2 of an inch (12.5 millimeters) in diameter, the eardrum's cone-shaped membrane is ultrasensitive and vibrates no more than 2 billionths of an inch (less than 5 billionths of a centimeter) at the threshold of hearing.

If ideal conditions of sound propagation existed, without wind deflection or conversion of sound to heat energy, the human ear could hear a sound source of 100 watts, about 1/8 horsepower, from a distance of some 2,000 miles (about 3,200 kilometers)—about the distance between Boston and Denver, or between London and Moscow.

Beyond the Sound of a Pin Dropping

The human ear is so sensitive that it can perceive sound waves with an energy of only 1/10,000 trillionth of a watt (0.0000000000000001, or 10^{-16}, of a watt). And the pressure of this barest audible sound is 10 billion times less than the atmospheric pressure at sea level.

This threshold value is so low that it is close to the energy of thermal motion. If our ears were just slightly more sensitive, we would constantly hear as background noise the collisions of molecules in the air!

The Energy of Music

The full force of an orchestra's fortissimo can be felt physically by everyone in the audience—the sound surrounds and vibrates the entire body, not just the eardrum. But the real power of a symphony orchestra is more in the music's and musicians' ability to move the audience emotionally than it is in the sound's raw energy.

How much more? Well, the sound energy from a 2-hour concert, if converted to mechanical energy, is about equal to the conductor's last 6 steps to his podium, and the thunderous applause after the finale is equal to the conductor raising the baton once over his head.

The Ear's Limits

For very short periods of time, our ears can withstand surges of sound that are 100 trillion times louder than the softest sounds detectable at the threshold of hearing. Such loud sounds, in output of acoustic watts, are comparable to the electrical energy consumption of a small city. Yet only a fraction of this sound energy is caught by the ear, and the scale of sound intensity is compressed by the human auditory system to about a 10,000-fold change. This scale compression allows us to hear over a broader range than would be otherwise possible.

The noise from a revved-up motorcycle represents sound that is 1 trillion times louder than the ear's lowest threshold level. And the blasting staccato of a pneumatic drill from across the street is 10 trillion times the barest audible whisper of a slight breeze against meadow grass. Still, for our ears to reach the threshold of pain (pain which warns that permanent damage may result), they would have to be subjected to 10,000 times *more* sound energy than the pounding pneumatic drill. Such painful, damaging noise would be experienced if one stood close to the piercing engines of a jet airliner. These engines can emit noise 10,000 times louder than the pneumatic drill that puts out noise 10 trillion times louder than the barest whisper of the meadow grass in the breeze.

Bugging the Ear

An artificial ear? It's not yet here, but researchers at Stanford University have devoted the last 10 years to developing one. Such an electronic hearing system may someday allow severely deaf people to comprehend ordinary speech. There has been steady progress, but the perfected artificial ear is years away. Still, a simple, 1-electrode system may soon be available. It will help the deaf recognize general sounds, distinguish between male and female voices, and assist in lipreading.

Healthy hearing depends on transforming a sound's mechanical vibrations to electrical signals that the auditory nerve sends to the brain for interpretation. But with the profoundly deaf—people who cannot be helped by conventional hearing aids—the fine hair cells of the inner ear that translate vibrations into electrical signals are damaged or destroyed and do not function.

The first challenge facing the scientists was to develop tiny electrodes that could be implanted in the fluid-filled cochlea of the inner ear and that could directly stimulate the auditory nerve fibers. That proved not to be an easy task because these electrodes had to survive inside the ear for many years. They also needed insulation that would perform over extremely short distances—in the order of one tenth of the diameter of a human hair. Because of the microspace involved, there was no way these electrodes could be wrapped in plastic (insulation) sleeves!

The state of the art in electronic ear transplants allows the deaf to distinguish general sounds—a ringing telephone or someone talking. In experiments, individuals identified words from a short list, but that is hardly comprehending everyday speech—and that is the ambitious, long-term goal of the Stanford research team.

The latest device consists of a small receiving unit, worn outside the body, which picks up the sound vibrations, converts them into radio

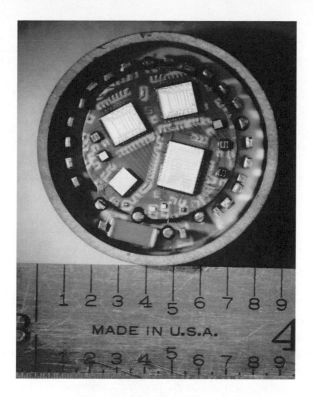

The 8-channel cochlear implant, a microreceiver developed by scientists at Stanford University, is a milestone in the development of a completely artificial ear that will someday allow the totally deaf to hear. Courtesy Stanford University Medical Center.

signals, and sends them to a tiny receiver implanted in the ear. The microreceiver then converts them into electrical signals that are sent to 8 microelectrodes in the auditory nerve. Eight electrodes are far from the 30,000 nerve fibers in each ear, and the Stanford team admits that the big challenge is learning how to encode speech into a set of electrical signals that the brain will interpret as speech.

Still years away, the perfected artificial ear may finally depend on future brain research and the next generation of microelectronic advances.

Human Hearing

A pin dropping on a wooden floor . . . a space shuttle blasting skyward—these events have one thing in common: They both create

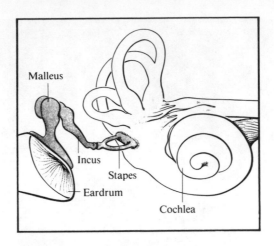

The stirrup (stapes) of the middle ear is the smallest bone in the human body, weighing about 1/2,500 of an ounce. Courtesy National Institutes of Health.

vibrations in the air. These sound waves, although astronomically different in degree, are the beginning of human hearing. Without them, we would only hear the internal workings of our body—heartbeats, the flow of blood, the creakings of bones and joints.

Some of these waves, after they are cleansed of dust and other particles by hairs and wax in the canal of the outer ear, beat against the thin membrane (1/250 of an inch, 1/10 of a millimeter) of the eardrum.

When the eardrum vibrates, it sets in motion a chain of tiny bones in the middle ear, the names of which we have all learned in school—the hammer (malleus), the anvil (incus), and the stirrup (stapes). The stirrup, the smallest bone in the human body, weighs about 1/2,500 of an ounce. The base of this stirrup-shaped bone is attached to a small membrane opposite the eardrum. Called the oval window because of its shape, this small membrane rocks and vibrates to the rhythm of the tiny stirrup and is the entranceway to the inner ear. On their journey across the middle ear, from the larger eardrum membrane to the smaller oval window membrane, the sound vibrations are amplified and concentrated 22 times. This increase in pressure on the oval window membrane makes possible the conversion of sound waves in air to sound waves in the liquid of the inner ear.

The fluid-filled inner ear, the cochlea, is located deep within the skull and is composed of one of the hardest bones in the human body. Inside the snail-shaped cochlea bone is the cochlea duct and inside the duct are the sensitive receptor hair cells, some 25,000 of them in each ear, that pick up the fluid sound vibrations, convert them into a variety of electrical signals that represent different frequencies, and send

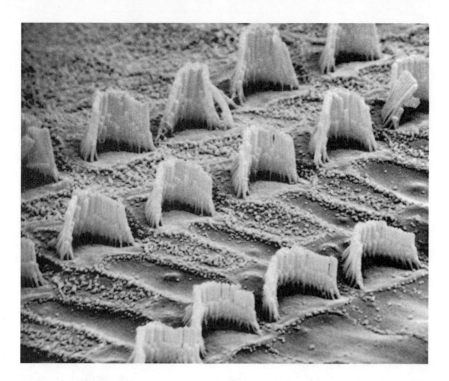

Inside the snail-shaped cochlea bone of the inner ear are sensitive receptor hair cells —some 25,000 of them—that respond to different frequencies and convert fluid vibrations into electrical impulses that are sent to the brain. The human ear is so sensitive that it can perceive sound waves with the energy of only 10,000 trillionths of a watt. Courtesy University of California at San Francisco.

them to the brain for interpretation via the auditory (also called coch-lear) nerve. This nerve contains 30,000 circuits in a strand whose diameter is no wider than a pencil lead.

The nerve cells that connect the hair cells with the auditory nerve can fire up to 1,000 times each second. These high rates are caused by loud sounds. A shotgun blast, for example, will no doubt make the inner ear's microelectrical sparks fly to the brain—an inner-ear Fourth of July.

Auditory Pops

Swallow or yawn, open your mouth wide, and the familiar popping sounds can be heard inside your ears.

These auditory pops occur in the middle ear and result from the

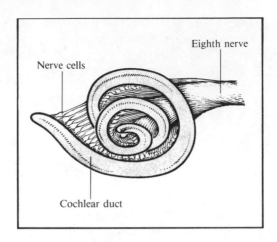

Nerve cells

Eighth nerve

Cochlear duct

The electrical impulses are sent to the brain via the auditory nerve. This nerve contains 30,000 circuits in a strand whose diameter is no wider than a pencil lead. Courtesy National Institutes of Health.

opening and closing of the Eustachian (auditory) tube, a 1½-inch (38-millimeter) canal of cartilage that connects the middle ear to the upper back part of the throat, behind the nose. The purpose of this inner passageway in our heads is to equalize the air pressure on both sides of our eardrum and to allow drainage. If it were not for this equal pressure, the eardrum would not vibrate efficiently, hearing sensitivity would be lost, and subtle sounds would not be heard.

Air pressure constantly fluctuates about 5 percent, but more extreme changes are experienced during such activities as mountain climbing, air travel, or riding an elevator to the top floor of a skyscraper. As the pressure difference builds up on either side of the eardrum's membrane, a swallowing or yawning response is initiated which opens up the usually closed Eustachian tube and allows outside air into the middle ear to equalize the pressure.

Passageways, be they in castles or in heads, can serve as entrances to foes as well as friends, and the auditory tube is no exception. Besides outside air, the route can be used by harmful bacteria, which can find a haven in the middle ear and cause serious infections, especially in young children.

By the age of 5, no less than 50 percent of all children have had at least one middle-ear infection, and this makes inflammation of the middle ear *(otitis media)* one of the most common childhood infections. Doctors attribute this to a poorly functioning Eustachian tube in those children who are prone to allergies or upper respiratory infections. Tube blockage inhibits drainage of fluid and mucus from the middle ear, and makes it susceptible to bacterial infection. In extreme cases of repeated infection, a vent tube can be surgically implanted in the eardrum to allow drainage and relieve pressure. In time, it naturally falls out and the eardrum heals itself.

Even though the Eustachian tube was first described by Bartolommeo Eustachio, an Italian anatomist, in 1563, biologists have traced the structure's evolution back to the first gill slit of the ancient fish.

Doctor's Office Vertigo

Physicians perform a very simple clinical test to determine if the semicircular canals are working properly. With the patient lying on his or her side, ice water is poured into one ear. The fluid in the canal adjacent to the ear is thereby cooled, its density increases, and it sinks. This results in a slight movement of the fluid around the canal, with the patient experiencing a sensation of rotating and the spasmodic movements of the eyeball also associated with vertigo. If the patient does not experience this ice-water-induced vertigo, the physician knows that something is wrong with the inner-ear balance organs and continues diagnosis. There is still a place, in this day and age of high-tech medicine, for ice-water-in-the-ear therapy.

Making a Deaf Ear Hear

The age of microsurgery has made it possible for deaf ears to hear again—for diseased and tattered eardrums to be reconstructed and for the tiny ossified or broken bones of the middle ear to be reconstructed or replaced.

One of the most common and successful microsurgical operations, available since the 1950s but constantly improved upon, is the stapedectomy—replacing the tiny frozen-in-place stirrup (stapes) bone, the body's smallest, with an artificial one made of a just-visible, soft plastic cylinder and a wire hook. It is the stirrup's footplate that attaches to the oval window, entrance to the inner ear, and through which sound vibrations travel from the air medium of the middle ear to the fluid medium of the inner ear.

To substitute the artificial stapes for the ossified natural one, the 2 tiny stirrup legs are broken off the footplate with a special surgical instrument, and the stapes—less its footplate—is removed. Next a tiny hole is drilled in the footplate. The surgeon, all the while peering through a binocular microscope, fits the base end of the artificial stapes into the drilled hole that meets the oval window and the inner ear. At the other end, a wire hook is attached to the tiny anvil bone. Suddenly, the ear can hear.

This operation, which enables thousands of deaf people to hear once again, is almost routine today. Still, it requires some of the most exacting movements in all of surgery, partly because the site is deep within the ear and partly because the stapes is only 1/10 of an inch (2.5 millimeters) in length—no longer than a grain of rice.

Baffled Balance

A chronic disorder of the hearing and balance senses is Ménière's disease, named after Prosper Ménière, the Frenchman who first described it in 1861. Its symptoms are high-pitched sounds within the ear *(tinnitus),* with a decreased sense of external reality; they can be buzzing, ringing, roaring, whistling, or hissing sounds, and they usually occur with hearing loss or deafness. Attacks of giddiness and more intense vertigo are common, the intense ones often followed by vomiting and sweating. If the victim is standing when loss of balance occurs, he or she will fall in the direction of the afflicted ear.

Famous victims of this inner-ear disease include Julius Caesar, Martin Luther, and Jonathan Swift. It most often occurs in middle age and is somewhat more common in men than in women.

The condition is caused by excessive fluid in the bony labyrinth of the ear, but the causes of this excess are not known for certain. Some possible causes are: a form of allergy; hardening of the ear arteries; toxic drug reaction; certain inner-ear infections; or hemorrhaging associated with a brain concussion. Regarding this last and most serious cause, if a sudden hemorrhage occurs in the semicircular canals, it produces an apoplectic-like fall that is often harmful.

Certain drugs are helpful, and limiting salt and fluid intake has also proven effective. Often, however, surgery is the only solution for severe cases.

Alan Shepard, the astronaut who became the first American in space with his suborbital flight in 1961, was a victim of Ménière's disease. After the flight, Shepard experienced unpredictable attacks of vertigo and was grounded as a result. A delicate operation, however, eventually corrected his condition. By inserting a small drainage shunt, surgeons diverted the excess fluid from the fluid sac through the small drainage tube and into the spinal fluid space next to the brain. This relieved the fluid pressure and enabled Shepard to get his wings again.

Alan Shepard eventually commanded the Apollo 14 mission to the moon in 1971. On that journey, he became the first golfer on the moon by swinging his club and sending a couple of golf balls sailing through the lunar vacuum. His sense of balance was definitely cured.

Unconscious Overload

Super loops, merry-go-rounds, and other amusement park rides play havoc with our sense of equilibrium, and it is a wonder that so many people really do enjoy confusing their senses and shaking up their bodies in this way.

Perhaps it has something to do with the fact that only a small amount of the sensory information about our orientation in space ever reaches consciousness; most of it is automatically transmitted to our reflex centers and acted upon without our ever knowing about it.

If we consciously felt the confusion of our senses, we might avoid such amusement park rides at all costs.

Our Balancing Act

Our sense of balance is housed in bony loops and chambers that are located next to the cochlea in the inner ear—the whole area often referred to as the bony labyrinth. Two separate sensing systems are found here, and each has a specialized role to play in keeping our bodies safely oriented in diverse situations.

Three semicircular canals comprise one system; they detect *motions* of the head and body. These bony canal loops emanate and return to 2 chambers, the utricle and the saccule, which contain the second system. Their main function is to constantly give the brain information about the *position* of the head.

The 3 fluid-filled semicircular canals of each inner ear are arranged at right angles to one another, and any movement of the head affects the fluid in at least 1 or 2 of them. Each canal has an enlarged end called an ampulla which contains receptor cells with fine hairs that record motion of the fluid and send it on to the brain to interpret. Any acceleration in any direction will be picked up by the fluid in the canals —a total of 6 in both ears. What this complex canal system finally does is communicate complex motions to the brain, which then tells other parts of the body how to respond. Twirling, spinning motions have the greatest effect on our balance because the fluid in the canals continues to move once the motions stop. As a result, we feel dizzy, unsteady, and have the illusion that we're still moving—vertigo.

The utricle and saccule chambers also contain sensory cells, but they

---

are unique. Each of their walls has a small area called a macula, slightly over 2 millimeters in diameter, which is the sensory area that detects the head's orientation with respect to direction of gravitational pull or other accelerating forces. The tiny macula is covered with a gelatinous layer in which many small calcium carbonate crystals (also called ear dust) are imbedded. Thousands of hair cells project into this soft layer, and their roots connect with nerve cells below. Because the calcium crystals are about 3 times heavier than the surrounding tissue, they bend the microscopic hair cells in response to the gravitational tugs that result from the head's movements and communicate their new direction to the brain. This makes it possible for a person to swim underwater with his or her eyes shut and still know which way is up. By substituting iron filings for the calcium crystals and using a magnet, animals have been made to swim upside down.

One of the most important functions of our balance organs is to help the eye muscles hold an object in view even when the head is moving. With vertigo, there is confusion of the reflexes between ear and eye. The ear signals that the head is moving when it isn't, and the eyes move rapidly to and fro in an attempt to keep the scene in focus. This well-known type of motion sickness results from an overstimulation of the inner-ear canal system, and it's not difficult to experience it. If you want to lose your balancing act, ride those most rigorous loops or dizzy-go-rounds at the amusement park. Or just spin yourself round and round in your own backyard.

There are many ways to self-induce a mild vertigo in your balancing act if that's what turns you . . . around.

Up and Down the Hearing Scale

The sense of hearing is functionally far superior to the sense of sight. Our ears can hear around corners and objects; not so the eyes. And we can hear in the dark, without light, when the eyes are blind.

About 1 octave of the frequency spectrum of electromagnetic waves is visible to the human eye, whereas *at least* 9 octaves of the spectrum—between wavelengths of 1.2 inches (3 centimeters) and 33 feet (10 meters)—can be heard by the human ear.

The range of a young and healthy human ear is about 10 full octaves —1/2 of an octave lower than a piano keyboard and some 2 1/2 octaves higher. (The piano ranges over 7 1/2 octaves.) Our most sensitive hearing range roughly corresponds to the upper 3 octaves of the piano.

Ordinary speech is in the 1,000- to 3,000-cycles-per-second range. A woman's speaking voice is around middle C, and a man's is about an octave lower, which means that the voices of both sexes are *below* the most sensitive range of the ear. (Is this why men and women so often don't hear one another?)

Babies have the most acute hearing of any of us. They can usually detect sound frequencies as low as 16 cycles and as high as 30,000 cycles per second. But this sensitivity range quickly narrows as we grow up, with 20 to 20,000 cycles each second representing the normal range for most young people. Then, as we grow older, it's downhill. Hearing sensitivity progressively deteriorates, especially with regard to high-pitched sounds.

One way to slow the inevitable hearing loss that comes with age is to quit the daily habits of coffee and nicotine consumption. Their use constricts arteries in the inner ear and adversely affects hearing. As we are constantly reminded by health professionals, kicking such habits will tremendously improve the body's general health at any age. If kept sharp, hearing and our other senses will stimulate the brain and keep us "younger" in our golden years. In retirement, who would not want to hear the voices of children playing or the songs of birds singing? Moral: Take care of your future hearing now.

TOUCH

Mother of the Senses

Touch, the dominant human sense, has been called "mother of the senses"—the largest and first-developed sense organ of the human body. The skin, in which the sensory receptors are located, commands the entire body, from the tip of the little toe to the hair on our heads.

During human gestation, when the embryo is about 1 inch in length and less than 6 weeks old, its skin is already well developed, long before the eyes and ears have formed. The newborn child can sense touch before it can see, hear, taste, or smell to any full extent. Its skin amounts to almost 20 percent of its body weight at birth.

The sense of touch gives us supreme joy; without it, a person often feels profound psychological pain. The skin's extraordinary sensitivity and ability to receive and transmit a wide variety of signals and to respond in many ways make it, as an organ system, second in importance only to the human brain. Indeed, the skin represents our external nervous system, the exposed portion that confronts the outside world, and it is the foundation for all other sensory organs—mouth, ears, eyes, nose—and no doubt evolved and over time differentiated into the other sense organs.

There are more nerve endings in the skin than in any other part of the body, and the nerve fibers are usually larger than the fibers for the other senses. The body of an adult has about 640,000 sensory receptors in the skin. This is 64 times more sense receptors than the sense of taste has on the tongue and in the mouth. Our fingertips are one of the most sensitive areas on the human body, with up to 50,000 nerve endings for every square inch (6.5 square centimeters).

A Magic Touch

Our fingertips are so sensitive that a single touch sensor can respond to a pressure of less than 1/1,400 of an ounce (about 20 milligrams), which is about what an average-sized fly weighs.

With training, the sense of touch can become highly developed. At the Bureau of Engraving and Printing, engravers use their hands to regulate the amount of ink that flows onto the plates. They can, it is claimed, detect a film of ink that is only one layer of molecules thick.

Russian scientists claim to have found a woman who has a magic touch. With her eyes closed, she can read ordinary printed material (*not* Braille) by finger touch.

The Touch Complex

Touch is really a complex of several skin-deep senses in which specialized nerve receptors detect contact, pressure, heat, cold, and pain. Like the sense of hearing, touch is stimulated by mechanical energy rather than light energy (vision) or chemical response (taste and smell). The individual tactile impressions, or syntheses of them, are then transmitted over special nerve pathways to the brain.

Seven anatomical types of touch receptors have been identified so far, and more will no doubt be discovered in the future. The specific receptor that detects heat, for example, has yet to be definitively determined. Scientists have learned that all the receptor types are present over the entire body, but they vary in number and density. The tongue, for example, has very high sensitivity while the center of the back is at the low end of sensitivity.

The touch receptors differ physically from one another, and researchers still debate some of their precise workings. Touch is, in fact,

FILLING UP THE FURROWS:

the least understood of the human senses. At various depths below the skin surface, sensors have been identified that detect delicate movement (the slightest deflection of a hair); movement (a moving touch that presses down the skin); vibration (a momentary touch or pressure that can be sensed even if it lasts only 1/10 of a second); steady contact (whenever the skin is pushed); cold (when temperature of the skin's surface drops by as little as 0.2 degree F); pain (which responds only to stimuli that could damage the tissue; and stroking movement (a touch which moves across the skin).

This last touch sensor, which detects stroking movements, is known as a Meissner's corpuscle, named after the German physiologist who discovered it in the nineteenth century. Most of us are happily familiar with its sensitivity to touch because it is in large part responsible for our sexual pleasure. These sensors are most highly concentrated in the hairless portions of the skin such as the fingertips, tongue, lips, nipples, clitoris, and penis. Their sensations provide some of the most joyous feelings in human life.

The Skin's Wings

Sensitivity to touch and pressure varies greatly over our bodies, depending on the density of nerve fibers in the skin. This sensitivity has been mapped by researchers who apply a standard procedure called a 2-point discrimination test, in which 2 pointed instruments (pairs of pins will do) are placed on the skin, the points at varying distances from one another, and the subject responds as to whether or not 1 or 2 points are felt. If the person feels the 2 points when they are very close together, then the skin is highly sensitive because the skin contains a high number of nerve endings. If the person feels only 1 point when the 2 points are separated by various distances, then the nerve endings are sparse and the skin is less sensitive in that area.

The tongue's tip, for example, tops the sensitivity list; it is rich in nerve endings, and the 2 points can be discriminated only 1/25 of an inch (1 millimeter) apart. At the opposite extreme of sensitivity is the center of the back, where the 2 points feel like 1 until they are about 3 inches (7.6 centimeters) apart. In between these extremes are the fingertips, a close second to the tongue's sensitive tip, and then the lips, the tip of the nose, the front of the torso, the thigh, and the lowly, relatively insensitive sole of the foot.

This list, of course, has left the best until last—the erogenous zones, which when stimulated during the right circumstances cause sexual arousal. The genitals and areas surrounding them, such as the thighs, the buttocks, and the abdomen, are of course the most sensitive, along with one nongenital area—a woman's breasts. But that's just the beginning. The nongenital erogenous zones extend over a large portion of the body—from the nose to the nipples, the earlobes to the armpits, the eyelids to the toes. In fact, after considering the long list of erogenous areas of the body, one is hard pressed to find a body area that isn't erogenous once it is associated with pleasurable sexual activity. Even a typical nonerogenous zone can become, through conditioning, an erogenous zone.

Few lovers would consider the nerve-barren centers of their backs excitable, but they can become so, especially if they are stroked just before the genitals are fondled and before intercourse begins.

No two lovers are alike in their touch sensitivities, which depend on prior conditioning and heredity (number of sensory nerves in a particular area). And the beauty of this is the continual sense of discovery that two lovers can share. After all, each is capable of giving the other his or her unique magic touch that can turn indifferent skin into soaring wings.

Losing Your Touch

You feel your clothes going on in the morning as you dress, but shortly thereafter you don't feel them against your body at all. The same is true for a pair of new shoes, a wristwatch, or a pair of glasses.

Why? All touch sensors adapt to some degree after they've been stimulated for a period of time. At first touch a very high impulse rate of nerve signals is sent to the brain, but the rate then slows until some sensors stop responding completely.

Hair receptors, wrapped around the hair's root, adapt in this way, and their signals become extinct in about 1 second. A specialized receptor called a Pacinian corpuscle measures rapid changes in pressure against the body. It responds when pressure is first applied against the skin and when the same pressure is removed, but not to the constant pressure in between. This receptor adapts and its initial response falls off to nothing within a few thousandths to a few hundredths of a second. These rapid-fire, on-off receptors that measure pressure are also located near the joint capsules and inform the brain about the different rates of movement for different parts of the body. Without their constant update to the brain and the resultant muscular response, runners would stumble, football players would fumble, and all Olympic competitors would become hopelessly uncoordinated.

TLC: Tender Loving Care

Touch is a vital sense, more vital to human welfare than anyone realized a century ago, and the amount of skin stimulation received by an infant or child is now known to strongly influence an individual's lifelong physical and mental health. Research over the last several decades has uncovered the powers of touch and has revealed that early touch deprivation can irreversibly damage personality, social skills, and the functioning of all the other senses. Without question, the sense of touch can be added to the list of basic human needs.

Increased handling of infants—be it cuddling or caressing—is known to stimulate respiration and blood flow. Touch—the first sense to fully function—is the foundation sense upon which the more complex sensory skills such as seeing and hearing are built. The stimulation of touch plays a key role in the growth of our other senses. Even physical growth is influenced by the normal or abnormal development of the touch sense.

In one study, a group of premature babies got routine care, while another group was stroked for 5 minutes every hour for a period of 10 days. The babies who were stroked and touched more often gained weight faster, were more active, and appeared to cry less. Even 8 months later, these babies were generally healthier than the routine-care group.

Touch deprivation, on the other hand, has serious consequences. Studies with infant monkeys have shown that, without normal tactile stimulation, they become very physically dependent, clinging to one another to the extent that they avoid normal activities. Older deprived monkeys exhibit many types of disturbed behavior, often avoiding other monkeys and becoming very aggressive when interaction occurs. Extreme deprivation of touch has even been shown to cause brain damage in animals by destroying nerve cells in the cerebellum.

Human infants who do not receive enough basic physical contact tend to develop psychosomatic disorders and generally experience retardation in physical and mental health. Inadequacies in later tactile behavior are also common—be it sexual dysfunction or an inability to demonstrate affection. Some prostitutes have admitted that they sell sex in order to be held. Even the skin of a touch-deprived individual can appear unhealthy—pale and toneless.

Some experts believe that serious mental health problems such as schizophrenia are caused by a lack of intimacy, including touch, between a mother and child. The consensus today is that no infant can receive too much tender loving care, and that too little can even prove life threatening or fatal, a fact that early twentieth-century statistics bear out. In 1915, a high majority of orphanages in the United States had almost 100 percent death rates for infants 1 year old or less. These institutions gave the infants adequate nutrition and clean surroundings, but the babies lost their appetites, were listless, and their bodies atrophied.

Why? This tragic death rate was later found to result in large part from touch deprivation and the absence of tender loving care. "Tender loving care" programs were soon initiated where the children were held and stroked daily. The result: mortality rates dropped, up to 70 percent in some institutions.

Ultimately, the touching sense is essential to our survival as healthy individuals and, through sex, as a species.

The Speed of Touch . . . and Tickle

All the skin's *specialized* sensory receptors send their signals at velocities of 98 to 230 feet (30 to 70 meters) per second, which give them a top speed of about 156 miles (250 kilometers) per hour. These are the more critical sensory signals which transmit specific information on location and intensity of the stimuli.

Free nerve endings, found everywhere on the skin and in other tissues as well (they are, for example, the only type in the cornea of the eye), can also detect touch and pressure. The velocities of their signals are generally much slower—sometimes less than 3 feet (1 meter) per second if they are sent along uninsulated nerve fibers. An example of such a slowpoke sensation is that of a tickle.

Itch and Tickle

Until recently it was thought that the itch and tickle sensations were caused by very mild stimulation of the pain nerve endings, but recent studies prove otherwise and trace them to sensitive free nerve endings in the superficial layers of the skin, the only tissue where itching and tickling occur.

The fibers that transmit these sensations are similar to those that transmit a burning type of pain (both types of fibers are very small and both are uninsulated), but they are distinct from the pain fibers.

If the itch receptors are excited in animals, the result is a scratch reflex, which should rid the skin of a flea about to bite or other irritant. If a pain nerve ending is excited, however, the result is a withdrawal

---

FILLING UP THE FURROWS:

reflex. These two entirely different responses demonstrate the distinction between pain and itch and tickle. Pain hurts and can produce tears or howls. An itch or a tickle irritates, and they can produce either annoyance or a giggle.

The Pain Beyond Touch

Beyond the pleasures and assurances of touch, there is always the looming possibility of pain. As a survival mechanism, pain warns our brains of danger and tells us to act to correct or avoid the cause. Who does not have vivid memories of burning one's hand on a hot stove and quickly withdrawing it? Pain is powerful. We remember. We learn to be more careful.

Still, pain does not always warn us of danger. It comes too late for us to avoid a bad sunburn, and a tumor in the brain can grow unnoticed because the tissue within our skulls has no pain receptors.

Pain receptors, free nerve endings, are spread over a larger area than any of the other sensory receptors. They completely ignore light contact, and only fire up if the stimuli threaten to damage the tissue. There are more pain receptors in the skin than other types of skin sensors, but they are not evenly distributed. For example, the neck and eyelids are densely covered, but there are few receptors on the sole of the foot and on the ball of the thumb, which is why the needle prick for a blood sample is often done on the thumb.

Unlike touch receptors, pain receptors do not adapt (or barely adapt in some cases)—the nerve continues to transmit as long as there is pain. After damage to the tissue has been done, however, the warning function is over and the pain falls off.

What's in a Pain?

Three different types of pain—pricking, burning, and aching—have been recognized, and 2 types of nerve fibers send their signals to the spinal cord, one much faster than the other. Pricking pain signals travel faster (up to 98 feet, 30 meters, per second), while burning and aching pain signals move more slowly (at 1.6 to 6.5 feet, ½ to 2 meters, per second). This variation in transmission speed for the types of pain is the reason pricking pains are followed by a slow burning pain. And while the pricking-type pain is localized to within 4 to 8 inches (10 to 20 centimeters) of the stimulated area, burning and aching pains are less well defined and are generalized to an area of a major limb or other large part of the body.

A standard test of pain response involves applying heat to the skin, and most of us perceive pain when the skin reaches an average critical temperature of 113 degrees F (45 degrees C), and everyone, with the exception of people with serious sensory dysfunction, perceives pain before his or her skin reaches a temperature of 116.6 degrees F (47 degrees C).

Even though there are 3 to 4 times fewer heat receptors than cold receptors in the human skin, freezing cold and burning hot sensations are both experienced exactly the same. Indeed, at 140 degrees F (60 degrees C) both the cold and heat pain nerve endings are stimulated, and after a point, there is no reason to make fine distinctions—all the brain has to know is: *very painful!*

TASTE

The Flavor Recipe

Taste and smell, contrary to what many people believe, are entirely separate sensory systems. The confusion results from a common failure to distinguish between the terms "taste" and "flavor." Flavor is much more than taste. It includes several sensory inputs: taste, smell, and texture-temperature-pain. All these inputs are independently stimulated to produce a distinct flavor when food enters the mouth. If one of these sensations is impaired, the flavor may change, but it won't disappear. The thousands of different foods and their flavors each of us can identify are combinations of all these factors.

An apple and a raw potato, without their distinctive odors smelled by the nose, have almost the same taste—a slight sweetness. Pepper and mustard stimulate the temperature receptors, sometimes to the point of pain. Ever have what seems like fireworks climbing up your nose after some hot green pepper? Menthol, in contrast, produces a cool sensation.

The tongue, our taste center, is more sensitive to touch, temperature, and pain than any other part of the body, and people who have lost their sense of smell still retain taste, but one very different than most of us possess. Such a limited taste sense would dramatically limit the flavor menu.

The Wilting Buds

Throughout life, the sense of taste changes. Newborns have more taste buds than adults, and the buds can be found throughout infants' mouths. Even premature babies, tests have shown, can taste the difference between sweet and salty substances. In adulthood, many of the taste buds disappear and those 10,000 or so remaining are concentrated on the tongue and throat.

After the age of 45, many taste buds degenerate, and the taste sense usually becomes progressively duller. Regeneration of cells on the tongue, as in all other parts of the body, slows for older people, and the elderly have only 20 percent as many taste buds on their tongues as the young. Postmenopausal women whose estrogen levels drop way down often lose a substantial degree of taste sensitivity. For both men and women, such a decline in sensitivity often results in poor appetite that in turn leads to improper nutrition and ill health. It certainly can't help the mental outlook either.

The elderly can often compensate for such taste loss by eating chewy foods, by not smoking, by brushing their tongues as well as their teeth, and by moderately seasoning the foods they eat. If you're daring, an occasional Mexican or Indian meal will let you know that you still have a lot of taste buds left.

The Tongue's Sensations

The Greeks recognized 9 varieties of taste, but they were probably including the sense of smell to make their distinctions. Today 4 primary tastes—sweet, salt, sour, and bitter—are accepted as the basic taste sensations that combine to create all others. Add to these possible taste combinations the sense of smell, as well as oral receptors for texture, temperature, and pain, and the thousands of flavors we experience are created.

Sweetness. Taste buds on the tip of the tongue are most sensitive to sweetness, and the sweet taste is the only one of the primary 4 that intensifies as the temperature of the food increases—at least up until it reaches body temperature. The sweet taste is not caused by any one chemical agent. Our tongue can detect a concentration of 1 part in 200 of table sugar when it is dissolved in saliva. This is the least sensitive and discriminating of the primary tastes. Because sugar is important for our metabolisms, it is welcomed into the body without much ado. The synthetic sweetener, saccharin, is more than 600 times sweeter than table sugar, and so 1 teaspoon of saccharin can sweeten 600 cups of coffee to the same degree as 1 teaspoon of sugar would sweeten 1 cup.

Saltiness. Salts dissolving on the tongue, especially on its rim, give us the salty taste, but researchers are unclear as to how salts subtly affect the taste buds. Different kinds of salts in equal concentrations do not taste equally salty, and this is probably because salts elicit other taste sensations. The salt taste is more sensitive than the sweet taste, and it can be detected in a solution of 1 part in 400.

Sourness. The sour taste is caused by acids—the more acidic the acid, the stronger the sour taste. Acids contain hydrogen, which dissociates in solution into free positively charged particles—hydrogen ions. The tongue is the only part of the human body that can detect hydrogen ions, and the taste buds on the tongue's rim are most sensitive to sourness. Sourness is the second most sensitive taste sensation and, in the form of hydrochloric acid, it can be detected in a solution of 1 part in 130,000.

Bitterness. Back-of-the-tongue taste buds are most sensitive to the bitter taste. They represent the last line of defense against dangerous food before it goes down the throat and into the body. Bitterness is not caused by any one type of chemical agent, but alkaloid substances, including quinine, caffeine, strychnine, and nicotine, always fire up this taste sensation. Because alkaloids in plants and by themselves are often intensely poisonous, the bitter taste is a danger signal throughout the animal kingdom. As a warning system on the human tongue, the bitter taste sensation is more sensitive than the other 3 primary tastes. Guardian against poison, the bitter taste is some 10,000 times more sensitive than the sweet taste. Bitterness can be detected in a solution with only 1 part quinine in 2 million parts of water. When in doubt, bitterness will tell you to spit it out.

Taste's Microcosm

Adults have some 10,000 taste buds on the tongue, the roof of the mouth, and the throat; children generally have more. The buds, clustered together in tiny bumps called papillae, are composed of about 40 cells each—some supporting cells and some taste cells.

Each taste bud is about 1/750 of an inch (1/30 of a millimeter) in diameter and about twice again as long. Under a microscope they appear similar to rosebuds ready to blossom. The taste cells of each taste bud are constantly renewed by mitotic division. Their life span is about 10 days, close to that of fireflies.

The taste cells surround a tiny taste pore, and several taste hairs protrude from the tip of each taste cell and point upward through the taste pore toward the mouth. These tiny hairs (microvilli) probably provide the receptor surface for taste. Food molecules in the saliva, sensed by these microhairs, trigger the creation of electrical signals that are sent off to the brain for interpretation.

There are about 1 million of these tiny "feelie" hairs in everyone's mouth, each one only 1/12,000 of an inch (1/500 of a millimeter) long.

The Zinc Link

A zinc deficiency impairs taste sensitivity, and this fact has been known for years among researchers in the chemical senses—taste and smell. When such a connection was first demonstrated, researchers hoped that most of the medical problems involving the taste sense—from a limited to a complete loss—could be attributed to a zinc deficiency, but that view has proven too simplistic.

Today a low zinc level in the body is considered one of several key factors in taste-sense disorders. About 25 percent of all the patients with taste and smell disorders are found to have zinc abnormalities. The zinc deficiency in these patients is not necessarily a problem in absorbing the trace mineral, but can involve problems with its transport, storage, or distribution within the body. Many victims of the chronic disease of the nervous system, multiple sclerosis, experience an altered sense of taste before treatment, and recent research indicates that these people share a defect in how zinc is stored in the body.

A sudden loss of the taste sense could reflect a serious medical problem such as a cerebral tumor or an endocrine disorder. If this happens, don't think that gorging yourself with foods high in animal protein—meat, eggs, seafood, and milk, which are all good sources of zinc—is adequate self-treatment. Instead, get to a doctor immediately, one who understands that the sudden loss of taste can be just as dangerous as a loss of vision.

The Flow of Taste

Taste buds, the sense organs of taste, are found predominantly on the surface of the tongue and are dependent on saliva to dissolve and absorb the food and carry its molecules to the taste-cell receptors within the buds. Without saliva, composed of 99.5 percent water, nothing can be tasted and no gustatory sensations can be translated into electrical impulses and sent to the brain.

It has been estimated that saliva flow in a 24-hour period amounts to about 45 fluid ounces (1,500 milliliters). The flow rate, however, varies tremendously. Without food in the mouth or thoughts of food in the mind, the saliva flow is low—about 6/1,000 of a fluid ounce. But once we take a bite or sip, there is a dramatic increase in saliva flow—up to 1/8 of a fluid ounce each minute—an increase of about 20 times.

In an average lifetime, more than 1.2 million fluid ounces of saliva are produced—almost 10,000 gallons. That's enough to fill a good-sized swimming pool.

Innate Tastes?

Do changes in our taste preferences throughout life correspond to the changing needs of our bodies for certain substances? All of us have heard it said that children go through food-preference changes based on the needs of their growing bodies. The parental attitude often is: Let the kids eat what they want because they will get what they need. Research in the 1930s gave some support to this viewpoint. Children with a vitamin D deficiency, one study claimed, chose to drink large amounts of cod-liver oil. As a rule, healthy children liked its taste, but they liked it less and less as they grew up, indicating that their need for vitamins A and D became less after their early growth spurt.

A growing body of research indicates that an involuntary taste preference based on body needs definitely exists. Laboratory research has shown that animals whose adrenal glands have been removed select water with a high salt content instead of pure water. This is also true of animals with their parathyroids removed. And the fact that animals in the wild seek out salt licks to build up a supply of mineral salts that grasses and plants lack demonstrates an innate mechanism that fulfills metabolic needs. The Mexican habit of taking tequila with salt and lemon may be a cultural adaptation of the body's need for more salt because of hot climate and perspiration resulting in salt loss.

Another experiment has shown that animals who are injected with excessive amounts of insulin choose the sweetest food from a large selection to get their blood sugar up after the insulin has depleted it.

Scientists do not fully understand how innate taste preferences work, but they agree that the mechanism is located in the central nervous system and not in the taste buds themselves. This also is borne out by the fact that past pleasant or unpleasant tastes contribute to a person's unique taste preferences. If you become sick immediately after eating a particular food, it's likely that you'll develop a taste aversion to that food. Your innate taste preferences may therefore enable you to keep down what you eat!

"Tasting" Alcohol

Because much of what we call "taste" is really the sense of smell, it is more accurate to talk about a substance's "flavor."

Often when food or drink enters the mouth, the odors stimulate the smell receptors in the nose thousands of times more strongly than they do the taste buds. Take alcohol, for instance. With our noses working well, we can detect the flavor of alcohol in $1/25,000$ the concentration required than when our noses are stopped up—when only our taste buds are working. All wine tasters, therefore, might be better called "wine smellers."

Fake Flavors and Taste Tampering

Flavoring additives, both natural and artificial, comprise two thirds of all food additives. Many natural flavors can now be duplicated synthetically and are less expensive than the originals. Vanillin, the major compound in vanilla flavoring, is a compound of ethyl chemicals and in its synthetic form is more stable and 3 times as strong as the natural form.

Even extremely bitter synthetic flavors find commercial use. For example, some are added to electrical insulating materials to keep rats from chewing on them.

Monosodium glutamate (MSG) is the best-known flavor modifier/ enhancer. It was discovered in Japan at the turn of the century and is used primarily in oriental foods. Because it is a "natural" substance, it was long believed to be safe. However, as recently as 1968 a reaction known as "Chinese Restaurant Syndrome" was identified and traced to MSG. The temporary burning sensations and headaches symptomatic of this condition are probably caused by excitation of nerve endings. MSG is not considered safe for infants, and manufacturers of baby foods have removed MSG from their products.

There are several other substances which, although not remarkable for their own taste, alter the taste of other substances. Miraculin, naturally found in the West African "miracle fruit," makes sour foods taste sweet. Natives chew the berries before consuming sour foods or drinking sour wine or beer. If one chews the leaves of the tropical plant

Gymnema sylvestre, the ability to taste sweetness is temporarily lost—the sweetest fruits taste sour and sugar tastes like sand.

SMELL

Scent Started It All

It is widely held that chemical signals helped to guide single-celled organisms to each other in the dark, vast, primordial seas billions of years ago. Without anything but scent to go by, other than what might be called Divine direction, these first organisms found one another and evolved into multicelled organisms.

Noses and Fish

Smell, a chemical sense like taste, is the least understood of all human senses. While it is 10,000 times more sensitive than taste and has an extremely low threshold, its range of detection is considerably less than for sight and hearing. Of the human senses, smell has been called the most primitive, indeed almost vestigial in humans, even though sensitivity varies greatly from one person to another. For most of the animal world, however, the sense of smell reigns supreme. A dog, for example, has some 20 times more tissue area filled with smell receptors than a person does, which is like comparing the surface of a handkerchief with a postage stamp. The dog's world is a sniff-and-smell world; ours is an image world, where the eyes dominate.

Smell receptors high in the nostrils are only about an inch (2.5 centimeters) away from the primitive brain—the limbic system—and some of the olfactory nerves that transmit the smell signals pass through the limbic system, a brain area responsible for generating fear, rage, aggression, and pleasure, as well as regulating sex drives and reproductive cycles. Certain smells can therefore readily stimulate the centers of emotion and sexuality, and their memories are often emotional and intense, eliciting either pleasure or repulsion. Research has confirmed that smell memories last longer than visual memories.

Just as the taste buds depend on saliva to detect the chemistry of food and liquids, so does the sense of smell depend on mucus, secreted by minute glands in the nose, to dissolve the odor molecules so the smell receptors can detect and code their chemistry and send the signals on to the olfactory bulb of the brain.

At this fundamental level of the sense of smell, there is no difference between a person and a fish.

Basic Odors

There have been many theories on the number of basic (primary, uncombined) smells. Plato recognized just 2: pleasant and unpleasant —not one of his strongest theories. His student Aristotle went on to name 6: sweet, bitter, acidic, astringent, pungent, and succulent. In the eighteenth century Linnaeus made his own list: aromatic, musky, garlicky, fragrant, goaty, repulsive, and nauseating.

Although the number of smells, when combined, is infinite, most physiologists believe that these can be reduced to primaries. Some have suggested that specific *molecular shapes,* which lock into specific receptors, determine the smell sensations. *Electrical charges* have also been observed—"pungents" carry a positive charge, "putrids" are negative.

Sherlock Holmes, the great fictional sleuth, advised that a good detective should be able to identify 75 different smells. Brewers, wine makers, and perfumers all have their own special terminology to describe aromas in their products. But again, these do not necessarily identify *basic* odors.

The most reliable current research, still in progress, predicts 32 basic odors. Only 7 have been positively identified so far, and of these, 5 coincide with human body scents: camphoraceous (from the camphor tree), musky, floral, pepperminty, ethereal, pungent, and putrid. An interesting "weakness" that exists in all of us is aiding this research: everyone has difficulty detecting at least one scent that would be obvious to the majority of other people. Thus, an elimination process is helping researchers to isolate basic smells.

Sniff, Sniff . . . What Is That Smell?

Two tiny yellow-brown patches of tissue, one in the upper half and one on the roof of each nostril, are what allow people to smell the odor molecules in the air they breathe through their noses. Unless air reaches this tissue, there can be no smell, as many stuffy-nosed people can confirm! This specialized tissue, packed with tens of millions of smell receptors and their microhairs, allows most of us to detect and recognize some 4,000 distinctly different scents (and up to 10,000 for a select group of human noses).

In humans, the sensory patches have an area of only 3/4 of a square inch (4.8 square centimeters), compared to a hunting dog with at least 10 square inches (65 square centimeters), or a shark with 24 square feet (2.2 square meters). And a rabbit, well known for its active nose, has a smell receptor area as great as the skin area of its entire body.

Smelling depends on breathing, which brings air and odor molecules into the nostrils. Sniffing is therefore a sure way of increasing the sensitivity of smell—the more air, the more odor molecules, and the more smell. Subtle smells, such as the bouquets of wines, are therefore sniffed. The body also responds to pleasant food odors with an increase of gastric juices and saliva for use in digestion.

But smell, usually considered the least important human sense, still retains its ancient, primary protective function. Dangerous and pungent smells still cause us to react immediately—often in a few thousandths of a second—to take action. A strong ammonia smell, for example, will send us scurrying for fresh air.

As an example of smell's protective mechanism in the extreme, our smell receptors can detect 1/400 billionth of a gram of methyl mercaptan in a liter of air—the substance that utility companies mix into odorless natural gas to allow us to detect the danger of leaking gas. Methyl mercaptan is more basic than its chemical name suggests. What is it? What is that smell? The product of decaying flesh—the essence of rotten meat!

Telesmell

The slow growth of videoconferencing as an alternative to face-to-face meetings has been blamed, by some experts, on the absence of human scents. According to researchers, people who confer by video find that it doesn't convey the "presence" of remote participants. "Something" is missing. Could the "something" be pheromones, message-carrying chemicals that are believed to play a role in attraction and warning?

If it's true that pheromones (pronounced fear-o-moans) play a part in communication and the establishing of relationships, new technology would be needed to transmit these body signatures around the globe. A serious telecommunications consulting report recently advised the use of "environmental fragrances" as substitutes, until the necessary technology is developed.

The Elusive Pheromones

Although research has identified specific chemical substances in lower forms of animals—particularly insects, which communicate essential messages through the sense of smell—the existence of human pheromones is still under debate.

There is no question that insects like moths, bees, and ants live predictable existences dictated by instinct and chemical communication. And no one would deny that individual humans emit chemicals that can be tasted and smelled. But do our body chemicals send definite, inescapable messages—signal aggression, fear, dominance, desire?

Recent evidence suggests that they do. Synchronization of the menstrual cycles of women who live together or are close friends or coworkers, has been linked directly to an olfactory response to body secretions. Of any two or more females sharing living quarters or seeing one another frequently, one of the females will be "dominant" in her level of pheromone output. Thus, over time, her body will cue the others to become synchronized with its menstrual timing. Reasons for this can only be speculated upon—whether to cause all to be fertile at the same mid-cycle peak, or perhaps to allow all to experience premense "blues," cramps, and irritability at the same time, thus excusing any disagreeable behavior or short tempers around *"that* time of the month."

Scentprints

In case you haven't noticed, male and female underarm scents differ. Men's are more musky because of the steroid hormonal compounds in their systems. In fact, every person and racial type has distinct, and individual, combinations of smells—much like a fingerprint.

Europeans/Caucasians have fewer and smaller scent glands than Negroids, and Orientals have the least of all. Japanese women rarely have genital scent glands; and in that nation underarm odor is so rare that it's considered a disease! In the past, a Japanese male could be exempted from military service if he suffered this malady, and could check into a hospital specializing in its treatment. Koreans have fewer scent glands than any other group on earth; in fact, 50 percent have no scent glands at all.

So distinct and definite are individual human scents that bloodhounds and other dogs have gained our respect for their ability to track or detect the slightest scented remainders of our presence. In laboratory tests dogs have been able to choose correctly from a set of glass slides the one that was slightly touched by a fingertip 6 weeks earlier. Some dogs can do it after the slides have been exposed to weather for a week. But even a bloodhound can't tell the difference between identical twins; the only way to alter their duplicate scentprints is to put them on radically different diets for a period of time—one spicy, one bland.

Although humans can't compete with the smelling skills of many animals, we don't do too badly when we set our minds to it. There have been several "T-shirt" studies in which blindfolded participants had to select their mate's dirty T, or separate the males' from the females'. Most people (usually 75 percent or better) perform these feats quite ably. Tests have also shown that most people can tell each other apart from the smell of their hands. In such tests, it was more difficult to distinguish between sisters than between two unrelated women.

Cravings and Copulins

Women have a better sense of smell than men or children because the female hormone estrogen activates the nose and olfactory receptors. They are particularly sensitive to the odor of musk—a scent associated with male bodies—and at mid-menstrual cycle, when estrogen levels are at their highest, their ability to detect musk is 100 to 100,000 times greater than during menstruation. Perception of other aromatics, such as clove, sandalwood, or cinnamon, also increases at mid-cycle.

During pregnancy, when estrogen is at a low level, taste and smell are affected. Thus, many women crave unusual foods or enjoy tastes that they disliked before becoming pregnant. Progesterone, the "pregnancy" hormone, causes redness and swelling of mucous membranes. A woman's sense of smell can be as much as 2,000 times more sensitive before her pregnancy than during it.

Vaginal copulins, specific scents sometimes referred to as pheromones, also peak at ovulation. Nonpill users at mid-cycle produce about 7.5 times more copulins than women who take the pill. Some fragrance researchers have isolated these "pheromones" in an attempt to find an irresistible ingredient for perfumes. It's possible that these researchers have been "barking up the wrong tree"; women, not men, are the prime responders to sexual scents such as the musk and aromatics mentioned earlier. One study showed that a majority of healthy, heterosexual males identified vaginal copulin scents as "mildly unpleasant." A woman scientist present at the reading of that report rose to suggest that the laboratory environment and absence of visual and tactile stimuli may have adversely affected the males' perceptions. Her point was well taken: Women *do* respond better to fragrance and may be able to detect subtle clues such as "aggression" or "desire" in sexual scent signals. Men respond more to visual sexual clues, such as body shape and stance, facial expression, or clothing.

For males, scent seems to be more a matter of "marking off territory" to repel other males.

Odor Memory and Aroma Therapy

Visual details can be recalled with nearly a 100 percent accuracy over short periods of time, with memory dropping to 50 percent after 3 months. Although memory of *smells* averages 80 percent recall after a brief time, this level does not drop—even after a year has passed! People have difficulty naming smells, because smell is a nonverbal experience. Reactions are emotional and polarized (pleasure, neutrality, or repulsion), and frequently are connected to some prior exposure. A woman, for example, might remember and visualize her mother every time she smells baking bread. A man jilted by a former girlfriend might become irritable and uncomfortable when he smells her perfume on someone else years later.

Smell *is* the sense most closely tied to our emotions, because some of the nerves that travel to the brain from olfactory receptors must pass through the limbic system, thus stimulating it and its centers of emotion and sexuality each time a smell is received.

It is possible to use scents to deliberately alter moods or control emotions. In Europe, some psychoanalysts have been using "aroma therapy" for years. Patients of a French analyst sniff vanilla-scented cotton to aid in the recollection of childhood memories.

In the United States, the International Flavors and Fragrances firm is studying a number of fragrances, each with a history of use in various cultures. According to folklore, extract of orange flowers can help you relax . . . rose oil also may be massaged on tense muscles. It is said that sniffing lavender can help you sleep, and that peppermint oil sniffed from a cotton ball helps dispel depression.

Because various scents are perceived differently as "pleasant" or "unpleasant"—Mediterraneans celebrate the smell of garlic, while Northern Europeans tend to dislike the smell—no absolute set of mood-altering fragrances should be expected from even the most vigorous scientific research. Each of us responds to many smells in our own way, a fact that makes life more interesting and maintains the element of surprise.

Putting On the Animal

Animal musks were applied by humans as attractants a thousand years ago and are still used as ingredients in modern perfumes. The glandular scent of the male musk deer of the Himalayan Mountains is the key ingredient in today's quality perfumes. One grain of dried musk secretion can fill several million cubic feet with its scent, which will last for several days. Because the deer is threatened with extinction, a musk scent produced from plants and a chemical synthetic is now being widely used. In fact, most "musk oil" perfumes are synthetic.

Civet, a soft secretion the color and texture of butter, can be extracted from the exotic Civet cat, male or female, without killing the animal. The substance alone has a revolting smell, but in small quantities it enhances perfumes and creates a sexual signal. *Castoreum,* taken from a male or female beaver, also has an unpleasant odor but reacts favorably with other perfume ingredients.

Ambergris, considered to be the world's strongest external aphrodisiac, is not really a sexual secretion. It is actually a growth caused by the irritation of cuttlefish beaks in the stomach of a male sperm whale. It is usually found in the form of a black, malodorous material floating on the ocean in chunks weighing just a few ounces. Good quality ambergris is grayish, aged, and free of the blood and fecal matter that make the black variety smell horrible. The real prize is silver-gray ambergris, which smells musty, musky, and "of the sea." Ambergris makes perfumes last longer, and sends out a seductive undertone. A substitute called lebdanum has been created from the leaves of rock roses, certainly more romantic-sounding than a purged stomach growth.

Eau de Antiseptic

Does peppermint merely mask mouth odors, or does it kill germs that cause bad breath? Are your cosmetics and colognes protecting you from disease? Biochemical researchers in the U.S. and India recently released evidence that certain fragrance materials have a measurable antibacterial and antifungal effect.

Peppermint oil was shown to be one of the most potent flavorings, and was reported effective against a fungus that causes lung disease and ear infections. It also works well against fungi that cause animal diseases and spoil food. Tests showed that peppermint oil is twice as strong as quintozene, a chemical used to protect seeds from fungus, and up to seven times as strong as other antifungal chemicals. It is *not* effective against bacteria, such as those causing mouth odor.

People have used spices and perfumes against microorganisms for centuries, even when the connection between germs and disease was unknown. Burning incense during religious ceremonies began as a way to eliminate the stench of animal sacrifices; and it is still practiced today as an act of purification. In the seventeenth century physicians treating plague victims wore leather beaks filled with cloves, cinnamon, and other aromatics, or wrapped perfumed rags over their faces. Such practices not only made their work less offensive, but—depending on the fragrance materials used—may have helped to prevent infection.

Clove flavor, musk, sandalwood, lemon scent, and a few others of the 500 tested by U.S. researchers were found to be as strong as carbolic acid, a common antiseptic. At least 200 of the 500 proved somewhat effective against microorganisms; and 64 fragrance materials significantly suppressed microorganisms that cause body odor, yeast infections, and staph infections. None of the antibacterial fragrants were as strong as disinfectants currently used in deodorant soaps; but, as studies continue, we may find safe, fragrant ways to rid our bodies and environments of odor- and disease-causing germs. "Eau de Antiseptic" may become m'Lady's favorite toilet water.

A Religion of Scents

Shunammitism, an ancient religion based on the belief that the body scents of the young have a healing effect on the old, was founded by a man who surrounded himself with the virgins of Shunam. He lived to the age of 115 and credited his longevity to the healthful air—the virgins' exhalations and body scents—which he regularly breathed.

There is reference to this religion in the Old Testament of the Judaic-Christian Bible. The elderly King David, frail and ailing, was supposedly rejuvenated when a young virgin was brought to his side. Moderns might have a somewhat different explanation for this effect, but the ancients' explanation—healthful fragrances—seems to support current ideas on the effect of the pheromones.

Hello, I Love You

The nose kiss, still practiced in many countries, is a form of greeting in which one inhales the scent of another person in order to "receive a portion" of him.

In several living languages, as well as in ancient Sanskrit, the verb "to greet" is the same as the verb "to smell." In Persian, the word *bujah* means "smell," but also means "love, yearning." The French *sentir* means both "to feel" and "to smell."

Not That Hungry

Primitive man seldom, if ever bathed, and was covered with matted odor-trapping hair. Because he had to compete with wild animals for food, his terrible odor was a protective mechanism. He smelled and tasted so bad that many predatory animals would not make a meal of him unless they were desperate. Even today, only one carnivore in 100,000 will deign to eat human flesh—and then only if the animal is old or sick. Even vultures won't touch human flesh until it has been cleansed and ripened by the sun. If it's any consolation, most monkeys and chimpanzees are similarly eschewed.

Aaa Choo, I Do!

Early Latins and Romans associated the length of a man's nose with his virility—and punishment for a sexual offense was amputation of the nose. The association is really not farfetched. At the onset of male puberty, there is a corresponding spurt of nose growth, and indeed the mucous lining of the nose assumes characteristics of erectile tissue (flared nostrils). Comparatively speaking, the nose and the penis are the only 2 organs that lie on the body's midline, and both protrude.

There are further evidences of a unique connection. Some physicians treat severe nosebleeds by applying ice to the genitals. There's also a connection between *nosebleeds* (or other nasal problems) and female menstruation. In one study, 83 percent of adult females who'd failed to have menstrual cycles because of underdeveloped ovaries also tended to have an impaired sense of smell. Among women with normal menses, only 2 percent had a poor sense of smell. Women who have menstrual problems also may experience nosebleeds; physicians can sometimes cure *both* problems simultaneously by applying cocaine to certain spots in the nose.

Still another sex-related nasal problem is the common disorder known as "Bride's Nose"—excessive sneezing and congestion experienced before, during, or after sexual intercourse. This usually lasts for only a day or 2, adding a bit of change from the usual, romantic honeymoon. On the other hand, there have been many reports of *relief* from stuffiness after sexual intercourse. Certainly worth a try!

Overload

Only 1 percent of all the sensory data our 5 senses constantly receive is processed by the brain. The other 99 percent is screened out as irrelevant.

If this were not the case, our minds would be constantly distracted by sensory overload. As a result, there could be no mental concentration or specialization and, ultimately, no survival.

Chapter Three

Signals and Switchboards: The Nerve Network

Access to Power

A single nerve cell in the human hand, as narrow as 1/25,000 of an inch (1 micron), can be sensed by the human brain.

Extension Cord

The body's nerve network, if stretched out in a straight line, would measure some 45 miles (72 kilometers). This unraveled length is about 42,000 times the average person's height.

Messages Through the Soup

As in a city's communications network, some of the body's signaling systems have several points of origin and numerous addressees. In a process which is similar to mailing and delivering letters or magazines, glands and other specialized transmitters send out messages in the form of genetic and chemical codes. These are broadcast through the bloodstream or pass directly from cell to cell. Special codes enable organs and cells to receive and act upon certain of these messages and ignore the rest.

These chemicals, floating through the body's delicately balanced fluids—the internal "soup"—are totally sufficient for plants and very simple animals, and meet a majority of the human body's communications needs. People and other higher animal forms also need communications systems which provide constant news about the world outside, transmit directions, and organize information for making decisions.

The nervous system carries out these crucial functions. This remarkable, versatile network of transmission lines and switchboards links the brain with the world in which we live. It reports events, sensations, pain, and pleasure. It organizes and orders most of the functions of the body, especially its motion and movement.

Billions of cells process tens of billions of pieces of information every few seconds. The means of communication inside the body are much more varied and complex than even the most technologically advanced "external" systems designed by humankind. If the body's internal communication is interrupted, life ceases almost instantly. Indeed, death could be defined as a complete breakdown of communications.

The Electric Tree

A diagram of the human nervous system looks remarkably like a picture of a tree without leaves. Most evident are the nerve branches over which the messages travel, but central to the system—the tree's "trunk"—is the spinal cord. Rooted in the lower part of the brain, the spinal cord consists mostly of the same kind of gray cells which process and transmit information within the brain itself.

Unlike the trunk of a tree, however, the spinal cord is not thick and rigid. It is the same size as the index finger—about 1/2 of an inch (1.3 centimeters) in diameter. It is less than 2 feet long, ranging from 15 to 18 inches (37 to 45 centimeters) in adults, and weighs only 30 to 40 grams—just a few ounces—or less than a hen's egg.

The spinal cord resembles a slender rubber hose, and bends as easily. It runs through the rounded central openings of the spinal column, a stack of 32 remarkable bones.

There are over 10 billion cells in the spinal cord and the nerves, extending to the farthest points of the body—about half the 20-plus

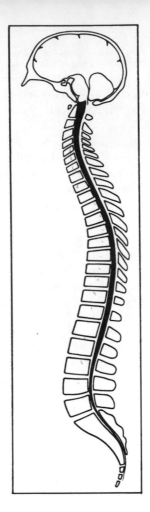

The spinal cord resembles a slender rubber hose, about as thick as an index finger and less than 2 feet long. It weighs just a few ounces, less than a hen's egg, but contains half the 20-plus billion nerve cells in the human body. Courtesy National Institutes of Health.

billion *nerve* cells in the body. The other half are in the brain. These vital nerve cells comprise only 1/5,000 of the 100 trillion cells in the human body.

Considering all that this "tree" within us means to our functioning as human beings, it is worthy of greater awe than the mightiest oak, or the most magnificently lit holiday evergreen. Ours, too, is an "electric" tree—switched on before we are born, and remaining charged with electrochemical impulses throughout our lives.

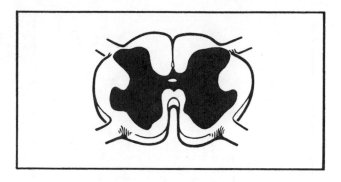

The same kind of gray cells that process and transmit information within the brain make up most of the spinal cord. Courtesy National Institutes of Health.

Branching Out

Like a spruce or other tree whose branches begin close to the ground, the nervous system divides into major branches which then subdivide again and again.

Some of the major branches lead to the head and face. Originating in the upper part of the spinal cord and in the brain itself, these signal circuits serve the specialized senses that provide the brain with such a large part of its news: vision, sound, smell, and taste.

These nerves control the muscles which we use to frown or smile, and direct the extremely complex activity of talking—one of the major outputs of the body's communications system.

Immediately below the head, major branches lead off to the arms, dividing again and again. The smallest nerves reaching the fingertips and other final destinations are far thinner than the most delicate hair; they are only 1/300 of an inch (0.8 millimeter) in length.

Next, other major nerves lead away from the spinal cord, passing between the thoracic vertebrae and along the ribs. These provide feeling to the chest area and control the heart, lungs, and other organs of the chest and abdomen.

The 2 most physically prominent branches, the sciatic nerves, lead downward to the legs from the lower part of the spinal cord. They spread and subdivide into fanlike extensions of smaller nerves which monitor and control the complex tasks of standing, walking, running, and maintaining balance. The sciatic nerves are the largest in the human body—about as thick as a lead pencil. This is some 3,000 times thicker than a fine nerve fiber.

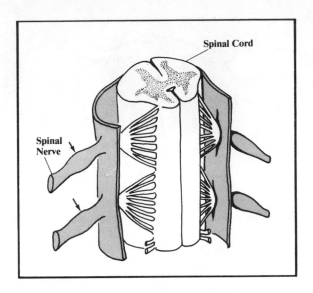

Major spinal nerves lead away from the spinal cord to the head and face; arms; chest, heart, and abdomen; and the legs. The sciatic nerves that branch off from the lower part of the spinal cord are the largest in the human body—about as thick as a lead pencil—some 3,000 times thicker than a fine nerve fiber. The arrows show where viruses such as herpes hide out. Courtesy National Institutes of Health.

Your Personal Network

Switchboards and relays in our nervous system route the messages through the network and maintain quality control, making sure that there is no loss in signal volume or clarity.

A telephone circuit essentially will handle messages of any kind, from any source, indifferently. Voices or the digital tones of a computer, good news or bad news, are accepted by a telephone wire, moving in either direction. The human nervous system is much more selective and specialized.

Messages travel over telephone lines at the speed of electricity—that is, the speed of light. A telephone message will travel across a city so quickly that only the most sensitive and precise instrument could measure the time elapsed.

The electrical impulses which travel over nerves are slower, but the body is a much smaller system, so nerve signals can travel between any 2 points in the body in a fraction of a second. Nerve cells, neurons, are thin but longer than other cells. Some—branches of the sciatic nerve,

SIGNALS AND SWITCHBOARDS:

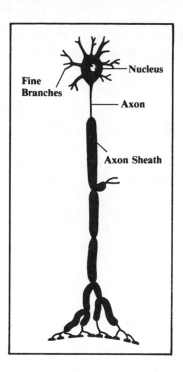

Some nerve cells, those from the spinal cord to the toes, are exceptionally long. Up to 3 feet (0.9 meter) in length, they are by far the longest cells in the human body. Courtesy National Institutes of Health.

which go from the spinal cord to the toes—are exceptionally long, up to 3 feet (0.9 meter) in length—by far the longest cells in the body.

These long filaments look like wires. More strikingly, they look like the extremely fine glass fibers which are now used to transmit information in the form of light pulses. Long, slender stems called axons are the principal part of a neuron. These end in fine extensions, called dendrites, which look like the roots of a plant or the frayed tangle of tiny wires at the end of a light cord minus its plug.

The dendrites of a nerve cell are adjacent to the dendrites of the next but do not quite touch. The space between the 2 cells is called a synapse. A message traveling up one axon is not immediately transferred across the synapse to the next in an uninterrupted electrical current. Instead, the message is relayed chemically.

Subtle alterations in the sodium and potassium ions between one set of dendrites and the next send the message on to the next cell. Other chemical processes, still not fully understood, also affect the handling of the message.

The process is repeated as the message continues up the axon of the next cell and on to the next synapse. The message crosses the synapse in less than 1/10,000 of a second—some 20 times faster than it takes a balloon to pop.

A Nerve for Every Occasion

Unlike telephone lines, nerves are specialized. Each transmits only one kind of information, and in only one direction.

The sensory nerves gather data that are sent back through the progressively larger nerve branches, up the spinal cord to the brain. Nerve endings scattered throughout the body provide the sense of touch, enabling us to feel pleasure as well as pain, a light touch or intense pressure.

Functions are specialized. Some nerves report only on heat or cold; some respond when the skin is stroked gently or jabbed with an object. Other cells acquire information from our eyes, ears, and nose. Still other nerves transmit instructions: The motor nerves direct the muscles and other organs, telling each fiber and joint of a finger or foot where to go and how fast. Each of these different kinds of nerves has its own reserved channel back to the intermediate switchboards in the ganglia stations or plexus networks and in the spinal cord, and then to the central processing unit in the brain.

Nerve fibers responsible for various specialized functions are concentrated together in nerve bundles. A nerve bundle only 1/25 of an inch (1 millimeter) in diameter typically contains hundreds or even more than a thousand separate nerve filaments, each carrying its own signal.

The sensory endings in the skin are also specialized. For example, one variety, known as Meissner's corpuscle, is exceptionally sensitive to touch. They are found on the fingertips but are also present in large numbers on the genital organs, especially the clitoris and the tip of the penis.

The World's Best Communications System

Different types of nerve cells carry messages at different speeds. Touch, pleasant or painful, is reported through the neurons at about 135 miles (216 kilometers) per hour. The fastest impulses, in large nerve fibers such as in the sciatic nerve, reach 325 miles (520 kilometers) per hour. Athletes depend on these, especially runners.

An electrical engineer contemplating the design of the nervous sys-

---

tem might consider these specialized circuits and electrochemical relays extremely complicated and slow. Compared to a system of silicon chips and circuit boards in an arcade game or home computer, the human nervous system does indeed operate slowly. However, the living components of the body's nervous system are so compact and efficient, and perform so many functions, that the added complexity is not a disadvantage. All things considered, the system as a whole operates very rapidly. How much faster, after all, could we jerk our fingers away from a hot object?

Fast and Cool

Although messages traveling over the neurons move much more slowly than digital data passing over a telephone wire, the entire system operates at extremely high speed.

If you have used a computer you know that many operations, like implementing a program or searching for something on a memory disk, take several seconds and may take much longer. The computer must work its way through a fixed sequence of instructions, which takes time. When a mechanical device like a disk drive is involved, that takes more time.

The nervous system operates under extremely sophisticated, flexible "programs" which seem to skip "unnecessary" levels of instructions. The brain and indeed the entire nervous system are extraordinarily compact, much more so than even the most advanced machine. A computer may be able to perform specialized tasks like calculations more rapidly and accurately, but for most purposes the equipment that everyone is born with is superior. Even the most optimistic enthusiasts working with supercomputers and artificial intelligence admit that they have a long way to go to match the human nervous system.

The body's system has another advantage. Engineers developing advanced high-capacity computers are finding it difficult to dispose of the heat generated by the flows of electrons within the chips and other components, especially when they are packed closely in the most powerful machines. Operating in its unique electrochemical way, the nervous system seems to have no difficulty staying cool, while processing enormous volumes of information.

Body Software

Most people like to think of themselves as being "in control." We want to do everything just the way *we* decide to do it. We are inclined to forget that a very large proportion of the functions controlled by the nervous system occur automatically, without our conscious attention.

You can decide you want a hamburger, rather than a cheeseburger or just the diet salad plate. You can control whether you eat quickly or slowly. But you can't tell your body how to digest that hamburger.

You can decide to stand up, but you won't be telling your heart, veins, and arteries to adjust your blood supply to accommodate the movement. Nor will you consciously instruct your body to keep its internal temperature at almost precisely the same level, despite your decision to lie on a beach in the hot sun or to later plunge into a cold ocean.

If everything that happened to us was put under our conscious control, our ability to decide what to do next would be all but lost—and we'd accomplish very little. The thinking part of our brains can do fantastic things for us; but in order to make this possible, the brain relies on the rest of the nervous system to "simplify" our lives.

The autonomous nerves function as the body's full-time "housekeeper." They ensure the continued functioning of essentials such as breathing and controlling levels of internal warmth. This subsystem also aids your sex life, as in the case of those autonomous nerves in the pelvic area that seem to have a "mind of their own," especially in initiating ejaculation and orgasm.

Beyond the sheer volume of functions to be controlled, the conscious mind would have further difficulty in maintaining smooth operations. Even the most brilliant mind is imperfect. Attention wanders. The mind forgets. It makes mistakes. These imperfections are the inescapable side effects of the brain's capacity to consider alternatives, examine new facts, and think about a problem until a fresh idea appears. The housekeeper or "secretarial" capabilities of the autonomous nervous system remind us of more important things than meeting times or anniversary dates. They "remind" us to breathe—an activity that is not automatic in some prematurely born humans.

The nervous system does many things that we take for granted. Unless abused or damaged, it continues to do us very well until death do us part.

SIGNALS AND SWITCHBOARDS:

Hammer on the Knee

Have you ever wondered why a doctor giving you a physical examination usually taps you just below the kneecap with a rubber hammer? The doctor is not checking your knee itself. He is testing the responses of a main branch of the sciatic nerve which runs close to the surface of your knee on the way to the lower leg.

The tap of the hammer causes the nerve to send a report up to the spinal cord. Nerve centers there should respond immediately, telling the muscles in the leg to jerk upward. This shows that the reflex ability of the nerves is functioning well to achieve important automatic reactions.

These reflexes help to protect the body. If you are walking through the woods and a twig springs back suddenly toward your eye, the eye will blink protectively before you are consciously aware of the danger. Full-term infants are born with this instinctive reflex, and under normal conditions adults never lose it.

If you unwittingly grasp a pot handle which is too hot, your hand will let go and pull back before you realize your mistake. This may spill the soup, but it reduces the risk of a serious burn.

This emergency response depends on switchboards below the brain which recognize danger signals and react directly. They relay the message on to the brain, but at the same time send immediate instructions down the motor nerves so that the muscles will pull back without delay.

This avoids the small but significant fraction of a second needed for the warning message to travel farther up the spinal cord. It also provides a simple, prompt, preprogrammed response without requiring the time which the brain would otherwise need to recognize a danger, decide what might be done, and send the signal to take action.

Basic reflexes such as the knee jerk or the Achilles tendon reflex can be influenced and modified by the brain. Emotional tension, for example, causes a person's knee to jerk higher than it otherwise would.

The Body Adjusting to Itself

Managing the motions that seem simple to us—such as walking or lifting small objects—is in fact a very complex business. We become fully aware of this complexity only when something goes wrong, because of fatigue, dizziness or sickness.

Much of the communications traffic over the nervous system is concerned with keeping the temperature of the whole system at the right level, breathing, keeping the blood moving at the right speed and pressure, extracting energy from food, and disposing of waste materials. This work is carried out by a special network, the autonomic system, which controls all the involuntary bodily functions.

Internal monitoring is also critical every time we reach toward something to pick it up. If the messages traveling over the nerves are too simple—just "go" and "get," for example—your fingers would miss or overshoot. If you are reaching for an egg or fragile cup, it might be broken.

This process, known as feedback, is so effortless a part of our daily life that it seems too obvious to require mention. In the early days of research into computers and robots, however, scientists encountered many difficulties because they had not realized the importance of feedback.

Through feedback circuits and devices called servomechanisms, researchers learned to make their machines less clumsy, less likely to spin around and fall flat. In order to do this, it was necessary to increase greatly the information-processing capacity of the system as well as the sensitivity and variety of sensors.

Using the human body as a model and resource for researchers, engineers have imitated certain aspects of the nervous system in the latest robotics technology. In just decades, they have selectively imitated a living system, one that took millions of years to evolve. It's a good thing that the human body is not patented.

Consciousness of the Unconscious

Biofeedback enables people to gain a limited, specialized degree of deliberate control over their autonomous nerves and the unconscious processes of feedback.

So far, this new method is applied mostly to cases in which the ordinary housekeeping functions of the body are not going well on their own. The subject is wired up to sensors which keep track of poor temperature control in some part of the body, excessive blood pressure, a feeling of "stress," or other problem.

Watching dials and cathode-ray terminals which look like TV sets, the patient can learn by trial and error to exercise conscious control—perhaps only on a limited and occasional basis—over the function which has gone wrong.

All of us can do something like this when we realize that too much tension and anxiety have built up. A deliberate effort to slow down, relax, and take it easy can often help—even by reducing rates of breathing and heartbeat. Through training and frequent sessions involving this kind of deliberate relaxation, many people learn to exercise considerable control over the general state of tension and state of mind.

Biofeedback teaches us ways to deal with stress more effectively and to learn to assist the self-regulating nerves of the body to do their jobs even more efficiently.

Biofeedback techniques have helped heart patients control their heart rates and blood pressure. Migraine sufferers have learned to control blood flow to their brains and reduce pain. Asthmatic children have been taught to correct their breathing problems. Patients have also learned to control stress by inducing their brain's alpha waves that signal inner peace and well-being. Even victims of strokes or serious accidents have regained partial control over injured skeletal muscles through biofeedback training.

And after successful training the biofeedback hardware can be sold or go into the closet. This doesn't make graduates authentic Indian yogis, but it does mean they can obtain relief without the electrodes and the humming, buzzing, or ringing devices that have helped them control some aspects of their involuntary nervous systems.

The Competitive Human

The complex interactions among the conscious and unconscious functions of the nervous system are shown most conspicuously in the performance of a trained athlete.

Champion long jumpers, for example, think in terms of getting the best possible performance from their muscles. It is easy to overlook that this also means optimum performance by the motor nerves and feedback mechanisms which guide those muscles and control their timing.

The nerves involved most directly in a long jump are the sciatic nerves which control the legs. A championship jump also requires perfect performance from the 30 other pairs of nerves which branch out from the spinal cord. For this reason, the lives of athletes call for self-discipline that goes beyond exercise of key muscles.

The sacral and lumbar nerves which lead away from the lower back are involved in maintaining balance and in giving added power to the leap.

Higher up, the thoracic and cervical nerves of the chest and neck ensure that the arms and head will provide the right balance and momentum during the run and the final jump. Autonomous nerves attend to the appropriate cueing of heart and lungs, although the responsiveness of these organs is determined by the individual's total lifestyle and habits.

The innate capacity of these nerves, enhanced through long training, enables athletes to focus mentally on a target, to concentrate on exceeding a personal "best"—or an accomplishment of another record holder.

When the starting command is given and the athlete begins to run, the involved nerve centers operate in essentially the same way as do similar nerve centers in a leopard or cheetah as they make running leaps while pursuing a gazelle.

Getting the Hang of It

Anyone who has ever tried to put the ball into the basket more often or lower his golf handicap knows that training the body to do some specialized form of physical activity is one of the most frustrating forms of learning.

This is not surprising because you are trying to train the spinal cord and peripheral nerves to learn new patterns or apply reflexes in an unfamiliar way. The brain can do only so much in instructing the other nerves, and sometimes too much thinking gets in the way.

We are especially conscious of this because an unprecedented number and variety of people are trying to succeed in some sport or athletic competition at a fairly serious level. More sedentary people face similar problems when they try to master a new dance step or learn how to type or drive a car.

In all these activities, learning to do something well takes time and repetition—practice, practice, practice. Conscious analytical attention by the athlete or a coach can help, but is no guarantee of progress.

What is happening? The nerves, including the switchboards and information-processing centers, are required to transmit and manage information in new ways and to work with the muscles in new patterns. The nerves learn to discriminate, to pay special attention to certain kinds of news and to ignore or suppress insignificant signals.

Learning of this kind tends to progress unpredictably. The athlete in training or the student driver experiences ups, downs, long periods of getting nowhere, and sudden breakthroughs.

An afternoon of perfect coordination, of flawless execution, can be followed by days or even months of stumbling mediocrity. We are frustrated because there seems no way to get at the problem and fix it. If frustration becomes too acute, performance is likely to become even worse. The remedy: Get away from it, if possible, and relax. Do something different. Then, when the time and feeling are right, try and try again.

Setting Your Mind to It

Can the thinking part of your mind help to improve your physical skills? Yes—in several ways. However difficult it may be, the body should be allowed to proceed with the complex process of learning in its own way, at its own pace. Worrying and feeling guilty do no good.

As every coach and exercise book tell you, a consistent routine of practice and repetition is fundamental; but this can fail if too much is expected too soon.

Concentration is also extremely important. Paradoxically, this is not only a question of focusing your thoughts on what you are doing. Even more important, concentration involves shutting out distractions so that the conscious mind will allow the rest of the nervous system to do what it has learned to do.

The Oriental masters of martial arts such as kung fu, judo, and karate place great emphasis on this kind of concentration. Training in concentration receives as much attention as conditioning the reactions of nerves and muscles. As a result, the accomplished expert in the martial arts can move with extraordinary speed, smoothness, and power.

Killing the Pain

For many people, especially the growing proportion of older persons, genuinely painful conditions like arthritis or back trouble weigh down every minute of their lives.

Marathoners and professional athletes sometimes sound like they are celebrating a cult of pain. Coping with the pain of running or playing on despite a painful injury is considered proof of dedication and toughness.

In fact, pain plays a crucial protective function. Pain is an alarm bell, a warning. When a bone or muscle is injured, pain tells us to use that part of the body very carefully or not at all while the body goes on about healing itself.

If a wild animal or your family dog has been hurt, it will respond to the pain by finding a safe place to curl up. Instinctively, it conserves its resources and avoids movement which could make the injury worse.

This is often the most sensible cure for people, but rest and care are not always enough. Modern medicine has devoted a great deal of attention to pain and to ways to reduce it—especially severe or chronic pain which does not serve any practical purpose as a warning.

Effective means for controlling pain temporarily or in one place have been available for more than a century. This has helped transform surgery from a crude, harsh craft into the precise, versatile science it is today.

A local anesthetic like Novocain is injected into the area next to a selected nerve or set of nerves. For a short period, it interferes with the neurons' signal-carrying ability, affecting motor nerves as well as sensory nerves. If, for example, a dentist has used a local anesthetic, numbness in the cheek and lips may make it difficult to speak clearly because the muscles will not respond.

Similar drugs, injected into the area of the spinal cord, will block all feeling throughout the body below the point of the injection. General anesthetics administered as a gas or into the bloodstream operate mostly on the lower levels of the brain, suspending certain functions of the entire network of nerves. Some cause a deep sleep and total unconsciousness. Others, like nitrous oxide, or laughing gas, usually put the patient asleep or into a state between consciousness and unconsciousness, depending on dosage, but only for a relatively short period. The short duration of its effects makes nitrous oxide good for extracting teeth. Instead of pain, the patient has a few laughs.

My Aching Back

In the timetable of evolution, the upright, two-legged condition of humankind is a recent innovation and perhaps an unwise one. It causes especially severe problems for the nervous system, which depends upon the vertebrae of the spinal column to support and protect the spinal cord.

For more conventional vertebrate animals, the spine is a sensible horizontal linkage of bone, sinew and muscle, hung like a clothesline between the main bony frameworks of the forequarters and hindquarters. In people, however, the spine, shoulders, neck, and head are all balanced perilously.

If a person is active and reasonably careful, it is possible to avoid damage to these vulnerable, sensitive systems. Hard physical work or steady exercise will maintain a sturdy tone in the muscles which hold the whole improbable structure together.

Trouble usually comes from a sedentary life and soft beds. It is often brought about by unaccustomed heavy lifting, shoveling snow, or an ill-considered impromptu softball game. Such activities exert a strain on the muscles of the lower back which may stiffen and tighten up, or go into spasm. These protective reactions result in pain, especially if the stiffness causes direct pressure on the main nerve branches in the lower back. The pain can be severe, even disabling.

In industrialized societies, some 60 percent of the male population between the ages of 25 and 69 have had back pain at one time or another. This amounts to millions of aching backs at any given moment.

Damaged Discs

In industrialized societies, back pain ranks second only to the common cold as a cause of time lost from work. About 4 hours for every worker each year go down the drain because of low-back pain, much of which is due to damaged areas of the spinal column.

The space between each bone of the spine is occupied by a pad of tough gristle, shaped like a flattened doughnut, called a disc. When a disc is damaged or slips out of place—a condition known as herniated nucleus pulposus—it may press on the spinal cord or upon one of the main nerves leading away from it, usually causing severe, even paralyzing, lower back or leg pain. Between the ages of 30 and 40, a man or woman, especially one who sits more than 50 percent of the time, is more susceptible to the condition because his or her discs are in the process of losing their water content. Below age 30, the discs have

When damaged or out of position, the discs between the vertebrae press on the spinal cord or spinal nerves and cause lower back or leg pain. In industrial societies, some 60 percent of all men between the ages of 25 and 69 have back pain at one time or another. Courtesy National Institutes of Health.

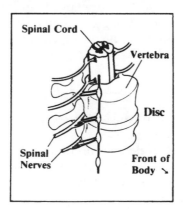

enough resilience to protect them from damage; above age 40, they acquire more stability from tough fibers that replace the water.

If damage is severe, a disc can be surgically removed, and the bones of the spinal column can be fused together. But surgery of this kind means the cutting of bone and tissue, accompanied by a recovery period of a month or more. There is a new technique called chymopapain which eliminates the risks of conventional surgery and allows some patients to leave the hospital the day of the operation. With the chymopapain treatment, doctors insert needles in the vicinity of the spinal injury. The needles deliver an enzyme which dissolves the damaged fragments of the disc, restoring smoothness and relieving pressure on the nerve.

Chymopapain has a 70 percent success rate. Its enzyme is very similar to your everyday meat tenderizer.

It Hurts Right There, Doctor

As a fever indicates that the body is fighting infection, pain has its purpose in reporting injury or internal problems. Unfortunately, pain is not a reliable indicator, and it is of limited help to a physician in forming a diagnosis.

The perception of a pain's very source may be incorrect. The tooth that you point out as the one that hurts may not be the one that's abscessed. That pain in your arm may not be caused by a strain or injury to that area but could be the result of a problem in your heart or other organ. These are examples of a phenomenon known as referred pain.

Pain is also a subjective experience, both to the degree that it is felt and in the psychological response to it. Anxious, fearful people may exaggerate pain—both in perceiving its intensity and describing it to a doctor. If we have been warned to expect pain, we are more likely to feel the hurt and to a greater degree. People who have been taught to be "brave" or to feel guilty for inconveniencing others are reluctant to acknowledge pain.

When It Itches . . .

An itch is caused by a local irritation on the skin, such as a mosquito bite or small scrape; or it may be simply the equivalent of static in the nerves themselves. The natural reaction, almost a reflex, is to scratch.

The pain caused by a fingernail scratching the skin is usually minor, but it can be fairly severe, accompanied by redness and swelling. In any event, scratching produces deliberate pain. It overrides, masks, and usually relieves the unpleasant, distracting sensations of an itch.

Scratching an itch—applying pain against an irritation—is another paradox which underlines the subjective, often vague nature of pain and the uncertainties of dealing with it. People are as suggestible about itches as about pains. If we see another person scratching, it is difficult for us to control the impulse to scratch—even if we'd felt no itch.

Sending the Wrong Signals

Occasionally the nervous system errs and produces odd or misleading signals.

This can be benign, as in the case of ordinary hiccups. Of course, the autonomous nerves controlling the diaphragm and other muscles used in breathing are generally quite reliable—so reliable that, as angry small children discover, it is impossible to hold one's breath long enough to do any harm.

Hiccups occur when the nervous system cues the diaphragm to produce spasmodic contractions. The contractions push air into the pharynx, an air passage in the throat, and close the opening between the vocal cords (the glottis); the "hic" sound is created when sudden bursts of air strike the closed glottis. This may all be a reaction to such stimuli as sudden swallowing of hot liquids or laughing uncontrollably —but the hiccups do us no good whatsoever.

Usually, everyone near the victim of hiccups will suggest a different cure. All have the same purpose, however—to interrupt the cycle of spasmodic movement and restore the usual rhythm. With rare exceptions, this does not take long—whatever the remedy.

Other kinds of garbled messages from the body are more serious, indicating damage or disease in the nervous system itself. A person who has lost a limb may continue to "receive" phantom sensations— including, perhaps, severe pain—and think the limb is still attached.

Sometimes, twitches or tremors appear in the face or fingers, or a person becomes unable to walk or talk normally. These symptoms may be brought on by extreme fatigue, severe psychological strain, or the numbing of a nerve by exposure to cold.

Tremors may also indicate nerve damage or the beginning of an illness, such as multiple sclerosis or Parkinson's disease. The quavering walk of very old people is a sign that the nervous system, along with other systems of the body, is wearing out—the "electric tree" is fading.

Nerves of Passion

The nerves involved most directly in the act of love branch off from the sacral area in the lower back, toward the lower end of the spinal cord. The sexual organs are served by a variety of sensory nerves as well as the autonomic nerves which march to their own drum.

Nerves serving the sex organs include those of the pelvic plexus, or pudendal nerves. In women, fine branches reach into the vagina and uterus. In men, the greater and lesser cavernous nerves control the parts of the penis that fill with blood to bring about an erection.

The nerves involved most directly in the sensations and excitement of sexual intercourse are the dorsal nerves, reaching to the clitoris and the end of the penis. Many of these nerves are very fine and difficult to find in conventional anatomical dissection. These slender filaments, however, can transmit an extraordinary intensity of signals.

The pace and nature of excitement differ between male and female. The male usually reaches a faster climax of sensations, the moment at which the autonomous nerves take over and call for ejaculation. The female's response tends to be more diffuse and subjective, but the location of key nerve endings—outside the vagina, as compared to the male's concentrated on the tip of the penis—often explains her relative slowness to reach a peak of pleasure.

A Pacemaker for Love?

Psychological impotence can be cured by relaxing and permitting the autonomic nerves of the pelvic plexus to do their spontaneous work without interference from anxiety. If, however, the pudendal nerves are damaged by illness or injury, the loss of sexual potency is not corrected so easily. Older men requiring surgical removal of the prostate gland, which can involve cutting key nerves needed for sexual functioning, often found their sex lives cut short also.

After close study of the fine nerves in the pelvic plexus, doctors developed new surgical techniques that permit removal of a diseased prostate without damage to the nerves passing near the prostate and rectum—those which control erections.

Other research is developing an electric pacemaker for lovemaking, similar to the pacemakers implanted in the body which send electrical signals to control the heartbeat. The pacemaker, attached to damaged nerves near the prostate, would provide a full erection and all the

SIGNALS AND SWITCHBOARDS:

pleasure that comes with it. Research on monkeys has demonstrated that the electrically stimulated erection can last for several hours!

East to West, Earlobe to Arm

Traditional Oriental medicine assumes that pathways or channels not evident in dissection link different parts of the body. These pathways play an important part in sensation and pain as well as other functions of the body. Stimulation of one site causes a response in the area to which it is linked. The association of body parts often seems incongruous.

For example, a carefully placed stimulus to the earlobe is said to affect feeling in an arm or lung; and the palm of the hand is said to influence the liver. These and other relationships have been mapped in detail over the centuries, and the traditional training of an Oriental physician is devoted in large part to mastering knowledge of the different pathways and their areas of influence.

Chinese doctors generally use finger pressure or electrical currents to apply the stimulus. In the West, the greatest attention has been devoted to acupuncture, an ancient Oriental technique in which slender needles are inserted carefully into selected spots on the body and then moved or twirled precisely.

Although many doctors outside the Far East remain skeptical, acupuncture seems to be effective in many cases and is used at times for anesthesia during major abdominal, throat, head, and neck surgery. Doubters explain this as an extreme case of suggestibility.

Some physicians in the West, however, have observed that pain centers—which they prefer to call "gateways"—may indeed affect sensations elsewhere in the body. Recent research suggests that the inserted acupuncture needles may generate nerve signals that override the pain sensation. Other researchers think that the needles may release the brain's own painkilling chemicals as they puncture the skin and flesh.

What cannot be denied is that the technique works for thousands of patients who have had some of the body's 500 to 800 acupuncture points pierced with thin steel needles.

Regeneration and Repair

Although our stock of nerve cells is fixed at birth and declines steadily thereafter, those running through our arms, legs, and most of the rest of the body are relatively well protected and insured against irreversible damage. These peripheral nerves are covered with a tough, white fatty sheath, called myelin, which serves as a protective insulation and also assists in recovery and repair after injuries.

Peripheral nerves with myelin sheaths—such as those in an injured leg—can regenerate themselves—in effect, they grow back, although slowly. Most nerves of this kind are long, and regeneration proceeds at only a millimeter or 2 each day, requiring 2 weeks or so to repair just 1 inch of nerve fiber. Regeneration of nerves from knee to toe could therefore easily take a full year. In time, however, full feeling and control can be restored. If muscle tone has been retained through massage and determined effort, full recovery is possible.

In more severe cases, where a nerve on an arm or the face has been cut by a wound or damaged by a badly broken bone, surgery may be needed. Although thousands of nerve cells with different functions may be packed into a single fascicle or nerve bundle, neurosurgeons often can locate the break, clean up the damaged ends, and sew the nerve back together. Microsurgery and new techniques involving laser beams fuse nerve ends together, using the red cells of the blood as a kind of glue. Today such techniques can repair peripheral nerve tissue that would have been lost just a decade ago.

A Tragic Loss of Control

So far, repair of the damaged spinal cord has largely defeated neurosurgeons. Most of the nerves in the spinal cord are gray cells, like those in the brain, which lack myelin sheaths, and so are unable to regenerate themselves. The spinal cord, like the heart and the liver, is one of the few organs absolutely necessary to life which has no duplicate and not much spare capacity. (Even the brain has 2 hemispheres, one of which can take over from the other after a stroke or other accident.) Both the heart and the liver can endure considerable abuse, but the vulnerable spinal cord can not—it has no backup system. This is the price humanity has paid for standing upright.

If the spinal column is cut through or crushed, the result is complete paralysis of the muscles and other conscious functions below the point at which the spinal cord is severed. If the damage is relatively low on the spine, only the legs are affected. But a break close to the skull can cause complete paralysis of all limbs.

One of the harsh paradoxes of modern times has been an increase in paralyzing injuries of this kind. Many infectious diseases such as polio, which used to kill or cripple so many children and young people, have been controlled almost completely. During the same period, however, accidents on the highways and, occasionally, in competitive sports have been paralyzing great numbers of people for the rest of their lives. Some 12,000 serious spinal cord injuries occur in the United States alone each year. About 75 percent of these result from motor vehicle accidents. Diving accidents and gunshot wounds are the second and third most common causes.

Sensational Chemistry

New and significant discoveries about the electrochemistry of the nervous system in the last decade promise new treatments for mental and nervous disorders.

In the early stages of studying the nervous system, scientists tended to assume that the synapse, the gap between the dendrites of one neuron and those of the next, functioned essentially like a simple electrical switch. The synapse was disconnected, or it was on—it "fired" as the signal was sent onward. It was presumed that the whole process was as neutral and passive as a telephone wire.

Now it is known that dozens of specialized chemicals produced in the body influence and control the transmission of signals across the synapse. These chemicals, neurotransmitters, function somewhat like the editor of a magazine or the producer of a TV news show. They shape and guide the tone and content of the transmissions—not just in a single synapse, but everywhere in the body.

Neurotransmitters can affect mood, tension, alertness, and feelings throughout the body, reduce pain, or make sensations more acute. Learning, emotions, perhaps even romantic attraction may be influenced by these potent chemicals.

Scientists are working to synthesize these natural chemicals. Used as medicine, these artificial substances could operate upon different kinds of cells selectively, making it possible to treat nervous diseases with unprecedented precision.

Treatment with neurotransmitters could reduce dependence on addictive drugs which cause long-term damage to the body. Reaching into the brain, drugs which imitate neurotransmitters may provide successful treatment to those who suffer from serious depression or schizophrenia. Because these medicines would be so similar to natural substances, the side effects caused by present medications could be avoided. In our daily life, such medicines could help us improve our performance or overcome difficulties of emotion or mood.

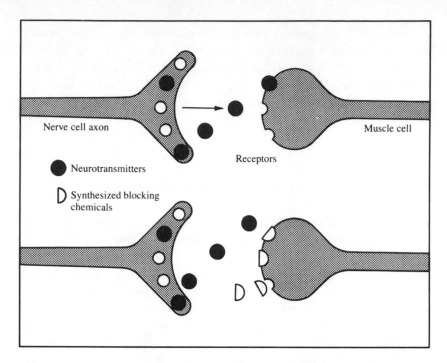

New discoveries about the electrochemistry of the nervous system hold great promise in the next few decades for treating disease. This diagram depicts how control of the nervous system at the microlevel takes place. A synthesized chemical blocks the action of a natural neurotransmitter, thus inhibiting muscle contraction. Wildlife experts use this knowledge to immobilize animals. Courtesy National Institutes of Health.

Partial Service May Be Restored Soon

Scientists seeking ways to repair the nonregenerative cells of the central nervous system are experimenting with man-made parts and computerized controls.

Working with animals, researchers have developed plastic inserts that function like the myelin sheath. Used to bypass a break, these nerve patches appear to be able to give the nerve tissue an opportunity to grow along the new pathway and regain function.

Doctors have also developed experimental systems which involve computer control of the muscles through artificial nerves, extremely thin stainless steel wires attached to the leg muscles of patients paralyzed by spinal injury. The computer's microprocessor sends signals in the right sequence, providing adequate feedback so that the injured person may walk. Before too long, at least some people who have suffered paralysis will be able to walk—with some difficulty, perhaps, but freed from constant dependence on a wheelchair.

Chapter Four

That Layered Look: Skin to Bone

SKIN AND HAIR

Counting Skins

The largest human organ is the skin, with a total surface area of about 25 square feet (2.3 square meters) for a large person. All of us completely change our outer skin about every 27 days. This adds up to almost 1,000 new outer skins in a lifetime.

Skin Revitalized

What holds our skin together? Mainly collagen, the protein of fibrous connective tissues. It is the most abundant protein in the human body and is present in skin, bone, and cartilage. Collagen is composed of protein molecules in bundles of coils.

Through an electron microscope, at very high magnifications, individual collagen fibrils resemble the steel reinforcing rods around which concrete walls are poured. The analogy has meaning because both the collagen and steel rods reinforce and strengthen surrounding

---

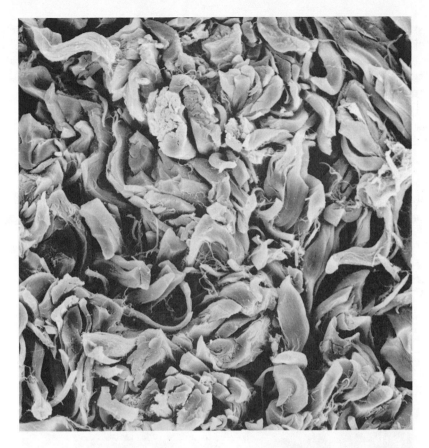

Collagen, the most abundant protein in the human body, is present in the skin, bone, and cartilage. It is what holds our skin together. Courtesy Dr. Karen Holbrook, University of Washington.

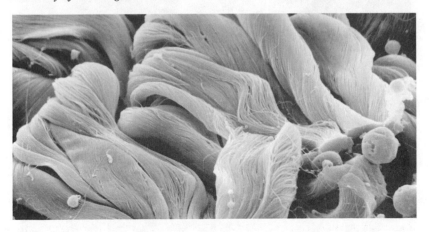

structures. Collagen bundles, at a lower magnification, resemble skeins of yarn.

A new skin treatment that smooths out wrinkles and scars involves collagen injections. Eternal youth—skin deep, at least—may become a reality for many of us in the not-too-distant future.

Shedding Skin

A good-sized man or woman sheds about 600,000 particles of skin every hour, which amounts to 1.5 pounds each year. By 70 years of age,

A close-up of a human skin particle flaking off. We are constantly shedding our skins. A good-sized man or woman sheds about 600,000 particles of skin every hour. Courtesy Dr. Karen Holbrook, University of Washington.

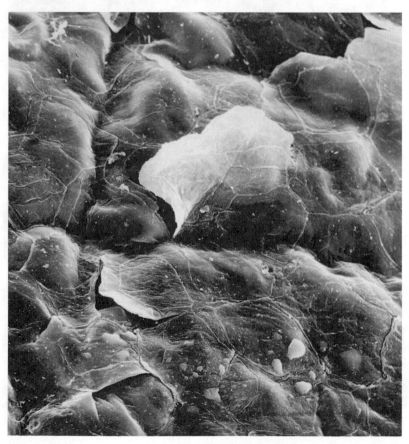

THAT LAYERED LOOK:

that person will have lost 105 pounds (48 kilograms) of skin—equal to about two thirds of their entire body weight.

Thin-Skinned

The human body has 6 pounds (2.7 kilograms) of skin, about 4 percent of its average weight. The skin's thickness varies, but it averages about 1/20 of an inch (1/50 of a centimeter) thick. Our eyelids contain the thinnest skin—less than 1/500 of an inch (1/200 of a centimeter) thick. This is more than 2 times thinner than a human hair.

Man-Made Skin

Skin transplants for badly burned victims with large burn areas have traditionally come from pigs or cadavers. The big drawback: They are rejected by the body's immune system. Also, cadaver skin has a limit of 25 days.

Recently, after years of development, nonrejectable artificial skin has become available—there are at least 3 skin substitutes available to save the lives of thousands of burn victims each year.

The first type of man-made skin is a clear polyurethane film, which is placed over the burn like a piece of gauze. It keeps the burn area moist and is permeable so that oxygen can reach the white blood cells that protect the wound from dangerous, often lethal, bacteria. But this substitute skin has a drawback also; it cannot be used for second- and third-degree burns, wherein the blood vessels have been destroyed.

Two other man-made skins can be used to treat more serious burns. The first is a compound of nylon and silicone rubber, which is coated with chemicals taken from collagen (a protein of fibrous connective tissues which is found in the second layer of normal skin). This artificial skin is not rejected by the body and is not perishable—it can be stored indefinitely. Only 1/100 of an inch thick, this dressing can remain over the wound for as long as 2 months before a graft from the patient's own skin is made.

The most promising artificial skin, with 2 layers just like human skin, has been developed by scientists at MIT. The top layer (epidermis) is made of rubberlike silicone. The bottom layer is porous and made of a mixture of proteins and chemicals. Like real skin, it can "breathe" and let moisture out, the body does not reject it, and the fibrous bottom layer promotes growth of the patient's own collagen and the rejuvenation of nerve fibers. After about a month, the protective top layer is removed and replaced by grafts from other parts of the body. After several months, the real skin has grown and replaced the artificial skin.

What is the recipe for the all-important bottom layer? A mixture of cowhide, shark cartilage, and plastic.

Skin Farms

Even though the future of artificial skin seems assured, and there will continue to be significant advances, the best covering for burn victims is still their own skin—always in short supply if the burn covers most of the body.

Recent research has pioneered ways to supplement a patient's skin supply—by growing it in the laboratory. In one method, cells are taken from the patient. These fibroblasts (from the inner layers of skin) are cultured in a solution of collagen and become a tissuelike lattice. Then epidermal cells from the outer skin layers are added, cultured, and both layers are eventually grafted.

Outer skin (epidermal) cells can also be cultured separately. In 2 to 3 weeks, the cells will form a sheet across the culture dish, which is then placed on the wound.

While the surface area of such lab-grown skin was small at first—less than 1 square inch (2 square centimeters) for a successful human graft —Boston researchers have successfully cultivated 1 square yard (0.8 square meter) of cells to treat burn victims. The future no doubt will have laboratory farms growing human skin and skin banks to store it.

Host to Billions

You could wash your hands vigorously for hours and hours with soap and water, but countless bacteria would still remain. The hands, or any other part of the body for that matter, cannot be made sterile this way.

Every square inch (6.4 square centimeters) of the human body has an average of some 32 million bacteria on it, with a grand body total of 100 billion—over 22 times the human population on planet earth. These 100 billion bacteria could fit inside a medium-sized pea.

Fairies' Intestines

Eighty percent of our body heat escapes through the skin, the rest through our breathing. Skin is the human radiator and regulator of body temperature. When the body gets really hot, the microscopic sweat glands (once referred to as "fairies' intestines" by Oliver Wendell Holmes) go into action and secrete water containing salt and small amounts of other substances such as ammonia. This is sweat. It is odorless and sterile until bacteria begin to act on it. Every day our bodies secrete at least a pint of sweat—even when we are relatively inactive and are unaware of it. The water in the sweat comes from the blood.

An English coal miner is on record as having sweated 1.8 British gallons (8 liters) in 5.5 hours. He lost 18 pounds as a result.

Skin Vents

There are over 2 million sweat glands in the adult body. They are tightly coiled tubes buried deep in the inner layer of skin, the dermis. Their ducts rise to the skin's surface through the pores, and if their coils were unwound, each one would be about 50 inches (127 centime-

A sweat pore magnified 125 times. There are over 2 million sweat glands on an adult's body, releasing 80 percent of our body heat. Courtesy Dr. Karen Holbrook, University of Washington.

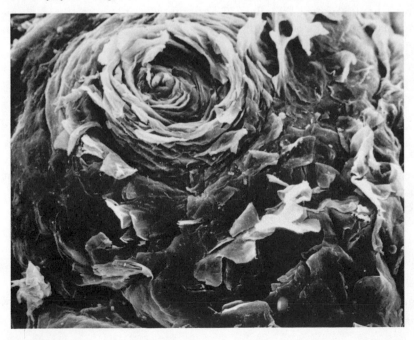

ters) in length. Everyone therefore has upwards of 2,000 miles (3,218 kilometers) of this ducting.

The Crowded Skin

Just 1 square inch (6.4 square centimeters) of skin, about twice the area of your thumbnail and no thicker than 2 pennies, contains about:
645 sweat glands
77 feet (23.5 meters) of nerves and over 1,000 nerve endings
65 hair follicles
97 sebaceous glands (they provide the lubricating oil for skin and hair)
19 feet (5.8 meters) of blood vessels

Down the Drain

People lose about 45 hairs every day; some of us as many as 60 hairs. But because the average scalp contains about 125,000 hairs, this loss is insignificant. Over a lifetime, though, an individual can lose more than 1.5 million hairs. At an average length of 3 inches (7.6 centimeters), this adds up to over 70 miles (113 kilometers) of hair scattered about our daily lives. It is one of the main reasons that Roto Rooter stays in business.

The Head's Harvest

Each hair follicle on the scalp grows almost 30 feet (9 meters) of hair during an average lifetime or about 5 inches (13 centimeters) every year. It takes 6 years to grow hair long enough to sit on. The longest hair on record belonged to Swami Pandarasannadhi of India; it was 26 feet (7.9 meters) long.

Avoiding Baldness

The sure cure for baldness? Castration. Most men prefer to lose their hair.

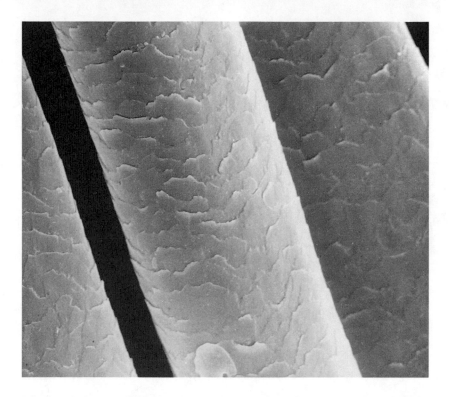

A human hair magnified 600 times. The average scalp contains about 125,000 hairs, and over a lifetime we lose some 1.5 million strands. Courtesy Dr. Karen Holbrook, University of Washington.

MUSCLE

Muscle Weight

A man who weighs 170 pounds has about 81 pounds of muscle—68 pounds of skeletal muscle and 13 pounds of cardiac and smooth muscle.

A woman has about 10 percent less muscle tissue for her body weight. If she weighs 120 pounds, all her muscles—including the inter-

---

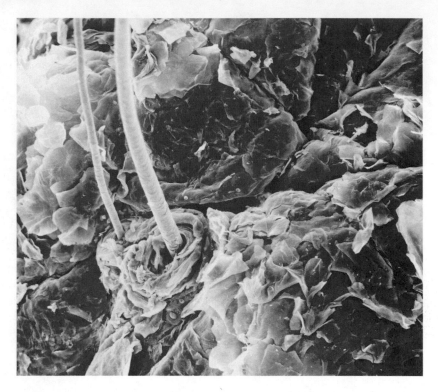

Each hair follicle grows almost 30 feet (9 meters) of hair during an average lifetime. Courtesy Dr. Karen Holbrook, University of Washington.

nal, involuntary smooth muscle of her heart and intestines—would weigh about 45 pounds.

Muscles are made up of fibers—some 6 trillion of them in the entire muscular system. They are thinner than a human hair and can support up to 1,000 times their own weight.

Minimuscles

The smallest muscle in the human body is located in the middle ear and activates one of the 3 small bones, the one commonly known as the stirrup, that sends vibrations from the eardrum into the inner ear. Less than 1/20 of an inch in length, the stapedius muscle is shorter than a dime is thick.

Connected to every hair follicle on the human body—and brunettes, for example, have about 100,000 on their heads alone—is a tiny involuntary muscle called the arrector pili. These minimuscles are stimulated by cold or emotional responses such as fear. When the body is cold, they raise the hair and produce goose bumps on the skin to help retain body heat. Researchers also believe that the hair-raising effect also once had the function of making our ancestors appear larger, thus discouraging potential enemies from being aggressive.

Muscleless Fingers

Your fingers have no muscles at all, only strong ligaments attached to muscles in the hand and forearm which activate all the wonders of human dexterity.

Bigger than Biceps

We sit on the most powerful and largest muscle in our body, the gluteus maximus (buttock muscle), which moves the thighbone away from the body and straightens out the hip joint. The large flat muscles of the back, the latissimi dorsi, are larger in terms of body area. They give our arms their motion by moving them down and back—competitive swimming pushes these muscles to their limits.

The longest muscle in our body is the sartorius, a long strap running from the waist to the knee. It flexes the hip and knee, and allows us to sit cross-legged, Buddha-fashion.

These 3 large muscles have been neglected because the biceps have always gotten more attention than they deserve—probably because we don't sit on them and they are therefore in a good position to be seen.

Slow and Fast Muscles

Depending on what function a muscle performs, it is either slow or fast or somewhere in between. Eye muscles, for example, must have a fast contraction time in order to keep the eye fixed on specific objects. Less than 1/100 of a second for contraction is common for eye muscles. The muscle that flexes the foot and leg, the gastrocnemius, which helps us run and jump, takes about 1/30 of a second to contract—fast enough to do its specialized work. Then there are the slow muscles such as the soleus of the lower leg, which helps support the body against gravity.

Like other muscles that must perform work over long periods, it contracts in about 1/10 of a second—slow but sure.

One-Way Muscles

Every time you push something—whether it's against the floor to do push-ups or against a car to get your neighbor out of the snow, your muscles are actually pulling (contracting) to do their work. Muscles work only this one way.

Computer Muscle

A mechanical engineering team at the University of Wisconsin has programmed a computer with every conceivable human motion—a feat that took more than 10 years. The program's hypothetical muscles

Electron micrograph of muscle tissue (top) interacting with a nerve cell. The small bubblelike structures in the nerve cell are vesicles that contain neurotransmitters that signal the muscle to contract. Courtesy University of California at San Francisco.

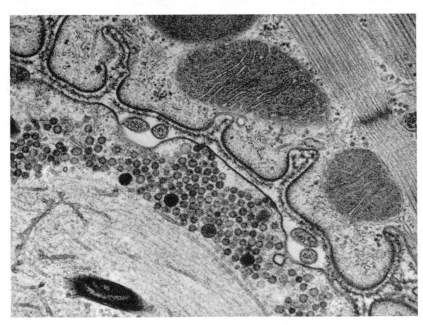

THAT LAYERED LOOK:

and bones can be altered and the result shown on a video screen. This so-called simulated surgery will help surgeons make the best decisions to treat a patient's specific problem.

Robotics will also find this human motion program invaluable. By knowing the muscle sequence of specific finger, hand, and arm movements, engineers can create the counterpart hardware to muscles and bones and produce a robot with more efficient humanlike motions.

Beneath a Face

That familiar face in the mirror each morning has some 30 facial muscles attached to the bones beneath the skin. Without these muscles, we would be expressionless—no smiles or laughter, no frowns, no surprised or squinting eyes.

Each time we smile, the risorius muscle draws the corners of the mouth outward, compressing the cheek muscles, and its neighbor, the zygomaticus muscle, draws the upper lip upward and outward. For that extraspecial smile, the orbicularis oculi muscle comes into play, narrowing the eyes and putting those wrinkles around them. There are 17 smiling muscles in all.

We have more facial muscles than any other animal.

Cold Down There?

The penis and clitoris contain no muscular tissue at all, even though there is some pornographic prose to the contrary, but a nearby muscle (the ischiocavernosus) helps to maintain erections in men and women during sexual arousal.

Below the penis, the cremaster muscle envelopes the testicles and helps to protect the sperm inside; it lowers them if the body is too warm and pulls them up toward the body for warmth if they get too cold.

Aging Muscles

The strength of our muscles declines as we grow older, from about the age of 25 on, at which time they are at their peak. Different muscles lose their strength at different rates. Back and hand muscles weaken first, followed by wrist and elbow muscles.

In general, men have more muscle strength than women at comparable ages. The muscular strength of a man at age 65, however, is about equal to that of a woman's at age 25.

BONE

Breaking Down Bones

Men and women have the same proportion of bone to their body weight, about 14 percent. A person weighing 150 pounds (68 kilograms) would therefore have 20 pounds (9 kilograms) of bone.

Bones are composed of 50 percent water and 50 percent solid matter. The solid matter is cartilage (mostly collagen fibers) that has been hardened by inorganic salts such as carbonate and phosphate of lime. Phosphorus is a major bone component and accounts for over 6 percent of bone material. Eighty-five percent of our body's phosphorus, some 20 ounces (560 grams), is found in bone. That's enough phosphorus to make 2,000 matchheads.

The Calcium Cache

Bones also contain 99 percent of the body's calcium, more than 2 pounds of it. Nerve impulses, muscle contraction, blood clotting, heartbeat are all very dependent on just the right amount of calcium in the bloodstream. The bone store of calcium is ever ready to be released. The parathyroid glands in the neck send the release signal by secreting a hormone if the blood level of calcium gets too low. If the level gets too high, calcium is absorbed back into the bone.

The mineral crystals of the bones interface directly with the blood flow, and this is where the calcium exchange takes place—from bone to blood or blood to bone. The surface area that these mineral salts expose to the bloodstream is surprisingly large—equal to 100 acres of land.

The Lonely Hyoid

At the base of the tongue, above the larynx, is the horseshoe-shaped hyoid bone, the only bone in the human body that does not meet up with another bone. This small bone anchors various muscles, including some attached to the tongue.

The hyoid was often broken in the early American West—at the town hangings. When someone is hanged, the hyoid breaks and chokes the victim to death. This isolated bone is also important in forensic medicine. When it is found to be fractured, this is good evidence of murder by strangulation.

The Leg's Kingpin

The thighbone (femur) is the heaviest, longest, and strongest bone in the human skeleton. As a rule, it is 27 percent of our total height, so a 6-foot man's thighbone would be about 1.6 feet long, and a 5-foot woman's would be 1.3 feet.

Collagen fibers, the tough protein found in all connective tissue including bone, have great tensile strength. Bone calcium salts have great compressional strength, just as the rock and sand of cement do. In fact, a bone's compressional strength is greater than reinforced concrete, while its tensile strength is about the same—some 20,000 pounds (9,000 kilograms) per square inch. This interlocking structure of collagen fibers and calcium crystals makes bone, ounce for ounce, stronger than steel and reinforced concrete, and bone is living tissue that repairs itself.

The Out-Front Kneecap

Sesamoid bones, which vary in number, are not counted in the average 206 bones of the adult skeleton. These small bones are imbedded in the tendons of pressure points such as the fingers and toes.

The kneecap (patella) is a lens-shaped sesamoid bone in the tendon of the knee that protects the knee joint. It is the largest sesamoid bone in the human body. Because it's right out front, it is also the most vulnerable.

Jumping sports such as basketball and volleyball are tough on the

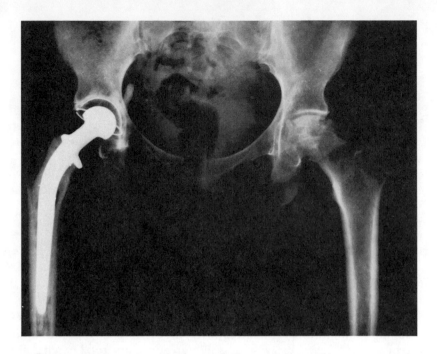

The thighbone (femur) is the heaviest, longest, and strongest bone in the human skeleton—be it a natural or artificial one. Ounce for ounce, it is stronger than steel or reinforced concrete. Courtesy National Institutes of Health.

kneecap and injuries often occur. Horseback riding, too, often causes kneecap pain. Even so, broken kneecaps are not common. When they do occur, they are often caused by taking a false step while going downstairs.

The modern-day arthroscope has revolutionized knee surgery. Outfitted with fiber-optic technology, this surgical instrument fits through a 1/4-inch incision and allows the surgeon to see details inside the knee. It avoids all the drawbacks of open-knee surgery and will soon replace the traditional surgery completely. Even broken kneecaps can be treated and repaired as the surgeon peers through his multilensed scope and uses a selection of microinstruments to probe and remove unwanted bone chips.

Two Marrows

All of our bones are filled with red marrow at birth, but as we grow to adulthood, the red marrow in the bones of our limbs is replaced by yellow marrow, which consists mostly of fat cells. Red bone marrow remains in the center of skull bones, pelvic bones, the ribs, and the vertebrae throughout life and actively produces red blood cells, white blood cells, and platelets.

The yellow marrow is a reserve for the human body. If the body's fat stores are used up, the yellow marrow comes to the rescue. If the blood becomes anemic, the yellow marrow becomes red marrow to produce more of the needed red blood cells.

Because 180 million red blood cells die each minute in our bodies, the marrow must constantly replace them. Each day of our healthy lives the red marrow produces over 200 billion red blood cells—a total that would take you at least 65 years to count.

Baby Face

There are 22 bones in the human skull—8 cranial bones and 14 facial bones. Only one of these bones moves, the lower jawbone (mandible) that enables us to chew food and talk.

The cranium is the only bone in the body that completely and closely encases an organ, the brain. In newborns, as all parents know, the cranial bones are not joined, and there are 6 gaps (fontanelles) in the skull at birth that allow the brain to grow to full size. The most noticeable of these soft spots is at the top of the skull, an easy place to take a baby's pulse.

The infant brain develops faster than the rest of the body, and that is why a baby's skull is one fourth the size of its entire skeleton as compared to an adult's, which is only one eighth the size of the body.

For all babies, brainpower is more important than beauty because the face is only one eighth the size of the cranium. This has changed by adulthood, however, and the face has grown to one half cranium size. But size is not everything. The 8 cranial bones may protect the brain, but the 14 bones of the face and their muscles allow us to express ourselves, with and without words, and often we communicate better without them. Baby faces prove that.

Beneath the Nods and Shakes

The atlas and the axis are the first 2 vertebrae in the spinal column and are distinctly different from the other 24 in the adult skeleton. (Children have 33, but during growth, the 9 bottom vertebrae fuse into just 2—the first 5 become the sacrum and the lowest 4 become the coccyx.)

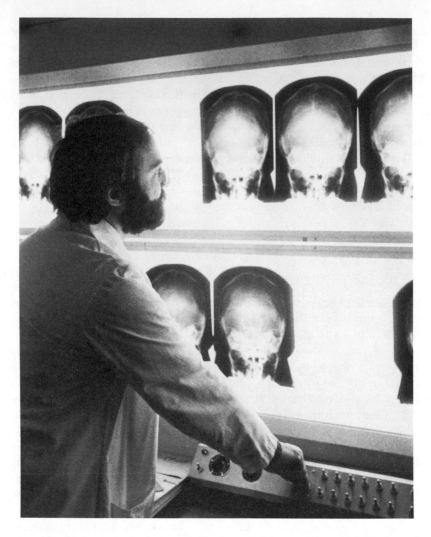

There are 22 bones in the human skull—8 cranial bones and 14 facial bones. The cranium is the only bone in the body that completely encases an organ. Courtesy National Institutes of Health.

What the atlas bone does is hold up our head. It is a ring of bone, with a large central opening, and has 2 large hollows into which fit projections from the base of the skull.

The second vertebra of the neck, the axis, has a central peglike projection that fits into the central opening of the atlas—nature's nut-and-bolt arrangement that keeps our heads on straight.

Whenever we nod our heads *yes,* the pivotal point is between the atlas vertebra and the base of the skull. When we shake our heads *no,*

THAT LAYERED LOOK:

the motion takes place between the atlas and the axis. *Yes* is therefore, physically, at least, a higher gesture than *no*.

New Bones About It

Bone tissue transplants and grafts have been commonplace for many years in correcting face and skull bone birth defects, fractures that won't heal, or holes left from removed tumors. But these procedures have several drawbacks. Because bone often is taken from the patient's own body—a piece of rib, pelvis, or shinbone—the surgery can lead to chronic pain and sometimes infection. Also, the success of the treatment depends on the cells from the intact bone migrating to the surface of the transplanted bone, a process called osteoconduction. The problem is that the grafts can be absorbed by the bone region under repair and this often means several operations are necessary.

What's the answer? Recently there have been encouraging results from a new method of treatment that will avoid most of these problems —the demineralized bone implant. Here's how it works. Bone is crushed into chips or ground into powder and then washed in hydrochloric acid to remove all minerals. (If the minerals were not removed, the bone would be resorbed by specialized cells.) The prepared bone is then dried and sterilized.

Next the demineralized bone is surgically implanted and causes growth of new bone through a process called osteoinduction, wherein fibroblast cells (which usually form scar tissue) produce cartilage in a period of about 2 weeks. Over the next few months, this new cartilage is transformed to bone, once new blood vessels have penetrated it. New bone can thus be grown even in the areas where no bone existed before.

Many children born with cleft palates have been treated successfully with the new demineralized bone. It was also used on a 6-year-old boy who had a deformed, "cloverleaf" skull that was completely fused. A neurosurgeon removed almost all of the skull, waited 3 weeks for the boy's brain to take a new shape, and then added demineralized bone powder over the thin lining of the brain. One year later the boy had a new, properly shaped, skull.

Another child got his first nose through the implant process; he was born without one.

Once the complexities of the process are more fully understood and techniques improved, many more uses will become apparent. For example, if new bone growth can be chemically programmed to stop at the cartilage stage, some of us could sprout new noses. There will be no more transplants or grafts, just the use of easily stored demineralized bone that surgeons can fit into any hard-to-get-to places of the body. It could eventually be used to reshape even the most grotesque deformities of the human body and cure all the degenerative diseases of bone and cartilage. Demineralized bone has the potential for rebuilding our bodies.

Losing Bone

Bone loss—it happens to almost all of us as we grow older. Many people believe it's just a natural and inevitable consequence of aging. This most common bone disease, called osteoporosis, has become a serious and widespread medical problem just in the twentieth century. Why? Because people are living longer than in earlier centuries, and osteoporosis is almost always a disease of middle and old age.

Calcium salts are taken from the bone in response to an increase in the parathyroid hormone that responds to inadequate levels of calcium in the blood. There appears to be an excess of this hormone as men and women get older. Bones weaken as a result of the calcium loss, becoming increasingly porous and brittle. They are therefore extremely susceptible to fractures, which is why 200,000 hips are broken in the United States each year. Most of these hip fractures occur at about age 75.

When osteoporosis attacks the spine, the vertebrae collapse and the person becomes shorter and a hump often develops in the upper back.

Women, especially Caucasian and Oriental, are more susceptible to bone loss and fractures than men. Recent studies have shown that women over 50 have higher levels of the parathyroid hormone than men. After menopause, women have lower or no amounts of the female sex hormone, estrogen. It is estrogen that regulates the amount of hormone flow, and when there is less or no estrogen, the parathyroid hormone pulls calcium away from the bone at a faster rate. A woman's bone mass drops about 1 percent each year after menopause, and because women have lighter skeletons, they therefore have less bone to begin with. Any bone loss is therefore a serious problem for them.

What can be done to prevent or retard the loss of bone? Exercise and an adequate supply of calcium are important, and treatment with sex hormones and vitamin D may prevent the disease from getting worse.

The next decade will no doubt bring about important advances in treatment. Meanwhile, remember that (and this is contrary to common belief) older adults need more calcium than children, and one of the easiest ways to take in calcium is to drink milk with your cookies or eat lots of cheese with your crackers.

Chapter Five

Going with the Flow: Heart to Heart

HEART

The Little Pump that Could . . .

Lub-dub . . . lub-dub . . . lub-dub . . . so beats the human heart from its first beat 4 weeks after conception to its last beat before death. At rest, the human heart beats an average of 72 times a minute, 4,300 times each hour, 104,000 times each day, 38 million times each year, and some 2.8 billion times in a lifetime of 74 years. But no heart is at its rest pace for a complete lifetime. It speeds up with exertion—be it lovemaking, jogging, or taking out the trash. The human heart therefore beats at least 3 billion times in an average lifetime.

The volume of blood the heart pumps through the body adds up to a staggering total over a period of years. An adult's heart, at rest, pushes almost 1½ gallons (5.7 liters) of blood through the circulatory system every minute, 87 gallons (330 liters) every hour, 2,100 gallons (8,000 liters) every day, 766,600 gallons (2.9 million liters) in a year, and more than 56 million gallons (213 million liters) of blood in a 74-year life span.

This means that just one human heart, pumping for 74 years, could completely fill the first-, second-, and third-stage fuel tanks of *56*

Saturn V moon rockets—the total volume of which would weigh some 332 million pounds (150 million kilograms). This is 530 million times the heart's own weight of about 10 ounces (280 grams).

Lub and Dub

When the healthy heart is heard beating through a stethoscope, 2 sounds are heard, represented as "lub" and "dub." These are called the first (lub) and second (dub) heart sounds.

When the heart valves open, no sound is created because this is a relatively slow process. Instead, it is the closing of the heart valves and the vibrations in the surrounding fluids and tissue that cause these 2 normal heart sounds.

Lub, the first heart sound, is that of the tricuspid and mitral valves, also known as the AV or atrioventricular valves, closing. These valves connect the upper and lower chambers (atria and ventricles) of the heart, and when they close, a low-pitched sound is heard.

Dub, the second heart sound, is created by the aortic and pulmonary valves (also known as the semilunar valves) closing. Dub is slightly shorter and not quite as low-pitched as lub.

While lub lasts slightly longer than dub, it amounts to only 1/30 of a second. Together, these normal first and second heart sounds only add up to 1/4 of a second. If the doctor doesn't listen intently, he or she will miss the message of the lub and dub show.

Heart Power

Your heart expends enough energy each day to lift almost 2,000 pounds (907 kilograms) to a height of 41 feet (12.5 meters). By the age of 50, your heart has done an amount of work equal to lifting more than 18,000 tons to an altitude of 142 miles (227 kilometers), a weight which is more than 100 times that of the heaviest payloads ever put into earth orbit.

Heart Watts

The human heart puts out about 2½ watts of power, only one eighth of what the brain does. Most of this—about 2 watts—is generated by the more powerful pump chamber, the left ventricle, which pushes blood into the aorta. The other pumping chamber, the right ventricle, pumps blood to the lungs. It puts out only 1/2 watt.

Two and a half watts of power output is about 3 times less than a small Christmas tree light bulb.

Thin Red Line

The amount of blood the heart pumps in an average lifetime could fill an artery, about the diameter of a drinking straw, stretching 12 times around the earth at the equator—some 300,000 miles (480,000 kilometers).

Different Beats

Inside the womb, an unborn's tiny heart sometimes beats as fast as 150 times a minute, but at birth it slows down to about 130. The normal pulse rate for infants at rest is 90 to 130 each minute, while the normal range for adults is between 60 and 100 beats every minute.

A man's resting pulse rate, on the average, is 72 per minute; a woman's 75, which adds up to over 1.5 million more beats for a woman's heart each year. While asleep, a person's pulse often falls to 55 beats a minute.

Just by walking, an average resting pulse of 72 beats a minute can jump to 94, but this is far below what is considered a high heart rate of 200 beats per minute for a person who is 25 years old.

As a group, highly conditioned athletes, whose powerful heart muscles can pump a lot of blood per beat, have the lowest at-rest pulses— as low as 35 beats per minute and commonly in the 45- to 50-beat range.

Emotions affect our heart rates and health. Anger and fear increase our heart rates 30 to 40 beats a minute.

The Self-Feeding Heart

To nourish itself for its never-ending work, the heart pumps 5 percent of its own blood through the left and right coronary arteries, which branch off from the base of the aortic artery. With the exception of the brain, no other organ requires as much blood. This means that 5 percent of all the oxygenated blood pumped from the upper left chamber serves the heart muscle, which is only about 2 hundredths of the body's mass. In comparison, the skeletal muscles, which constitute somewhat over a third of the body's mass (some 70 times more mass than the heart), receive only 15 percent of the heart's output—only 3 times what the heart sends to itself.

The heart therefore feeds itself by pumping some 100 gallons (380 liters) of oxygen-rich blood to its own muscle tissue every day.

The Magical Muscle's Beat

The heart, a hollow muscle, is the strongest muscle in the human body, with one very occasional exception—a woman's uterus. But while the uterus is more powerful as a muscle, it is only called upon to perform at childbirth, no more than a few times in a woman's childbearing years. The life-sustaining heart muscle, however, beats some 3 billion times during the average person's life. It is, without doubt, the supreme muscle of the human body.

Heart muscle, myocardium, composes the thick middle layer in the heart wall and is in between the smooth inner and outer layers that lubricate the heart against friction. The muscle cells are surrounded by connective tissue; some fibers circle around the entire heart and others loop around one chamber, then another.

Cardiac muscle tissue is unique, unlike any other in the body. While skeletal—also called striated—muscle is controlled by the voluntary nervous system, cardiac muscle is involuntary and spontaneously contracts on its own, without any stimulation from the central nervous system or hormonal system. A specialized group of cardiac muscle cells in the right upper chamber (the SA node) generate their own electrical current and command the rest of the heart fibers to contract. This cluster of special cells acts as the heart's pacemaker.

Heart muscle cells are not separated like skeletal muscle cells. Instead, they form an interconnected latticework, and each wave of contraction spreads throughout the whole mass of muscle, so that the heart contracts as one. Cardiac muscle cells are also much smaller than the skeletal muscle cells—only a few hundredths of an inch long versus inches—and they contain many more mitochondria, the cells' converters of food into energy, to support their prodigious energy output. The heart's muscle fibers are so different from other muscles in the body that many scientists view them as a unique combination of nerve and muscle cells.

As in all muscle, however, proteins give cardiac muscle the power to contract. Thin bundles of threads, myofibrils, run the length of each muscle fiber, and within each bundle are filaments of proteins ar-

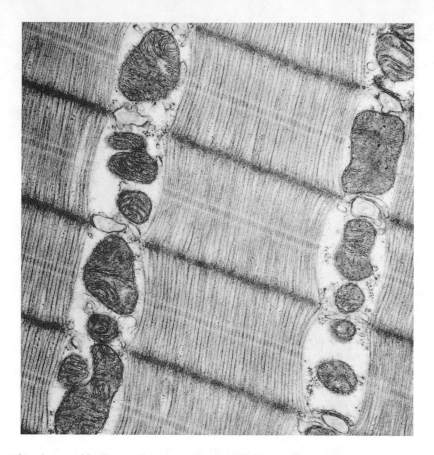

The microworld of human heart muscle, magnified more than 51,000 times. Cardiac muscle is involuntary and contracts on its own. Filaments of 2 proteins, actin and myosin, interact, causing the heart muscle to contract. It remains a mystery as to how the heart begins to beat in the womb. Courtesy Stanford University Medical Center.

ranged in a repeating pattern called sacromeres. They contain 2 proteins: actin and myosin. It is these threads of proteins, interacting with one another, that cause the heart muscle to contract.

The complete answer to the mystery of the heartbeat lies in this microcellular realm. Human hearts begin beating in the embryo about 4 weeks after conception, before it has formed any nerve cells at all! Specialized cells, similar to those in the heart's own pacemaker tissue, may be involved, but exactly how these first cells start to beat remains a mystery. But once begun, the heart's muscle is not easy to completely stop. For centuries, doctors and scientists have witnessed the phenomenon of disembodied hearts that keep beating, and even strips of heart muscle cut from a heart will continue to beat in a test tube filled with

GOING WITH THE FLOW:

saline solution. In fact, individual heart muscles will pulse if grown in a tissue culture. The human heartbeat, we now know, emanates from these magical, microscopic cardiac muscle cells.

Sex and the Heart

The heart soars in love—and so does the blood pressure. During sexual intercourse, the heart rate increases and blood pressure jumps about 50 percent.

One study—done in Middlesex, England—showed that blood pressure rose 48 percent for men during coitus and 57 percent for women. This increase also held true for a female subject who suffered fainting spells during sex and for a male who suffered massive headaches during the act.

Heart failure during the heights of sexual excitement is not all that rare. And keep in mind that sexual adventures have their price: intercourse-associated death occurs more often to people during extramarital sex.

Heart of Anger

Three separate studies have shown that anger can lead to heart problems. They show that angry people are more prone to coronary heart disease than more laid-back, go-with-the-flow people.

Anger was measured by how high the participants scored on the hostility scale of the Minnesota Multiphasic Personality Inventory (MMPI) test. When the scores of subjects who later died were examined, they were found to predict coronary heart disease as well as other causes of death. This strong relationship between the hostility score and death was independent of other high-risk habits known to contribute to heart disease such as smoking and high cholesterol, high blood pressure, and alcohol use. In fact, the hostility score more highly correlated with blocked arteries than did the well-known type A behavior personality.

One of the researchers believed, based on subject responses, that what was really being measured was the personality trait mistrust, which results in anger-hostility, a more easily measurable emotion. Individuals who are not prone to constant mistrust and anger may therefore be protected from ill health, including heart disease. The Japanese, with the lowest incidence of coronary heart disease of any industrial nation, present a strong argument in favor of this view. Their mores stress depending on others, trusting in their benevolence, and harmony.

If you're a person who often gets angry, consider making a sign and placing it in a visible location at home or in the office. It should read: WARNING: ANGER IS DANGEROUS TO YOUR HEART AND HEALTH.

The Hearts of Apollo

The traditional cardiovascular risk factors (cigarette smoking, high blood pressure, high cholesterol levels, for example) account for only half the cases of heart disease. Modern medicine has neglected the fact that emotional reactions can damage the heart and circulatory system, but in recent years that attitude has changed dramatically. In the near future, stress may be considered the most important risk factor of all.

Stress and its physical consequences may, in fact, explain why more than 1,200 Americans die each day of sudden cardiac death, which is usually caused by a highly irregular heart rhythm called ventricular fibrillation. These victims may be very calm outwardly, but outward behavior is often not a good indication of how a person's heart and blood vessels respond to stress. Studies have shown that 1 in 5 healthy-appearing and outwardly calm people are really "hot reactors"—individuals whose cardiovascular systems overrespond to stress. In severe reactions, surges in cardiac output, blood pressure, and blood-vessel resistance occur. As a result, the heart pumps very hard against great resistance—the stuff of which heart attacks are made.

The heightened interest in stress-induced heart disease is another little-known benefit from the Apollo moon program, a benefit that wasn't without high price. There was an extraordinarily high incidence of sudden deaths and heart attacks among the young men who worked at Cape Canaveral in the 1960s. An 8-year study revealed that these men were under tremendous pressure to perform and reach the national goal of putting men on the moon before the end of the 1960s. Later, autopsies revealed that the heart muscle of 85 percent of the dead men had lesions known as contraction bands—a kind of damage that can result from a high amount of stress-induced chemicals from the adrenal glands.

The push toward the moon took its toll on the human heart. The danger, it turns out, was higher on the ground than it was aboard a Saturn V or on the surface of the moon.

Bypassing the Bypass?

Some 170,000 coronary artery bypass operations were performed in 1982 at a total cost of more than $2 billion, and still the medical profession debates the risks and benefits of the surgery. The techniques for this open-heart surgery were developed in the late 1960s as a way to correct blocked coronary arteries that were not carrying enough blood to the heart muscle—a potentially fatal condition.

The invention of the heart-lung machine was essential to the operation; it allowed surgeons to operate on a stilled heart, and kept the patient alive during the hours of surgery. Finding the vessel material for the grafts was also a major breakthrough—it turned out to be a part of the human body, an expendable blood vessel in the leg, the saphenous vein. Its removal does not impair body function and, in fact, is commonly removed in varicose vein operations.

Heart surgeons expose the heart by opening up the chest, hook up the heart-lung machine, and then sew one end of the saphenous-vein graft to the aorta, which feeds fresh blood through the coronary arteries to the heart muscle. The other end of the vein is sewn to the blocked coronary artery on the other side of the obstruction, thus bypassing it. (High-tech optical systems and hair-thin needles make such minute stitching possible.)

With new surgical techniques such as balloon and laser angioplasty and revolutionary new drugs, coronary bypass surgery may eventually become relegated to the medical history books as a surgical technique that was especially popular in the 1970s and 80s, but which was made obsolete by new discoveries. If the future bears this out, at least the skills of heart surgeons will have been greatly enhanced by performing this demanding and delicate surgery. As Dr. Denton Cooley, the famous cardiovascular surgeon, once remarked, smiling, "You practice for this procedure by circumcising gnats."

Balloons and Lasers for the Heart

Balloon angioplasty has been used since the late 1970s to unclog heart arteries. Laser angioplasty, however, is still under development.

Both techniques involve making a small skin incision, usually in the groin, thigh, or elbow area, and threading a catheter up through the body—in the case of insertion in the elbow, the catheter goes through the arteries of the upper arm, the shoulder, into the aorta, and then

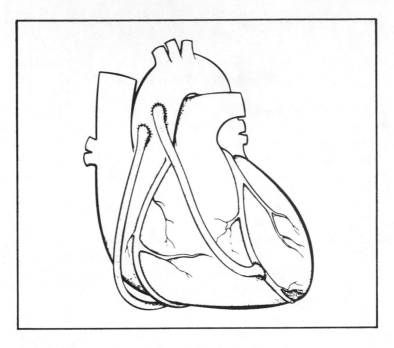

Some 170,000 bypass operations (diagram above) were performed in 1982 to correct blocked coronary arteries (photograph on facing page). New surgical techniques and drugs may eventually relegate coronary bypass surgery to the history books. Courtesy National Institutes of Health.

into the coronary artery until it reaches the point that is clogged by fatty deposits.

The hollow catheters are only about 1/12 of an inch (2 millimeters) in diameter, but they can deliver several different devices into the human body. For these 2 techniques, the catheters deliver either a miniballoon or the fiber optics needed to provide laser light.

In balloon surgery, once the catheter reaches the blockage, a tiny sausage-shaped balloon is inflated with fluid against the arterial walls for a few seconds and is then deflated. This procedure is repeated 3 times, and the pressure of the miniballoon is increased each time. Eventually the plaque is compressed against the artery's wall, allowing oxygen-rich blood to flow once again to the heart muscle.

The miniballoon is about 4/5 of an inch (2 centimeters) in length, and when inflated its diameter of about 1/12 of an inch (2 millimeters) almost doubles to open up the clogged artery.

Balloon surgery succeeds in 4 out of 5 patients by relieving the symptoms of blockage such as angina, and 84 percent of the patients remain healthy after 3 years. The technique cannot, however, compress or remove the arterial blockages that have been hardened from

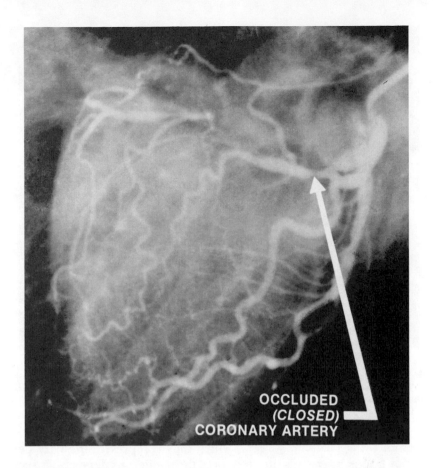

OCCLUDED
(CLOSED)
CORONARY ARTERY

natural calcification. Also, as easy as the technique may seem, it isn't. Doctors must learn the procedure, and they must be ready for a number of life-threatening complications such as the blood supply stopping in the artery. An open-heart surgical team must always be on standby. The most common problem is snaking the catheter through the tortuous artery system of some patients and up to the blockage. The real advantage of the balloon technique is cost—only one fifth the cost of bypass surgery, which was from $15,000 to $25,000 in the early 1980s. This cost factor includes less operating room time (1 hour versus what is often 8) and fewer medical support personnel.

While laser angioplasty is not yet in clinical use, in 1983 it was first used to unclog coronary arteries in patients by an American medical team working in Toulouse, France. The laser treatment unclogged the arteries in 4 out of 5 patients. In this technique, laser energy vaporizes blood clots and plaques, and the blockages are transformed into vapors and hydrocarbon molecules that are dissolved in the blood-

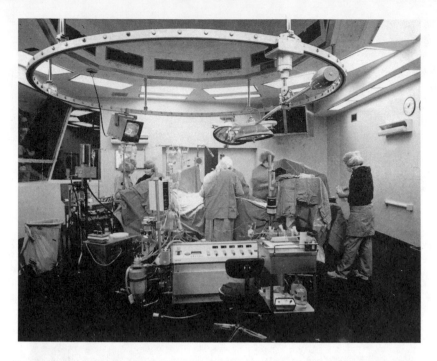

An operating room equipped for coronary bypass surgery, with heart-lung machine in foreground. Over $2 billion was spent in North America alone in 1982 for this operation. Courtesy National Institutes of Health.

stream. Unlike balloon surgery, which only compresses the fatty deposits, laser surgery rids the arteries of the dangerous deposits. Lasers can also scour the arteries clean of calcified deposits.

The future for healing the heart with lasers is somewhat speculative, but some experts believe it will be *the* tool of heart surgery by the early 1990s. Development of an imaging system in the catheter that will allow surgeons to see inside the artery and view the blockage is also under way. This also will provide more precise laser control and better results. Both balloon and laser techniques may someday be combined to treat coronary-blockage problems. The balloon would make the initial penetration and the laser would follow up and vaporize all the gunk.

Whether the cost of laser equipment can ever compete with the reasonable equipment cost of balloon surgery is another question entirely. It is far more costly now. Laser equipment costs from $50,000 to $100,000. The balloon catheter, however, is a modest $150 to $200.

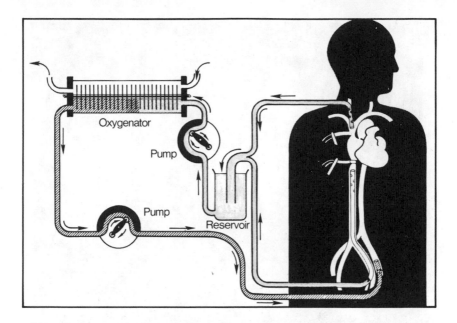

The heart-lung machine takes over the patient's circulation and makes heart surgery possible. This diagram shows how the blood is removed, oxygenated outside the body, and returned to the body, with the heart at rest during surgery. Courtesy National Institutes of Health.

Future Heart: Beyond the Jarvik 7

The artificial heart era has just begun, and its significance is enormous for the future of medicine and the human life span. Eventually millions of people worldwide could have reliable mechanical hearts implanted in their chests that would be supported by compact, portable equipment—not the unwieldy life-support system needed by Barney Clark. As Dr. Robert K. Jarvik has made clear, the artificial heart must eventually be more than reliable and dependable. Its owner must become oblivious to it and it must be unnoticed by others.

The most difficult problems associated with the artificial heart will not be technological or mechanical, but rather ethical (who gets an artificial heart?) and economical (can society afford the price?). In fact, some experts have suggested that the man-made heart could be the first major medical advance in history that is rejected by society as costing too much. But this is doubtful. Where there is demand, there is supply, and this should hold true for the artificial heart. Personally

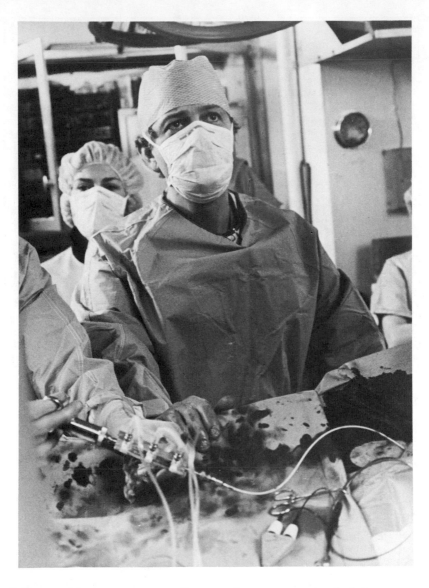

Balloon and laser surgery, as well as new drugs, may soon make bypass surgery obsolete. Here the surgeon watches the X-ray monitor as his colleague inflates the balloon at the tip of the catheter inside the patient's coronary artery. This compresses the plaque and allows blood to flow again. Courtesy National Institutes of Health.

tailored health insurance plans, for instance, might make artificial heart coverage an individual option, with genetic information and family medical history as major factors in the decision.

While the University of Utah Medical Center is well known for its state-of-the-art development of the artificial heart, the research is an international endeavor. Other research centers, located in Argentina, Austria, China, Czechoslovakia, France, Germany, Italy, Japan, and the U.S.S.R., are helping to shape the future of the artificial heart. Even in the United States, medical engineering alternatives to the basic Jarvik design are being pursued. The Cleveland Clinic, for example, is developing and testing a rotary-type artificial pump with only one moving part that is driven by a simple electric motor. Each of the heart's ventricles would be replaced by a rotary pump that would hum along instead of beat. Still, the Jarvik 7 total artificial heart is the only device to be implanted in humans, and its future design changes offer the best clues to what future artificial hearts will be like.

Barney Clark's artificial heart depended on a cart-mounted pneumatic driver that was about the size of a portable television set and weighed about 375 pounds (169 kilograms). But there was even more support equipment—an air dryer, air compressor, and standby emergency tanks of compressed air—enough to fill a room.

Those involved in its development agree that the future artificial heart must be miniaturized and self-contained. Plans call for a portable battery-powered heart driver to replace the bulky equipment used for the first human transplant. It would weigh about 8½ pounds (4 kilograms) and fit into a case about the size of a camera bag. Powered by rechargeable batteries worn around the waist, the unit would have an 8- to 10-hour power supply before the batteries had to be charged. Power to the artificial heart would be sent through the skin via a lead with a small cable inside. There would be no pneumatic tubes entering the body that would require tethering the patient to the bulky air-supply machinery. The patient would be completely mobile.

What makes this mobility possible is the development of a unique electrohydraulic power converter and blood pump (with only one moving part) that will be an integral part of this future heart. This self-contained drive system was under development by Dr. Jarvik and his colleagues even before Barney Clark had his Jarvik 7 implanted. However, years of testing and refinement remain before it will be ready for human use.

In this future heart, a miniature direct-current motor pumps hydraulic fluid (silicone oil) back and forth between the left and right ventricles. The fluid motion actuates the diaphragm of the blood pump, just as compressed air did for Barney Clark's man-made heart.

This precision miniature pump is an engineering marvel. It weighs only 3 ounces (85 grams) and occupies about the same volume as a

C-sized flashlight battery. What kind of flow can this mighty minipump generate? Some 48 quarts (45 liters) every minute! Your kitchen dishwasher, with a much larger pump, only generates 8 quarts (7.6 liters) of water in a minute.

The Jarvik Breakthrough

Development of the artificial heart has been a slow, steady process, spanning 25 years, and it still continues. Animals with implanted devices were surviving less than 3 days in the late 1960s.

A major advance came in the 1970s with a design that used a diaphragm as the pumping element. In 1974, Dr. Robert K. Jarvik fitted his Jarvik 3 experimental heart with a strong and flexible 3-layer diaphragm made of smooth polyurethane. This was a breakthrough. Earlier artificial devices only had a single-layer diaphragm which often ruptured. The new material had a long "flex" life, discouraged clotting and red blood cell damage, and was not rejected by the body.

The Jarvik diaphragm initially increased survival times to as much as 4 months, and continued to improve. What was the secret formula for the diaphragm's polyurethane? Dr. Jarvik chose Biomer, which is a medical grade of Lycra. This is an elastic material used in girdles and brassieres. Cross your heart. . . .

Barney's Extra Beats

During the almost 2,700 hours (112 days) that Dr. Barney Clark survived with the Jarvik 7 artificial heart (from December 2, 1982, to March 23, 1983) his new plastic-and-aluminum, man-made pump beat about 13 million times. It pumped approximately 7 quarts (6.6 liters) of blood each minute, a full 7 times more than his ailing heart, for a total of some 285,000 gallons—that's a workload!

It was surgeon William C. DeVries who implanted the first total artificial heart into a human being—Barney Clark, the tough dentist whose heart was on its last beats. Fifteen years earlier, as a graduate student in 1967, DeVries was inspired by a lecture that Dr. Willem J. Kolff gave about his invention of the kidney dialysis machine. They met for the first time after the lecture, and the human heart skipped a beat into the future.

Hearty Implants

Three lifesaving devices have been developed to aid the ailing heart, and together they have saved tens of thousands of lives that would have otherwise been doomed. Dependent on microtechnology, these devices regulate heart rhythms or assist a weak or incapacitated pumping chamber. They are used in heart repair before a patient is forced to shop for a completely new—donor or artificial—heart.

Assist Devices: A Time to Heal. Left-hand heart-assist devices (also known as ventricular assist devices or VADs) are really one-chambered, temporary artificial hearts that help to wean weak and ailing hearts back to health so that they can resume beating on their own. Often, after open-heart surgery during which the heart-lung machine keeps the patient alive, the stilled heart will not resume beating. This happens to about 2,000 patients each year.

The left-hand heart assist is an auxiliary pump which substitutes for the powerful left ventricle pumping chamber of the heart. It is positioned on the outside of the chest and is powered by external air power, just as Barney Clark's Jarvik 7 was. A portable electrical support system is being developed for the future, and this will avoid the bulky and unwieldy pneumatic support system. The assist device is gradually slowed over time, about a week in most cases, until the heart has had time to heal and can begin to pump again.

Defibrillators: Shocking the Heart. If the main pumping chamber, the left ventricle, starts fluttering wildly, it can be—and often is—fatal. Known as ventricular fibrillation, this condition kills about 300,000 Americans each year, often without warning. But once a patient is known to be at risk, prevention can be accomplished by implanting a defibrillator in the abdomen and connecting it to the heart with electrodes. This device, about the size of a pack of cigarettes and weighing 9 ounces (252 grams), constantly monitors the heart. When it detects irregular and potentially lethal heart spasms, the defibrillator delivers an electrical shock of 200-plus watts, which stops the dangerous arrhythmia and returns the heart to its normal rhythm. Implantation cuts the expected death rate in half. Specially developed lithium batteries power the device, and their projected life is 3 years or 100 shocks.

Pacemakers: The Transmitting Implant. More than 1 million pacemakers have been implanted worldwide to correct an electrical disorder in the heart's natural pacemaking tissue, the sinoatrial node. The disorder, called heart block, was first treated with an artificial pacemaker in 1952. Pacemakers deliver rhythmical electrical stimulation whenever it

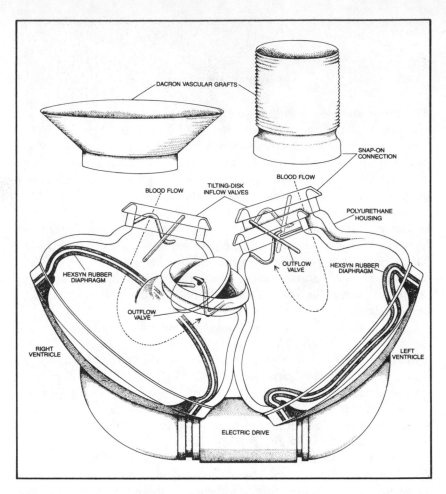

DACRON VASCULAR GRAFTS

SNAP-ON
CONNECTION

BLOOD FLOW

BLOOD FLOW

TILTING-DISK
INFLOW VALVES

POLYURETHANE
HOUSING

HEXSYN RUBBER
DIAPHRAGM

OUTFLOW
VALVE

HEXSYN RUBBER
DIAPHRAGM

OUTFLOW
VALVE

RIGHT
VENTRICLE

LEFT
VENTRICLE

ELECTRIC DRIVE

A portable battery-driven artificial heart will eventually replace the bulky support system that Barney Clark needed. This will allow the patient complete mobility. The C-battery-sized pump in this design can pump some 48 quarts (45 liters) every minute. From "The Total Artificial Heart," Robert K. Jarvik. © *1981 by* **Scientific American.** *All rights reserved.*

is needed, and it is delivered to the heart through electrodes attached to the inside of the right ventricle.

Because each unit costs about $3,000, it is a multibillion-dollar industry worldwide, and the competition is keen. There are more than 20 different makes to choose from in the marketplace, and they have become very sophisticated. Today's pacemaker can be recharged by placing a magnetic coil against the chest. It is also capable of sending telemetry to outside monitoring equipment, even over telephone lines to distant medical centers.

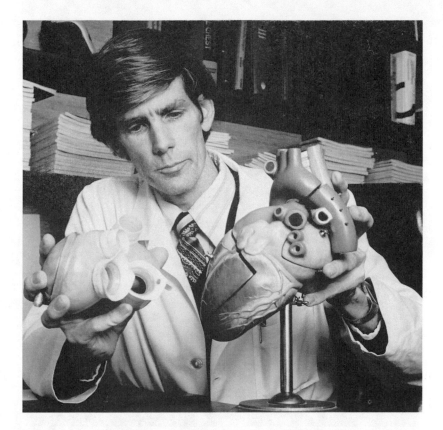

Dr. William C. DeVries, who implanted the first total artificial heart into Barney Clark, was inspired in 1967 at a lecture given by Dr. Willem J. Kolff, the man who invented the kidney dialysis machine. DeVries is currently at the Humana Heart Institute in Louisville, Kentucky, which has promised to pay for 100 artificial heart implants. Jarvik 7 is in right hand; human heart model in left. Courtesy National Institutes of Health.

Artificial pacemakers can transmit information on more than a half dozen factors, including voltage, pulse rate, electrode performance, and full electrocardiogram data. All this can be done with an extremely small amount of energy—about 25 microwatts. This electrical power is 10,000 times less than what a small transistor radio uses.

Controlling the Wayward Heart

Fifty years ago the only drug other than nitroglycerin that doctors administered to heart patients was digitalis, a drug derived from the

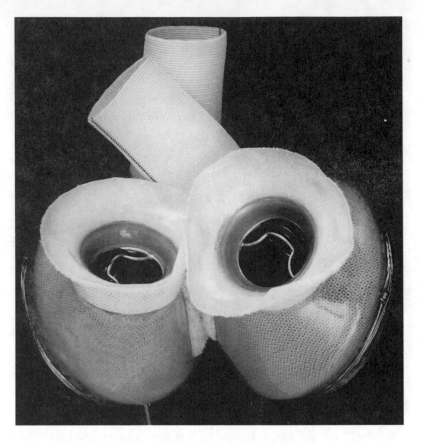

The famous Jarvik 7 implanted into Barney Clark, beat about 13 million times and pumped some 285,000 gallons of blood before Clark died.

leaves of the foxglove plant that causes the heart muscle to pump harder, thereby improving circulation and ridding the body of excess fluid. It is used to treat heart failure because it counters fluid buildup in the body—an early effect of heart attack.

Today a wide variety of heart drugs exist that can stabilize serious heart conditions and extend life: streptokinase, a clot dissolver, administered soon after a heart attack; the old standby nitroglycerin, which "lays back" the heart and reduces its oxygen needs, thereby alleviating angina pain; the newer blocking agents that slow down the heart by blocking its normal response to nerve impulses; various vasodilating drugs, such as the new prazosin, which block receptors in the peripheral blood vessels so that they dilate instead of contract. And research promises many more in the years to come—a cardiac medicine chest that caters to the ailing heart.

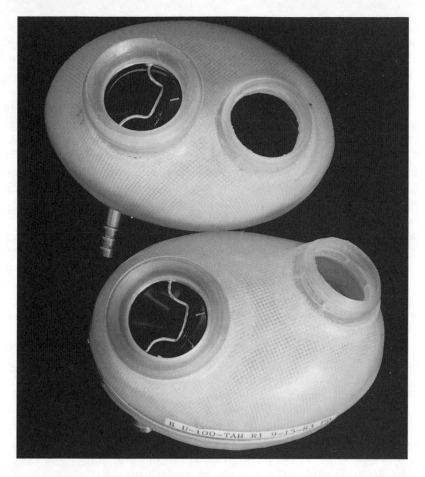

The Utah 100, a narrower and thinner model being tested, will fit into smaller men and women, and perhaps some children. Courtesy National Institutes of Health and the University of Utah Medical Center.

The 1970s brought forth the beta-blockers which slow down the heartbeat and also decrease the speed of the heart's contraction. Less oxygen is therefore needed by the heart muscles—at rest and during exercise—and this allows the heart more rest during its cycle. Beta-blockers such as propranolol protect the ailing heart against excessive work. They decrease high blood pressure, correct some serious rhythm disturbances, and reduce or eliminate angina chest pain. Studies also indicate that beta-blockers can prevent sudden death of patients who already have had a heart attack. Taken daily, this drug is often used in conjunction with nitrates.

The beta class of drugs works by occupying the nerve-receptor sites on the heart muscle and blocking the stimulating substances (for example, the hormone epinephrine, a heart stimulant and blood-vessel constrictor) released by the sympathetic nervous system. They don't, in other words, allow the heart to respond normally to nerve impulses, and this is good for a vulnerable heart.

An even newer class of heart drugs—the calcium blockers—became generally available to heart patients in the early 1980s. These drugs offer a completely new approach to the treatment of heart disease. Calcium is what normally stimulates heart muscle contractions. By inhibiting the flow of calcium ions across cell membranes, calcium blockers reduce the frequency of heart contraction. The speed and strength of contractions are reduced and less oxygen is needed. As a result, the coronary arteries are also dilated, increasing blood flow. The heart doesn't work as hard and is at less risk.

Calcium blockers such as verapamil, diltiazem, and nifedipine prevent arterial spasms by inhibiting contraction of the vessels' muscular walls and are used to treat hypertension, arrhythmia, and angina. In U.S. trials of nifedipine, which prevents spasms of the coronary arteries, 80 of 127 patients treated (63 percent) gained control of their angina, and an Australian study showed an even higher success rate. Evidence also indicates that these blockers help prevent second heart attacks and will reduce the need for coronary bypass operations. Unlike the beta-blockers, the calcium blockers do not adversely affect lung function and do not cause sodium retention.

The revolution in cardiac chemistry will continue during the remaining years of the twentieth century. No doubt, because of this new generation of wonder drugs, more broken hearts will be healed without resorting to sawing through the sternum, plugging in the heart-lung machine, and performing open-heart surgery.

Aspirin for Your Heart

Aspirin is the most widely used drug in the world, and its medicinal properties have been known for over 2,000 years. Hippocrates of Chios, the Greek physician and "Father of Medicine," recommended chewing willow bark to lessen pain and fever. Today it is known that aspirin and willow bark share the same chemicals—salicylates—the same substances that Friedrich Bayer used in the first mass-produced aspirin in the late nineteenth century.

Several rigorous studies have shown that a daily dose of aspirin reduces the threat of recurrent heart attacks and deaths that result therefrom. Another study demonstrated that daily aspirin cut in half the number of heart attacks and deaths from heart attacks in men with unstable angina caused by coronary blockage. The evidence is there, but how does it work?

Aspirin influences the platelets in the blood and acts as an anticoagulant by inhibiting the platelets from releasing substances that help form clots. It is therefore aspirin's anticoagulant properties that help to prevent heart attacks in people who have coronary or other arterial blockage. With aspirin in the bloodstream, the platelets are kept from sticking together and forming a plug—a deadly plug to some diseased hearts.

If the good news about aspirin's benefit to the heart and circulation continues to spread, it may well dramatically increase the annual worldwide aspirin consumption—as if 100,000 tons of aspirin swallowed each year isn't enough. (Note: Your doctor should be consulted before you take aspirin on a regular basis. Some patients with certain medical conditions should avoid taking aspirin.)

BLOOD

Blood Cells Galore

In just 1 second, as many as 8 million blood cells die in the human body —each and every second of our lives. But do not despair. For the healthy body, the same number are born each second.

A red blood cell is only about 1/3,000 of an inch (7.7 micrometers) in diameter, but the 8 million, lined up end to end, would stretch more than 2,000 feet (610 meters). In an average human lifetime, a person's red-blood-cell birth or death count, if placed single file, would stretch from the earth to the sun and back about 5 times. Just 2 1/2 hours' worth of red blood cells would stretch from New York to London.

A Drop of Blood

A needle prick of the finger will bring forth a tiny droplet of blood. If the droplet of blood equals about 1 cubic millimeter, it will contain some 5 million red blood cells.

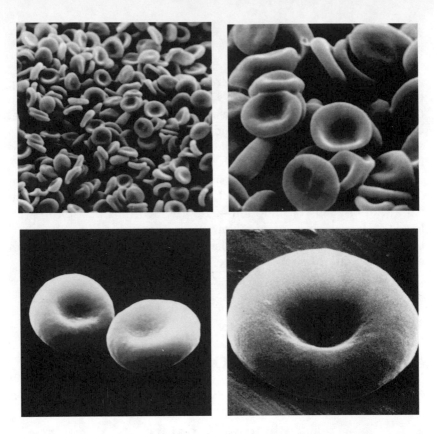

Zooming in on red blood cells, from a magnification of 1,800 to more than 10,000 times. As many as 8 million blood cells die in the human body each second, but the same number are created when we are healthy. Courtesy Ronald G. Cohn (Syntex Research) and National Institutes of Health.

Blood's Recipe

Human blood is mostly water, about 78 percent. The remaining 22 percent is composed of solids—proteins, salts, minerals, carbohydrates, hormones—and gases.

The blood's plasma—the pale yellowish clear fluid in which red and white blood cells float—dominates blood and represents 55 percent of the total. Besides cells and their contents, which make up the other 45 percent, plasma transports platelets for clotting, nutrients, hormones, and proteins. The dominant protein is albumin, which acts as a carrier for small molecules and gives blood its gummy texture. Albumin is to blood as cornstarch is to pudding. It is widely found in plant and animal life. Milk and egg whites contain high amounts of albumin, for example, and so some of your favorite dessert recipes share a major ingredient with human blood.

Blood Weight

The next time you carry a gallon of milk, you'll have a good idea of what your blood would weigh if you were able to carry it separately.

Blood, our liquid tissue, represents about 7 to 9 percent of body weight, men with a higher percentage than women. Women also have proportionately fewer red blood cells.

If you're a man and weigh 154 pounds (70 kilograms), your body contains some 5½ quarts (5⅕ liters) of blood, which would weigh about 14 pounds (6.3 kilograms). The body of a woman who weighs 110 pounds (50 kilograms) contains about 3.5 quarts (3.3 liters) of blood. Her blood would weigh about 10 pounds (4.5 kilograms).

If a large man and a petite woman suffer the same serious wound from which blood is lost, the woman is extremely vulnerable and at high risk because, with less blood and fewer red cells than a man to begin with, she loses proportionately more of her blood. The woman is, however, less likely to receive such a wound in the first place. She is also less likely than a man to be a victim of circulatory disease. All in all, a woman is healthier *and* lighter with less blood.

Blood's Mileage

A microscopic red blood cell travels about 950 miles (1,528 kilometers) in its short 4-month lifetime. To match this size-to-distance-to-time relationship, a person of average height would have to travel some 2 billion miles (3.2 billion kilometers) in the same time—a distance equal to 80,000 times around the earth.

A Short, Busy Life

It takes 6 days for red blood cells to gestate in the bone marrow before they are born at a rate of 480 million each minute. More than a half ton of red blood cells are created in an average lifetime.

Once born, they live for about 4 months, circulating throughout the body, feeding and serving the 60 trillion other body cells. Each circuit through the body takes about 20 seconds, and the red blood cells make some 250,000 round-trips before heading back to the bone marrow, their birthplace, to die. There—worn out from their short, busy life—they are eaten by larger white blood cells, the phagocytes.

Zooming In on Hemoglobin

The most abundant human body cells are red blood cells, some 25 trillion of them in all, and they make up about 45 percent of the volume of blood. Red blood cells contain about two thirds water and one third hemoglobin, the iron-containing protein that carries oxygen from the lungs to the body cells and removes carbon dioxide, the cells' waste product. Oxygen-rich hemoglobin is what makes arterial blood red. A person of average weight has about 1 pound (1/2 kilogram) of hemoglobin.

Hemoglobin molecules, each containing one atom of iron, are so densely packed in each red blood cell that they almost form crystals. In a single red blood cell, with a diameter some 20 times smaller than the width of a human hair, there are about 300 million hemoglobin molecules. Because of the size of the hemoglobin molecule, the number of possible arrangements of the amino acids in the simple protein component, globin, is enormous—10^{619} or 1 followed by 619 zeros. This represents a number some 50 times larger than the total number of stars in our Milky Way Galaxy.

Blood Aplenty

The amount of blood donated each year in North America—approximately 12 million pints (5.7 million liters)—is enough to fill the bodies of some 1.2 million people, the entire population of Detroit or Birmingham, England.

White Blood for Red

A white fluid, chemically similar to Teflon and derived from petroleum, is being injected into the bodies of patients in the United States and Japan in clinical trials. Fluosol, the so-called artificial blood manu-

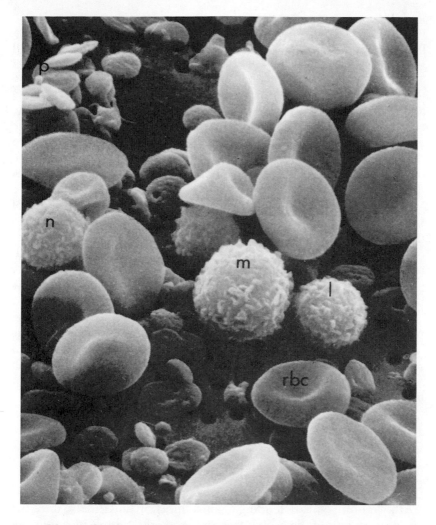

Normal human blood magnified almost 2,700 times by an electron microscope. In the scanning field are red blood cells (rbc), three types of white blood cells (n, m, and l), and platelets (p). Red cells outnumber whites about 600 to 1. Courtesy Bruce Wetzel and Harry Schaefer, National Cancer Institute.

factured by Alpha Therapeutic Corporation, is more accurately described as a temporary blood substitute that takes over one of the crucial functions of human blood—oxygen delivery to and carbon dioxide removal from body cells and tissues. Unlike real blood, however, it cannot produce antibodies and fight infection.

The oxygen-carrying liquid is expected to gain Food and Drug Administration approval, at least for some of its uses, in the near future, and its list of medical uses continues to expand. This is because of its unique ability to deliver 3 to 5 times more oxygen to the body than the natural red blood cells it partially imitates. This makes it valuable in treating patients with severe anemia (such as sickle cell), stroke, heart attack, and carbon monoxide poisoning. Fluosol has also increased the survival rate for patients undergoing major surgery because of its ability to deliver extra oxygen. It also enables surgeons to improve the results of coronary balloon surgery by inflating the microballoon at the end of the catheter for a few more seconds, thus further compressing the plaque against the arterial walls. The extra inflation time, when the oxygen is cut off, will not damage the tissue because Fluosol has delivered that extra boost of oxygen.

Diagnostic procedures can also be improved with the injection of Fluosol. The quality of coronary X-ray images can be enhanced, and the risks of the procedure lowered, when Fluosol is mixed with a radio-opaque substance. With a molecular change, it has also been animal-tested as a cancer-imaging agent. And experiments indicate that it may prove useful in preserving donor kidneys for a longer period of time before transplantation.

All these benefits are possible because Fluosol's perfluorocarbon particles are much smaller than red blood cells and slip through the capillary membranes at a much faster rate. How much smaller? About 300 times smaller than a typical red blood cell, which would make them about 1/300,000 of an inch (1/12 of a micron) in diameter. This is about 6,200 times smaller than the period at the end of this sentence.

The Wandering Whites

If red blood cells are the body's working class, then white blood cells are the fighting elite, defending against infection and disease once the invaders penetrate the body's largest organ, the skin. White cells defend us against bacteria, viruses, fungi, and parasites, often engulfing and destroying them by the millions. They also produce antibodies, specifically tailored proteins that destroy or render harmless the infecting foreign agent.

There are about 75 billion white blood cells in the human body at any one time, a small number when compared to the red cells, which normally outnumber them by about 600 to 1. Under normal conditions white-cell counts sometimes decrease even further, during rest, for example, or in response to certain foods.

The whites are true cells because, unlike the reds, they have a nucleus. The nucleus varies in size and shape among the several varieties. The whites are unique among blood cells in other ways too. They have mobility independent of the blood's current. This enables them to leave the circulatory system, travel through the capillary walls into tissue to fight infection, and gobble up the infectious microbes.

Even though the whites are often much larger than red cells, 3 to 4 times in some cases, they can actually squeeze through tiny pores between capillary wall membrane cells to stalk and attack invaders.

This squeeze-through process is known as diapedesis. Even though each white cell (for example, a neutrophil or monocyte) is tremendously larger than the pore, a tiny portion of it at a time squeezes through the pore until it has passed into the tissue. Figuratively, this is the body's camel passing through the eye of a needle.

Cellular Sacrifice

Most white blood cells, about 70 percent, are formed in the bone marrow, and most of these are stored there until they are needed by the body, at which time they enter the blood, patrol for invaders, and migrate to the infection site. About 3 times as many of these white cells, a 6-day supply, as are circulating in the blood are always ready and waiting in the bone marrow. Once these whites leave the marrow and enter the blood, they spend only about 7 hours circulating in the blood and then another 2 or 3 days in the tissue after leaving the capillaries. Their life span is therefore no longer than 4 days.

When these white cells live fulfilling lives, which is to say, when they do what they are intended to do, their lives are cut short. If they fight a serious infection, they may live only a few hours. These microdefenders rush to the infected area, gobble up the invaders, and die as a result —a case of sacrificial ingestion.

The Second Wave of Whites

White lymphocyte cells amount to about 30 percent of the body's white-blood-cell population. Together with the neutrophils, they add up to over 90 percent of the blood's entire defense force.

Lymphocytes are the second line of defense, the second wave of white cells to arrive at the front lines. The hungry phagocyte cells— macrophages and neutrophils—are the first to do battle by attacking and gobbling up as many invaders as they can. The lymphocytes are defender specialists which, through a complex sequence of interactions and changes, sensitize themselves to an invader and produce antibodies (protein compounds formed with 2 chains of amino acids) that bind to and coat the invader agents (antigens), thereby destroying or neutralizing them. There are 2 types of lymphocytes—B cells and T cells. Physically both types look alike, with nuclei that occupy most or all of the cell, and with clear, nongranular cytoplasm. They do, however, have different functions. The B cells produce the antibodies that are programmed to seek out and destroy the invaders. The T cells are more aggressive and attack the enemy directly with potent chemicals. They also prod their fellow B cells to produce antibodies, and they regulate the immune response to protect the body from the dangers of its own overreaction.

In response to an enemy, B-cell lymphocytes multiply quickly, forming hundreds of plasma cells. These in turn manufacture antibodies at a rate of about 2,000 a second—over 7 million in an hour.

The Clones of Lymphocytes

There are millions of lymphocytes in a lymph gland, but at first only a few of them can respond to a specific foreign invader. This group of specific sensitized lymphocytes (T cells or B cells) is called a clone. After they encounter an enemy, the clone cells multiply rapidly and increase their number dramatically.

The lymphoid tissue is capable of forming 10,000 to 100,000 different types of sensitive T-cell or B-cell lymphocytes, each of which can grow into a unique and effective clone group when just the right target enemy comes along. Every infectious enemy therefore has its very own lymphocyte clone group to confront, and each group can be traced back to one or a few original sensitized lymphocytes or their antibodies. But where did the first cells of any unique clone come from? No one is sure, but some researchers believe there is a separate gene behind the birth of each and every clone group.

Little Gobblers

The most abundant type of white blood cell, the neutrophil, makes up between 60 to 70 percent of the normal body's 75 billion total white count. This white cell, about $1/2,500$ of an inch (10 micrometers) in diameter, is distinguished from the monocytes and lymphocytes by minute granules in the cytoplasm. Neutrophils represent the infantry of the body's defense mechanism and, compared to the large and ravenous macrophages, are the little gobblers of foreign invaders. But even though the macrophages can swell up to 8 times the size of neutrophils, the sheer numbers of these smaller white cells clearly make them the dominant defenders against disease.

The body of a 150-pound (68-kilogram) person produces about 100 billion neutrophils each and every day—almost 22 times the planet earth's entire human population.

Slow but Sure

Both of the white neutrophil and macrophage cells ingest their enemy and travel through the tissue to do so. What's their top speed? About 1 inch (2.5 centimeters) every 10½ hours or 180 times their own length every minute. This may seem slow, but with this speed no area of the human body is more than a minute's time from any capillary—so help is always close by.

Gypsies and Stay-at-Homes

While some macrophages are gypsy cells that wander through the tissues, seeking out foreign invaders, the vast majority are stay-at-homes that find a particular tissue site and remain there after leaving a capillary. Unless the front line of battle comes to their area, they can remain attached to the tissue for months or even years.

The stay-at-homes are known as tissue macrophages, and they have different appearances depending on where they are located in the body —be it in the lymph nodes; the skin and tissues underneath; the lung; the spleen and the bone marrow; the brain; the liver; or other areas of the body that are especially exposed to infection.

Tissue macrophages are tough defenders of their home territory. Those in the liver, called Kupffer's cells, attack the large numbers of invading bacteria that enter through the gastrointestinal tract. Normally, all the bacteria are destroyed at this vulnerable entrance to the entire body's circulation. These macrophages of the liver can ingest a bacteria in 1/100 of a second!

Monocyte Metamorphosis

Monocytes, one of the several types of white blood cells, are generated in the bone marrow and also migrate through the capillary walls to fight infection. Unlike the neutrophils, however, monocytes are unable

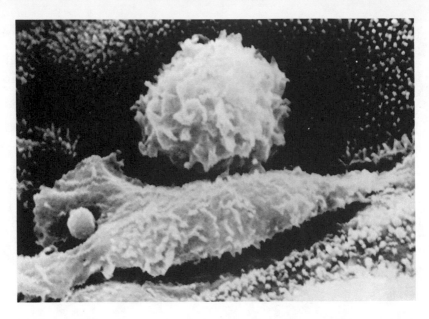

Two macrophage white blood cells, the bottom one about to gobble up a foreign object. Such white cells, found throughout the body, defend their territory against foreign invaders. The macrophages of the liver can ingest a bacteria in 1/100 of a second. Courtesy National Institutes of Health.

to ingest the enemy while in the bloodstream because they are immature cells at this time. But once at the injured site, they go through a metamorphosis. Swelling up, the monocytes increase their diameter by as much as 5 times—up to 1/300 of an inch (80 microns), just visible to the naked human eye. In doing so, they transform into tissue macrophages, the giant protectors of the body's defense system. Once in the tissue, they become the first line of defense, standing watch for the enemy, always ready to attack and destroy the intruder by ingesting it —a process called phagocytosis.

If they do not engage the infectious enemy, they can lie in wait for months or even years, the longest life span of any blood cell. But when they do battle, they become devouring warriors for the body, ingesting as many as 100 bacteria (5 times more than a neutrophil white cell can), even gulping down whole malaria parasites.

The Platelets: Squeezing Clots and Beating Hearts

Platelets are the blood's smallest cells, about 4 times smaller than red blood cells—1/12,000 of an inch (2 microns) in diameter. Their minute size is the reason they were not discovered for 200 years after red blood cells were identified. Despite their small size, however, they play a large role in protecting the human body and plugging up its small holes.

Literally "little plates," platelets are diskshaped, colorless bodies in the plasma that help in the formation of blood clots. They originate in the bone marrow, in large cells called megakaryocytes, which themselves break up into thousands of platelets. Adults have about 1 trillion platelets in their blood plasma. Some 200 billion are produced each day, while a like number of old ones simultaneously retire and die after a life span of about 10 days.

Microscopic blood-vessel injuries are repaired by platelets without

A blood clot forms on the surface of an injured artery. Platelets replace surface cells and fibrin strands congregate across the site, as the coagulation process begins. Courtesy Dr. James G. White (University of Minnesota) and the National Institutes of Health.

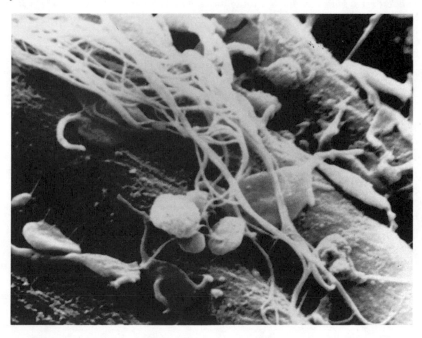

the more complex clotting process coming into play. They rush to the injury site, swell into irregular shapes, and stick together and to the rough edges of the injured vessel to form a plug. In this way, *millions* of small capillaries are repaired each day without clotting.

For larger injuries, platelets initiate a complex sequence of chemical reactions by releasing active compounds they have stored. Serotonin, for example, is released at the site and constricts vessels and reduces bleeding. Then solid fibrin strands, created from the soluble protein, fibrinogen, in the plasma, form a meshlike web across the injured site. This fibrin network entangles the platelets and other blood cells to form a clot.

In the beginning, the blood clot is 99 percent water, but after a few minutes, the clot contracts, squeezing out the blood's fluid—serum. It is the platelets, containing the proteins, actin and myosin, that initiate the contraction. Within an hour, the serum is squeezed out leaving the dense plug of platelets, fibrin, and other blood substances that stop the bleeding. When exposed to the air, this compressed clot is known as a scab.

The contractile proteins, actin and myosin, do more than squeeze clots dry and form scabs. They also cause the human heart to beat by

Platelets aggregate on the blood vessel wall to begin clot formation. The blood's smallest cells, platelets, are 1/12,000 of an inch (2 microns) in diameter. They were not discovered until 200 years after red blood cells were. Courtesy National Institutes of Health.

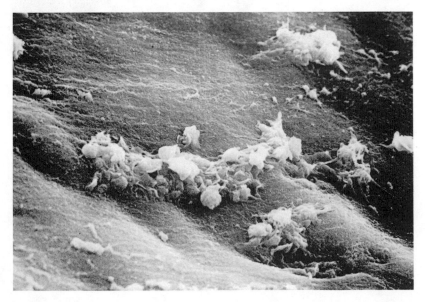

contracting the cardiac muscle fibers. Inside the platelets, these microproteins both move the blood *and* stop the blood.

CIRCULATION

The Arching Aorta

Arteries carry oxygen-laden blood *away* from the heart, while veins carry oxygen-depleted blood *toward* the heart. The only exceptions are the pulmonary arteries, which carry oxygen-depleted blood to the lungs, and the pulmonary veins, which carry oxygen-enriched blood from the lungs to the heart.

The aorta is the largest single artery in the human circulatory system, and it carries oxygenated blood from the heart to all parts of the body. It originates from one of the heart's two lower chambers—the left ventricle—which pumps 2 to 3 ounces (60 to 90 milliliters) into it with each heartbeat. Oxygenated blood spurts from the left ventricle into the aorta at about 80 feet (24 meters) a minute, or about 1 mile (1.6 kilometers) per hour.

As the aorta leads off the ventricle, it has an interior diameter of about 1 inch (25 millimeters). This makes it by far the largest artery in the human body—about 125 times larger than the smallest arteries, the arterioles, which are no thicker than human hairs and which lead into the microscopic capillaries.

Where's Your Blood?

Blood is not evenly distributed throughout the body as might be expected. The capillaries, surprisingly, where the all-important diffusion of substances takes place between the blood and tissues, contain only 5 percent of blood volume in the greater circulatory system (not including pulmonary circulation).

Where's the other 95 percent? The heart contains 7 percent and the lungs 9 percent of the blood. The arteries account for another 15 percent. But altogether, including the capillaries, these add up to only

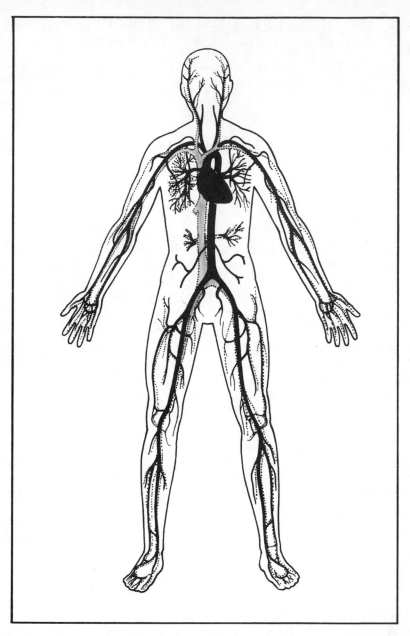

The human circulatory system, from head to toe. The aorta, the body's largest artery, carries blood from the heart to all other parts of the body. It is 125 times larger than the smallest arteries that are no thicker than human hairs. Courtesy National Institutes of Health.

GOING WITH THE FLOW:

36 percent of the body's blood. Most of our blood—some 64 percent— is in our veins, returning to the heart.

For decades, the veins were considered nothing more than passageways for returning the blood to the heart, but that view has changed drastically. Veins are capable of constricting and enlarging. This allows them to store large quantities of blood and release it when needed by the body. The veins therefore act as an emergency blood reservoir.

The human body can lose as much as 20 to 25 percent of its total blood volume yet the circulatory system can function almost normally because of vein constriction and their large reservoir of blood.

Capillary Capsules

Microstretch. There are about 62,000 miles (99,000 kilometers) of arteries, capillaries, and veins in the human body—enough to stretch 2½ times around the earth's equator or almost 9 round-trips from London to New York.

Dense Billions. Our bodies contain some 10 billion capillaries which feed our cells with fresh oxygenated blood and cart away the cells' waste products of uric acid and carbon dioxide. They are microbridges between the smallest arteries (arterioles) and the smallest veins (venules).

More than a million capillaries are in a square inch (6.5 square centimeters) of muscle tissue. In fact, no cell in our body is more than 1/500 of an inch (50 microns) away from a capillary.

Tiny Tunnels. The average diameter of a capillary is about the same size as a red blood cell—1/3,000 of an inch (8 microns). This often causes the red cells to line up single file in a capillary as they carry their oxygen cargo to the surrounding tissues. Sometimes they must even squeeze through a capillary that is smaller than themselves.

A Very Thin Spread. If all 10 billion capillaries in your body could be spread out flat, their surface area would equal about 700 square yards (585 square meters)—the square area of about 6 tennis courts. It would be a very thin spread, however, because the thickness of a capillary wall is about 1/50,000 of an inch (½ micron)—about 300 times thinner than a human hair.

Micromotion. In the capillaries, blood moves about 1/80 of an inch (0.3 millimeter) a second or 43 inches (109 centimeters) an hour. This is more than a thousand times slower than the speed blood flows in the aorta after leaving the heart. At this slow capillary speed, blood is only in the capillary for 1 or 2 seconds because of their microlengths. In about 1 second, therefore, our trillions of body cells are rejuvenated and cleaned with fresh blood in a space invisible to the naked human eye. This micromotion that no one thinks about is at the opposite end of a heartbeat.

Vasomotion

The capillaries do not receive a constant flow of blood, but instead receive it in a cyclical rhythm, depending on the tissue's need for oxygen—vasomotion. Micromuscles (precapillary sphincters) open and close the entrances to capillaries and this controls blood flow. Generally, they constrict and relax 5 to 10 times each minute, automatically regulating the blood flow to the tissue. This means that a single capillary sphincter flexes as much as 14,400 times each day—and there are 10 billion capillaries!

Tiny Tides

The movement of water and nutrients back and forth between the capillary membranes and the spaces between the tissue cells—diffusion—is a constant process, and the total amount of water exchanged is tremendous when this microcosmic exchange is applied to the entire body.

The rate of diffusion of water through capillary membranes of the entire body—*not* the flow *through* the capillaries—amounts to an amazing 62 gallons (236 liters) every minute because the same fluid moves to and fro tens of thousands of times through such a large surface area of membrane. This is 45 times the total blood volume of an average-sized man and almost 72 times that of a smaller woman.

Stand Still, Legs Swell

Blood returning to the heart can only flow in one direction because of tiny valves in the veins. When a person moves or tenses muscles, blood is pumped toward the heart. This pumping system is known as the venous pump, and it occurs every time muscles contract and the veins are compressed.

When a person stands completely still, this pumping system does not work. As a result capillary pressure increases, fluid leaks into the tissue spaces from the circulatory system, and the legs swell. Blood volume also drops. As much as 20 percent of a person's blood volume is lost from the circulatory system within the first 15 minutes of standing absolutely still.

Continental Varicose

Blood pressure in the veins is usually low, but during pregnancy or when one stands most of the time, pressure increases and the veins are stretched more than normally. The veins stretch, but their valves, directing the one-way flow to the heart, do not. As a result, the valves don't close completely and some blood reverses its flow. This increases the venous pressure even further, the veins continue to enlarge, and the valves stop functioning completely. Fluid leaks from the capillary blood into the tissue, and the veins become varicose.

One of the best treatments for varicose veins is elevation of the legs to a level as high as the heart. Needless to say, this is impractical for people who must stand all day or all night to earn their living. Tight binders on the legs are also helpful. Severe cases have traditionally been corrected with surgery, and this is still recommended for moderate cases. But an older treatment for serious varicose veins is making a comeback. A chemical compound, sodium moruate, is injected into as many as 20 veins in each leg to shrink them. The leg is then bandaged tightly to compress the veins and cause them to atrophy. The bandaging is continued for 1 to 6 weeks—until the veins are shut down.

The technique is called sclerotherapy and was used extensively in the 1930s and 1940s, but it fell out of favor in the 1950s because the varicose veins began swelling again after treatment. With improved bandaging techniques, however, European doctors improved the technique, and the veins remained shut down. This is a medical instance, where the European physicians held on to a traditional treatment and gave it a future, while American doctors were too quick to abandon it.

The Killer Sludge

Tens of thousands of people die each day throughout the world from heart attacks and strokes, both of which are caused by the insidious disease arteriosclerosis—the buildup of cholesterol (a steroid alcohol) and fatty substances in the arteries in the form of patches known as plaques. As the deposits accumulate, they block the flow of blood, and when major arteries of the body are involved—those serving the brain, heart, kidneys, and legs—a major medical problem results. The danger point is reached at 60 percent blockage.

The traditional medical consensus has been that the process of arteriosclerosis—which usually begins in a person's twenties—cannot be stopped or reversed, but just slowed down. Today, however, adherence to this attitude would be harmful to a patient's health. Several recent studies indicate there are effective ways (besides the standard advice to stop smoking, lose weight, reduce fat in one's diet, and exercise) to combat and perhaps eventually rid the body of the deadly sludge that kills so many of us.

In controlled studies involving animals fed high-cholesterol diets, it was found that vitamins C and E were lost from the arterial linings. When these compounds were added to the same high-cholesterol diet, however, the plaque buildup was either prevented or reduced. Future studies will demonstrate if this holds true for humans. If it does, buy vitamin stocks.

Another study involved human patients. The group receiving treatment with low-cholesterol diets and cholesterol-lowering drugs had less buildup of fatty deposits than the control group. Measurements of the size of plaques, especially in the main arteries to legs and the brain, are documented by analyzing special X-ray angiograms with computers—a technique originally developed by NASA to evaluate and enhance planetary photographs.

Dietary, vitamin, and drug research in the next 2 decades may well bring the mass killer, arteriosclerosis, under partial, if not complete, medical control, enabling doctors to stop or reverse the process in most patients. Some researchers even predict that a new generation of drugs may eventually make it possible for the heart to create its own bypass arteries to substitute for those that have been blocked or otherwise damaged by arteriosclerosis. But that probably is decades away.

Nevertheless, today there is new hope and real evidence that this killer can and will be stopped. But it will not happen next year. Keep in mind that doctors still do not understand why veins are seldom affected by arteriosclerosis. Nor does anyone know why leg veins, grafted onto the heart and aorta during bypass surgery, often *do* develop the dangerous buildup. Much of the mystery remains, but the sleuths pursuing the killer sludge will break the case in the end, keeping our lifelines of blood flow open.

Chapter Six

Ins and Outs: Lungs, Kidneys, Intestines

LUNGS AND BREATHING

A Breath for All Occasions

Just lying in bed, your body will require that you breathe about 8 quarts of air (7.6 liters) a minute. If you sit up and remain seated, you will consume 16 quarts of air a minute (15.2 liters). If you decide to go for a walk, 24 quarts (22.8 liters) a minute will be needed. And if you break into a run, your body may demand 50 quarts of air a minute (47.5 liters).

The winner of the 1982 Boston Marathon, Alberto Salazar, used about 60 quarts of air each minute (57 liters) to run the traditional distance of 26 miles 385 yards (slightly more than 41 kilometers).

A Breath of Air

Breathing is much more than taking air in and letting air out. Those actions actually are the beginning and end products of what constitutes "breathing."

Having no muscles of their own, the lungs are passive during breathing. They inflate much like a bellows, with the muscles that surround the chest cavity doing the work.

When we take in air (inspiration), the muscles over the rib cage contract and the ribs are lifted, increasing the internal space (volume) in the chest from front to back and side to side. The diaphragm—the strong muscle that separates the chest from the abdomen—moves down, lowering the floor of the chest to further increase the total space from top to bottom. These muscular actions produce a partial vacuum in the lungs, and outside air rushes in to equalize the lowered pressure.

When we breathe out (expiration), the muscles over the rib cage relax, the ribs drop down and the diaphragm returns to its rest position up under the lungs. Expiration reduces the total volume in the chest, increases air pressure, and forces air out of the lungs. Together, inspiration and expiration, alternating over and over again, form the act of breathing, or respiration, which means "to breathe again."

Artificial respiration, whether applied by one individual to another following an apparent drowning or other accident, or by an iron lung, is designed to simulate these muscular actions that force us to breathe.

The average person breathes 16 times each minute and takes in

An X ray of the human lung airways. In an average lifetime, we breathe over 75 million gallons of air (over 2.85 trillion liters), almost 1 1/2 times the total volume of the late great airship, the **Hindenburg.** *Courtesy National Institutes of Health.*

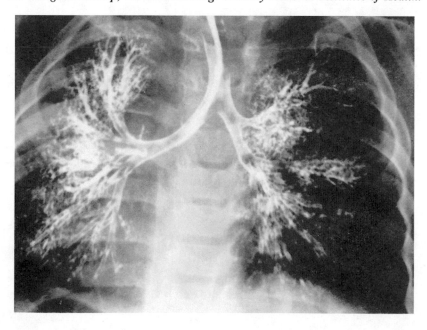

INS AND OUTS:

about one pint of air (0.5 liter) with each breath. In the average lifetime then, we breathe over 75 million gallons of air (over 2.85 trillion liters). This is almost 1½ times the total volume capacity of the late great airship, the *Hindenburg*, which contained about 52 million gallons (197 million liters) of lighter-than-air gas.

Breathing in Action

We breathe in and out 12 to 20 times a minute, depending on our size. Children breathe twice as fast as adults. Because oxygen can be absorbed from the air only at the surface of the lungs, the lung's volume is relatively unimportant; what matters is its surface area. Therefore, smaller people breathe faster to make up for their lungs' relative lack of surface area.

Other factors affect the rate at which we breathe. At a rate of 16 to 20 times a minute, women generally breathe more rapidly than men. We breathe faster while jogging or otherwise engaging in muscular activities, or when we have a fever or certain diseases such as an overactive thyroid gland (hyperthyroidism).

The older we get, the slower we breathe. At birth, the average person breathes 40 to 60 times a minute. By 5 years of age, the same person breathes 24 to 26 times a minute, and by age 15 the rate has dropped to 20 to 22 times a minute. By age 25, the rate of respiration stabilizes at 14 to 18 breaths a minute for men and 16 to 20 for women.

A change in the position of the body also can affect breathing. Lying in bed, we breathe 12 to 14 times a minute. When we sit up, the rate increases to 18. Standing upright raises breathing to 20 to 22 times a minute. Anger or other emotions also may cause breathing to speed up or slow down.

In the average lifetime, we take better than 600 million breaths of air.

The Breathing Machine

The lungs are only one part of the pulmonary system, the "breathing machine." The pulmonary system consists of the respiratory passages (nose, sinuses, mouth) and the lungs, 2 spongelike organs which are suspended in the chest cavity from the breathing airways by a series of successively smaller flexible tubes. Although relatively large, each lung weighs only 1 pound (2.2 kilograms).

The right lung has 3 lobes or sections and is larger than the left

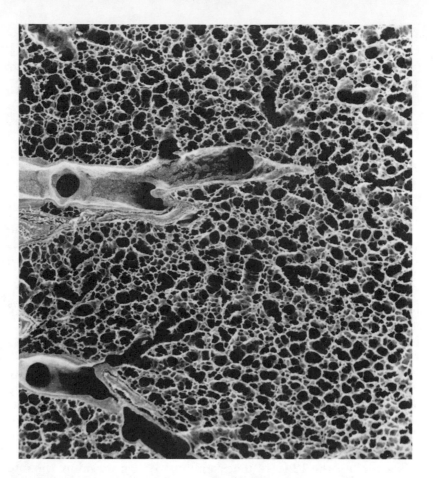

The tiny air sacs, alveoli, and airways of the lungs magnified 50 times resemble the intricate branches of a tree or bush. Each lung has 300 million alveoli, all of which have thin walls about 1/125,000 of an inch (0.2 micron) thick through which oxygen from the lungs and carbon dioxide from the cells are exchanged. Courtesy National Institutes of Health.

which has only 2. Each lobe in the lungs is self-contained to a certain extent so that one lobe can suffer a disorder or injury without affecting the others.

Air enters the body through the nose or mouth. It then travels to the farthest parts of the lungs through the subdivisions of a structure, the tracheobronchial tree—which looks like a tree turned upside down in the chest—its trunk extending to the throat.

The main part of this structure is the trachea (windpipe) which extends for about 4 inches from the top of the throat to its bottom, where it divides into 2 branches, one going to the right lung and the other to the left. The sides and front of the trachea are stiffened and the airway kept open with 10 to 20 C-shaped rings of heavy cartilage.

From each of the 2 branches below the trachea, the bronchial tree divides progressively into thousands of smaller branchlike tubes, and subdivides into millions of bronchioles, the smallest tubes in the tree. The smallest of these bronchioles is about 1/100 of an inch, roughly the thickness of a human hair. The air-absorbing area of the lungs is increased by this branching.

At the end of each bronchiole are clusters of tiny air sacs called alveoli. It is through the thin walls of the alveoli in the lungs (a mere 0.2 micron in thickness) that the exchange of oxygen from the lungs and carbon dioxide from the cells (transported by the bloodstream to adjacent capillaries) is made.

Each alveolus is microscopic, but because there are 300 million of them, their total surface area is great. If the tissue of the alveoli were flattened out, it would cover 1,000 square feet or about the area of 3 boxing rings.

The Sounds of Breathing

In examining their patients, doctors often listen to the patient's chest with a stethoscope. This examination is called auscultation. By listening to the air flowing in and out of the bronchi in the chest, the doctor can tell certain things about the condition of the lungs.

Crepitations, a harsh, crackling burst of sound, can mean the presence of an illness such as pneumonia.

Continuous, high- or low-pitched sounds occurring when you breathe in and out may be caused by asthma. If, however, you cough and the sound disappears, it was probably caused by a bit of mucus that collected in the larger bronchi.

Rales are harsher, disconnected sounds which may indicate bronchitis or edema (the collection of water in the lungs).

A crackling noise may suggest friction resulting from a disease such as pleurisy, an inflammation of the pleura that lines the chest cavity.

Breathing on the Right Foot

Runners who develop a leg pain while doing their thing often follow the advice in an old trainer's tale and switch their breathing pattern so they exhale when they land on the opposite leg. Scientists are now saying there may be some validity to this measure.

On the average, we take 4 steps with every breath we take, walking or running, and we almost always exhale when the same foot hits the ground. It has been suggested that the foot we exhale on takes a greater beating than the other, possibly because the diaphragm is in its relaxed position when we exhale and does not absorb the shock of impact, thus producing leg pains.

Runners in competition can tune in to the "breathing-foot" pattern of an opponent and put on a burst of speed when the competition's breathing pattern shifts down to 2 or 3 to 1 instead of the 4 steps to each breath. For the noncompetitive runner, pain in the exhaling leg may be a useful indication that you need to slow down—or at least shift your breathing to the other leg for a while.

Blue Blood

In the days of the landed gentry, the story goes that the landowners who did not work in the fields, and so were never tanned by the sun, were referred to as "blue bloods" because the superficial blue veins on their hands could be seen through their skin. Today, if you are said to have "blue blood" you probably are suffocating.

Blood carrying carbon dioxide from the body's cells is pumped from the right side of the heart through the pulmonary venous artery to the capillaries of the alveoli. This blood is blue because it carries very little oxygen.

When this blue blood reaches the alveoli, carbon dioxide passes through the thin capillary and alveoli walls to the alveoli sacs. At the same time, because there is more oxygen in the alveolus than in the returning blood, oxygen—being a gas—moves from greater to lesser concentration and passes through the 2 thin walls to the oxygen-depleted blood. There it dissolves and turns the blood red again.

Your blood will remain blue only if you are prevented from obtaining oxygen. Therefore, being a true "blue blood" would be an extremely undesirable condition.

The Oxygen Delivery Route

The lungs, the heart, and the blood are dependent on each other. The job of the lungs is to add oxygen to the blood going to the heart and to remove carbon dioxide from the blood coming from the heart.

The heart continuously pumps oxygenated red blood cells through the blood vessels (arteries and capillaries) to the cells in the tissues of the body. As the red blood cells reach the tissue cells, they deposit their cargo of oxygen and pick up the cells' main waste product, carbon dioxide. The carbon dioxide is carried back to the lungs by the red blood cells and the liquid plasma in the blood. In the lungs, the carbon dioxide is unloaded through a fine network of capillaries in the walls of the alveoli, after which it travels up the bronchial tree and is exhaled into the atmosphere. At the same time, oxygen is picked up by the red blood cells, returned to the heart through the pulmonary vein, and the process starts over again. The red blood cells pass through the walls of a lung capillary single file in about 1 second.

The capillaries in the 5 lobes of the lungs in a single strand would extend 1,000 miles (1,600 kilometers) in length and would stretch from Berlin to Moscow or from Washington, D.C., to Montreal and back again.

Heavy Air

People who work under abnormally high air pressure such as divers and others who work below water level sometimes experience a situation in which the blood and body tissues absorb extra amounts of gases from the air such as nitrogen, carbon dioxide, and oxygen. This is harmless as long as inside and outside pressures are equal. However, if the individual passes from an area of high pressure to one of low pressure too quickly, the extra nitrogen in the blood is released into the tissues and blood vessels as small bubbles of gas which cause dizziness, nausea, muscle pains, and joint pains—the reason for the condition's popular name, the bends. These symptoms can be avoided or relieved by passing the person through a series of "decompression chambers" gradually reducing the outside pressure. In this way the gases in the blood are brought slowly into balance with the atmospheric gases.

Catching Your Breath

Shortness of breath after running up a long flight of stairs or an active game of basketball is not unusual. Breathlessness under these conditions is your lungs' way of telling you they need more oxygen and forcing you to take deeper breaths more often (panting) to deliver the amount of oxygen demanded by the cells after your strenuous activity.

But, if you are winded by simply walking up that flight of stairs or doing other everyday activities, then you may have a problem. Surprisingly, that problem could be in your blood, not your lungs or your heart. Oxygen is carried to the cells of the body by the hemoglobin in the blood. People who have an insufficient amount of hemoglobin in their blood do not get enough oxygen delivered from their lungs to their body's cells. These people have the condition called anemia. Lacking an adequate supply of oxygen in the blood going to the cells makes the cells oxygen-hungry, and they complain to the lungs which then force you to pant in an effort to alleviate the oxygen shortage.

Self-Service Gas

Healthy lungs always take in the exact amount of air they need. Like the body's other important organs, the lungs function automatically. However, the lungs also can be controlled voluntarily, making it possible to "hold your breath" for swimming under water, trying to cure the hiccups, or projecting the voice.

When voluntary breath control threatens to harm the body, however, involuntary control takes over. When the carbon dioxide levels reach an intolerable point, the automatic breath-control center in the brain's medulla oblongata (located close to where the brain connects with the spinal cord) takes over, forcing you to take the next breath. Similarly, the act of taking a long drink—during which the breath is held—is always followed by the immediate intake of air.

The involuntary rate of breathing is controlled by the concentration of carbon dioxide in the lungs. Carbon dioxide is poured into the lungs as the result of chemical activities in the cells due to physical activity, anxiety, or nervous tension. The carbon dioxide in the alveoli of the lungs mixes with water to make the blood slightly acidic by forming carbonic acid. The respiratory center in the brain detects higher than normal levels and orders the lungs to work harder to lower the concentration of carbon dioxide. When the levels are very high, as during heavy exercise or athletic events, the brain orders the lungs to breathe even deeper—hence the common reference to a "second wind."

Because of carbon dioxide's effect on breathing, you can hold your breath longer if you breathe deeply for about 1 minute before you stop breathing. In this way you can hold your breath 3 times longer than if you exhaled all of the air in your lungs before trying to hold your breath, a fact put to good use by voice and athletic coaches.

When you are physically and mentally at rest, your breathing becomes shallow and can lead to sleep. If this happens when it's not appropriate to fall asleep, such as in a classroom or during a conversation, you may feel the urge to take a deep breath to cleanse the lungs of

166

carbon dioxide. Often this takes the form of a broad yawn, discreetly covered by a raised hand held in front of your gaping mouth.

Getting Oxygen Out of the Air

To live, our body's cells must receive a continuous supply of oxygen and have a means of disposing of the carbon dioxide they produce as a waste product. For humans, the problem of getting oxygen into the cells from the atmosphere is resolved in part by what we call breathing.

However, because oxygen exists as tiny molecules that can pass freely in either direction through the semipermeable membrane of a cell, it is necessary for the body to "trap" the oxygen inside the cell by combining it with substances inside the cell. The oxygen, as part of a larger molecule, becomes too large to pass back out through the cell membrane. The oxygen enters in one direction, is trapped, and remains inside the cell. Without the necessary oxygen, the cells in the vital organs of the body would die within 5 minutes.

Full of Hot Air

The lungs prefer warm, moist air. As air enters the body through the nose, it is humidified by a liquid (up to a pint a day) produced by the tear glands in the throat and nose. As the air enters the nasal passages and the throat, it is moistened by these secretions and simultaneously warmed by superficial blood vessels in the same area. These blood vessels open wide on cold days to provide more heat and close up on warm days when their service is not needed. Each day, 18.5 cubic yards (14.8 cubic meters) of air are cleaned, humidified, and warmed by the air passages, enough to loft a fleet of 320 balloons.

Filtered Air

Along with the air we breathe for its oxygen content, we sometimes take in other substances from the atmosphere. The exhaust gases from automobiles, factories, and other devices of modern living pollute the air we breathe with materials containing lead, sulfur and nitrogen dioxides, particulates (which can be smaller than red blood cells), carbon monoxide, hydrocarbons, and substances called oxidants.

As we breathe in air, hairs in the nose, together with mucus secre-

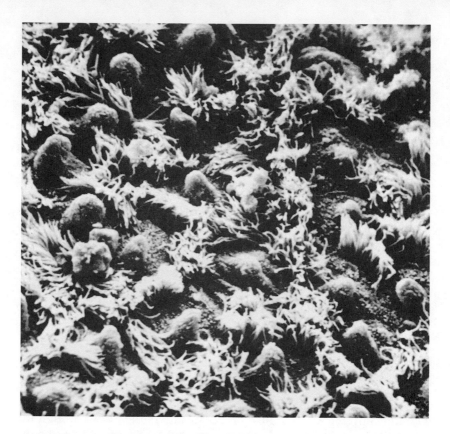

Two magnifications (above and on facing page) of the cilia in the lungs, the microhairs that protect the lungs and clean them, if the lungs' owner cooperates, of harmful foreign matter. Courtesy National Institutes of Health.

tions, filter out dust and other large particles that may enter. Farther on, the lungs protect us with the action of 2 types of cells that line the trachea. The bulged-out shape of the goblet cells that line the airways like a blanket, produce mucus. This mucus traps harmful pollutants that might be inhaled and some dangerous bacteria and other infectious agents.

The ciliated cells that line the air passages are microscopic, hairlike projections that sweep the mucus with a back-and-forth motion—about 12 times a second—that moves the mucus toward the throat where it is cleared out of the airways into the mouth and unconsciously swallowed.

Inhaled bacteria and viruses can be destroyed in the nose and throat by a powerful germ killer, lysozyme. In the farthest reaches of the alveoli are other cells that defend the body, macrophages. These scav-

INS AND OUTS:

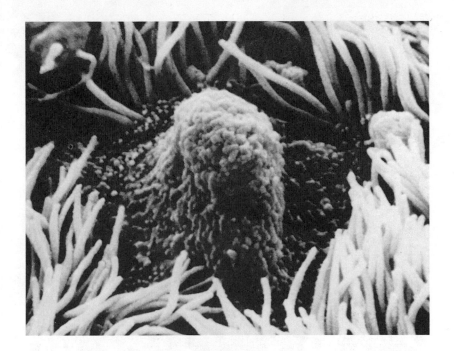

enger cells have many projections and are able to destroy harmful materials by swallowing them or by releasing enzymes that kill them.

Cigarette smoke interferes with mucus production and changes the consistency of the mucus by altering the mucus glands. Cigarette smoke can paralyze the scavenger or macrophage cells that line the throat so that they cannot swallow and destroy harmful lung invaders. Cigarette smoke also paralyzes the cilia cells so that they do not sweep unwanted substances from the windpipe. If the irritation to the cilia continues long enough, the cilia wither and die and are not replaced. With more mucus being produced and few if any cilia to sweep it into the mouth for swallowing, the mucus drops into the air sacs of the lungs preventing them from expanding to take in air. The lung literally fills with these secretions and the smoker is forced to cough to blow out the mucus to keep from drowning. The use of medicines to suppress the smoker's cough is therefore counterproductive as it prevents the smoker from using the only action left to clear the lungs.

There is some evidence that smoking marijuana may have the same paralyzing effect on the cilia and the mucus production in the trachea as cigarette smoking. There is additional evidence that marijuana might cause the lung cells to trigger other damage.

Deaths among smokers exceed the expected mortality by 60 percent. Statistically, a person who smokes one pack of cigarettes a day will take 7 years off his life expectancy. A man who smokes one pack a day may

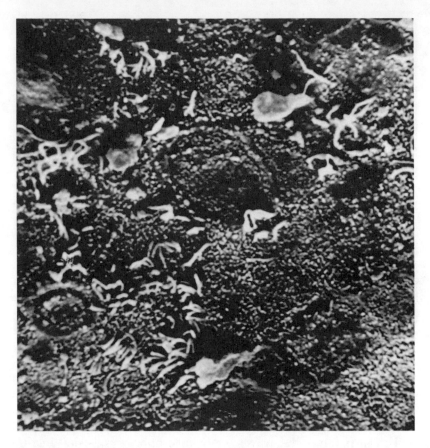

Cigarette smoking can eventually destroy the cilia, and the lungs become susceptible to disease. Courtesy National Institutes of Health.

expect to live to 67; the man who smokes 2 packs a day may make it only to age 60 as opposed to 74 for the nonsmoker.

Inflating the Lungs

The lungs are inflated for the first time by the newly born infant's gasp for air induced by the shock of exposure to the air outside the mother's womb or, traditionally, by the firm whack applied to the infant's bottom immediately after delivery. Either way, the reaction contracts the muscles that expand the chest cavity and lower its air pressure. When the infant opens its mouth, the weight of atmospheric pressure forces

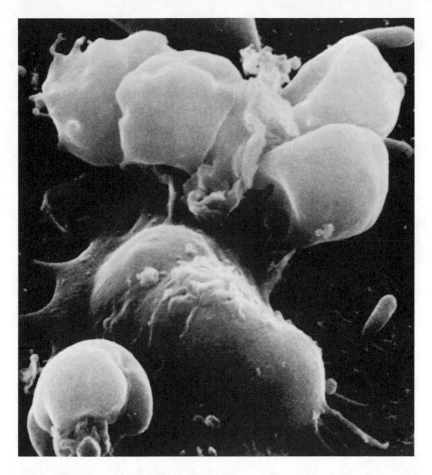

Deep inside the lungs macrophages defend their territory by destroying harmful lung invaders, either by gobbling them up or by releasing an enzyme that kills them. Courtesy National Institutes of Health.

air into the lungs and inflates them for the first time. Thereafter, breathing is a chemical reflex.

After birth, the nose is the natural passageway for the air we breathe. Some people, however, breathe through their mouths, perhaps because of bad teeth (making it difficult to close the lips over the teeth), or poor posture. Oral breathing also may be caused by a blockage in the nostrils of the nose from a cold or allergy creating swollen passages and an excess of mucus. Others may breathe through their mouths because of a nasal septum (the cartilage up the center of the nose) that is out of alignment (deviated nasal septum), or adenoids that block the back of the nasal passages. In bypassing the nose to take in air, mouth breathers increase their chances of inhaling more foreign particles from the air and also miss out on the "air-conditioning" provided by the nose.

Whether you breathe through your nose or your mouth, there are various ways of inflating the lungs with the air delivered. Professional singers and small babies practice "abdominal breathing." This method does not inflate the chest, but achieves a larger space in the chest cavity by lowering the diaphragm. The diaphragm pushes against the abdominal contents which push, in turn, against the abdominal muscles that give way, moving the abdomen outward. In this way, air is drawn into even the deepest alveoli.

The other alternative is chest or thoracic breathing in which muscles lift the rib cage and the sternum (the bone in the center of the chest to which the ribs are attached). The diaphragm then moves down and the diameter of the chest is enlarged front to back, side to side, and top to bottom.

No matter how you inflate your lungs, the oxygen in the air you breathe in is really outside your body—being directly connected with the air outside your nose through the air passages to the lungs—until the oxygen crosses the alveolar walls and enters the bloodstream through the capillary walls.

The Lung's Overcoat

The pleura is a closed, double-walled sac that lines the chest cavity around the lungs. Its architecture is like a piece of clothing without a seam or a paper bag without an open end. When the newly born infant takes its first breath, the pleura stretches with the inspired air and is pushed in contact with the inside of the chest and the top of the diaphragm. There it will stay for the rest of the individual's life—barring an accident or chest surgery.

A hole in the pleura can be produced by an accident, sometimes from inside by a disease like tuberculosis, or by the trauma of blowing on a musical instrument daily over a period of years. A hole in the pleura lets air seep in between the 2 layers of the pleura, creating a space between them and collapsing the lung. Air comes in on inspiration, but the torn lung tissue prevents it from escaping on expiration, and so it accumulates in the pleural space. A physician can extract this air through a needle.

Occasionally, a decision will be made to treat a disease of the lungs like tuberculosis by giving the lung a chance to rest and heal. The surgeon makes a hole in the chest cavity to let air in, or air may be injected between the pleural layers to create an artificial pneumothorax, collapse of the lung. In all cases, when the hole in the pleura heals, the lung reinflates.

Balancing Act

While the purpose of respiration (the act of breathing in and breathing out) is to supply oxygen to the body's cells and to remove the waste product of cell activity, carbon dioxide, our bodies need both of these gases in balanced amounts for good health.

Voluntary, deep, rapid breathing (hyperventilation) can cause a flushing out of almost all of the normal carbon dioxide from the lungs —and, therefore, from the bloodstream—causing dizziness and perhaps blackout. Hyperventilation is usually followed by a period in which breathing stops (apnea) that can last for 40 to 60 seconds. Cases have been reported of individuals suffering permanent brain damage when periods of apnea have been long enough to cause brain-cell death.

On the other hand, breathing 100 percent oxygen can cause dizziness too. Athletes who take a whiff of oxygen when they come out of a game have been poorly advised. At the atmospheric pressure of sea level, the oxygen in the blood going away from the lungs to the cells is at 98 percent saturation under normal activity. The addition of more oxygen to the lungs when you are exercising causes supersaturation and dizziness.

The best time to give an athlete a boost of oxygen is during competition when the oxygen levels in the lungs decrease. Administration of a 66 percent concentration of oxygen during competition can improve performance, according to Herbert A. de Vries, professor of exercise physiology at the University of Southern California.

Low Air Pressure

In passing through the lungs at sea level, the blood acquires an oxygen concentration of 97 percent (a volume percent of oxygen present in a given amount of blood). At altitudes above 10,000 feet (3,050 meters), however, the low air pressure of the atmosphere results in only an 85 percent oxygen concentration in the blood and can cause difficulty in breathing, nausea, vomiting, and give a blue tinge to the lips, nails, and finally the skin (cyanosis) because of low oxygen content in the blood. Because the brain and other vital organs are deprived of oxygen under these conditions, emotional disturbances can occur and decisions made during this time may lead to accidents. At very high altitudes unconsciousness may occur. The symptoms clear up on return to lower altitudes.

This condition can happen in other situations in which the blood does not receive its normal saturation of oxygen, such as when you are deep inside a mine where the quality of air is reduced, or when there is interference with the air supply to the lungs from an obstruction by a foreign object, or when the surface area of the alveoli has been reduced, as happens in tuberculosis.

The level of oxygen in the air may be reduced by one half without the rate of breathing being affected. Excess oxygen does not affect the rate of breathing, but it does have a bad effect on the lungs and can even produce growths in the lungs. An oxygen concentration in an atmosphere between 60 and 70 percent is the maximum that can be breathed with safety for any length of time.

It is possible for the body to adapt itself to altitudes of up to 20,000 feet over a period of time. Athletes competing in events at high altitudes often train for long periods before the event to increase their chest volume and the number of oxygen-carrying red blood cells.

Exercising the Lungs

Although the lungs have no muscle tissue of their own, they must exercise to remain in good working order. People who lie inactive in bed for long periods of time, such as patients in a hospital, can develop pneumonia if they do not exercise their lungs.

If you do not breathe as deeply as you should on a regular basis, parts of the lungs become unused and slowly fill with fluid, causing pneumonia. This condition is common in the elderly whose vital capacity (the total amount of air that can be inhaled and exhaled) may already be diminished because of a loss of elasticity in the muscles involved in breathing.

Periodic exercise of the lungs also can help to remove excess contaminants that can collect from breathing polluted air. The best method of exercising the lungs is deep exhalation. To do this, breathe out as much air as you think possible, then purse your lips and continue to blow out even more air. The lungs cannot be harmed by this kind of exercise. It may cause some people to feel uncomfortable, but it does not cause damage to lung tissue.

TEETH, MOUTH, AND THROAT

The Not So Wise Teeth

As the human diet has evolved from tough, chewy meats to softer foods, the need for a large jaw to accommodate 32 large chewing tools has decreased and, along with it, the size of the human jaw. Unfortunately for us, the size of our teeth has remained the same. For people with small jaws, this may mean crowding of some teeth, particularly the 4 large teeth at the corners of the jaws.

One or all 4 of these third molars may fail to appear for the lucky few, but most of us get some or all 4 of them. Because of their close proximity to the second molars, these teeth often have a hard time emerging and may become impacted in the jawbone, requiring surgical attention. Many dentists in the past have advocated routine extraction of these teeth, but modern practice recommends removal only if problems develop. When extraction is required for orthodontic reasons—correcting jaw and tooth alignment with braces—the third molars should be removed at as early an age as possible. The older the person, the greater the discomfort and the larger the dental bill.

The third molars usually erupt between the ages of 16 and 30, a time by which our ancestors felt the individual would have acquired some wisdom—hence the popular name for the third molars, wisdom teeth.

Gnash, Grind, Chomp . . .

In the still of the night you hear the sound of someone walking up creaking stairs—and then you remember, you live in a one-storied ranch house! The sound is coming from your bed partner's mouth, the sound of bruxism.

Bruxers involuntarily gnash their teeth either during sleep, or unconsciously during waking hours. This stressful grinding of the teeth exerts thousands of pounds of pressure on the teeth surfaces and can severely damage the teeth, the gums, and the jawbones.

During bruxism episodes, there is no food to cushion the blows of the teeth colliding. Bruxism therefore can upset the delicate pressure balance of teeth, wearing down the ridges of tooth enamel and loosening or moving teeth from their proper positions. All of this grinding and clenching of teeth can cause facial muscles to ache or tighten up with sharp pain. This can lead to pain and clicking or cracking sounds in the joint of the jawbones—and a severe headache.

Gum diseases may be aggravated by bruxism to the extent that the bone supporting the teeth is lost and they become loosened and fall out.

The most significant contributor to the habitual grinding of teeth is emotional stress arising from family or job situations. In addition, children moving from deciduous to permanent teeth may grind their teeth in an attempt to bring a greater number of teeth in contact. Some cases of bruxism have been reported to be hereditary.

Treatment includes grinding down spots on some teeth, repairing fillings or crowns, or moving teeth orthodontically to make them come together in better alignment. Some dentists prescribe a night guard of soft plastic—much like an orthodontic retainer—worn in the mouth to absorb the shock of teeth gnashing against each other. Dentists or physicians may prescribe medicines to relieve stress and relax muscles before other treatments are begun.

There are approximately 37 million bruxers in the United States alone gnashing their teeth away. Researchers at the San Antonio Metropolitan Medical Center believe bruxism occurs during the REM or rapid-eye-movement phase of sleep, the time of vivid dreaming.

Bad Breath

Bad breath, or halitosis, may be caused by an infection in the respiratory tract, the breakdown of bacteria in the mouth or air passages, or from eating large quantities of garlic or other strong-smelling foods.

True halitosis is the product of the body's inefficient metabolism of fats. Strong-smelling volatile substances from this faulty metabolism enter the bloodstream and are excreted through the lungs in the exhaled breath, giving it a foul odor. These signals of a disease process call for medical attention.

The solution for most of us, however, is to brush our teeth regularly and otherwise cleanse our mouths, particularly after eating odorous foods. Chewing on mints or other mouth fresheners also helps.

In 1982, Americans spent over $360 million in pursuit of a sweet breath.

INS AND OUTS:

Dry Mouth

Digestion starts in the mouth with the addition of enzymes to the food as it is being chewed. Saliva (spittle or, commonly, spit) has a number of other important functions including cleansing the teeth of food particles; controlling the growth of bacteria that contribute to tooth decay; and preservation of the teeth by bathing them with protective minerals such as calcium, phosphorus, and fluoride.

Saliva also moistens and lubricates the soft tissues that line the mouth and helps keep them supple. Without saliva, we would not enjoy eating as much as we do, for it is the moisture of saliva added to food in the mouth that stimulates the taste buds to produce taste sensations.

A deficiency of saliva causes a dry mouth and is a common side effect of numerous medications and other treatments. Dry mouth also can be a symptom of certain diseases. Researchers at the National Institute of Dental Research examining the problem of dry mouth have found over 200 drugs that list this sign as a side effect, including painkillers, sedatives, drugs used to treat high blood pressure, and even antihistamine drugs sold without prescription for allergies and blocked nasal passages. Some drugs used to treat Parkinsonism, usually a disease of the older age group, have been implicated as well. Although it is often assumed that saliva production changes and dry mouth occurs as a result of normal aging, this is an incorrect generalization. Most dry-mouth complaints in older people are related to the medications they are taking.

Other causes of dry mouth are treatments such as radiation to the head and neck, chemotherapy, nutritional deficiencies such as anemia, and conditions such as anxiety, mental stress, and depression.

Dry mouth is the bane of singers, actors, and anxious students called upon to recite in class.

The Superhighway

The throat is one of the busiest thoroughfares in the body. Through the mouth and down the throat, we consume 40 tons (36,000 kilograms) of food in a lifetime and inhale over 499,000 cubic yards (381,513 cubic meters) of air. The larynx, or "voice box," is located about 5 inches down the throat from the pharynx at the back of the nose. Just below the larynx, the throat divides into 2 tubes, the trachea going to the lungs, and the food tube or esophagus going to the stomach.

The larynx acts as a derailer to divert food, drink, and air down their respective tracks. When we swallow, the larynx rises causing a piece of cartilage called the epiglottis to move up and back over the glottis, the pathway for air through the trachea. This makes a tight seal so that we are prevented from "swallowing the wrong way." Because of this action of the larynx during swallowing, it is impossible to make a sound while you swallow.

Should the larynx be prevented from doing its work, food or drink can slip into the trachea, setting off a fit of coughing to dislodge the food before it blocks the airway and threatens to suffocate the individual. The old admonition, "Don't talk with food in your mouth," is one of the more practical rules imposed on children.

During swallowing a flap of tissue at the rear of the soft palate on the roof of the mouth moves up to cover the nasal passages above so that food and drink do not go up and run out the nose. This flap is the uvula which has nothing to do with projecting the voice as is sometimes assumed.

Because of the switching mechanism of the larynx, it is possible for you to defy gravity and swallow while standing on your head instead of drooling saliva from your mouth, an important esthetic consideration for gymnasts, yoga enthusiasts, and circus performers.

To Sleep, Perchance to Dream . . .

Not if you have a mouth breather for a roommate. The uvula, the flap of tissue that hangs from the back part of the roof of the mouth, was intended to cover the nasal passages when we swallow. When an individual sleeps on their back with their mouth open, a stream of air passes over the uvula and the roof of the mouth (palate) and sets them vibrating, producing that spoiler of sleep, the snore.

Research has demonstrated that a snore can reach 69 decibels as compared to 70 to 90 decibels for a pneumatic drill.

Breathing Interruptus

That embarrassing sound we often make at awkward moments, the hiccup, or hiccough if you prefer, is another form of breathing.

When the diaphragm goes into one of its occasional spasms, the body reacts by enlarging the chest cavity by moving the diaphragm down. This forces a sudden rush of air into the lungs. Nerve endings in the diaphragm send off signals to the brain which orders the epiglottis at the end of the tongue to clamp down over the glottis in the larynx to stop this rush of air. The air, suddenly started and suddenly interrupted, makes the sharp sound that we call the hiccup. It is more common in infants, possibly because distention of the stomach from overeating throws the diaphragm into spasm.

According to the *Guinness Book of World Records,* "the longest recorded attack of hiccoughs is that afflicting Charles Osborne," who started hiccoughing at the age of 28 in 1922 and was still hiccoughing in 1982.

First Line of Defense

A cough is another form of breathing. In coughing, we inhale to a greater than normal depth and follow it with a violent exhalation. Partial closing of the vocal cords causes air to rush past the larynx forcefully, producing the characteristic noise of the cough.

Coughing is our protection against the introduction of an irritant into the air passage—food, drink, mucus, pollutants in the atmosphere, or cigarette smoke. Coughing may be caused by irritation of the mucous membranes in the air passages, but stimulation of other parts of the body, or sometimes emotional factors, also will produce coughing.

The cough that accompanies a head cold and sometimes an allergic reaction is the body's attempt to get rid of excess mucus produced in an effort to counteract a disease process.

The cilia that line the throat help to protect us from choking on our own secretions and foreign particles that may enter the throat by sweeping back and forth vigorously to force out these inhaled bits.

When a bit of food or drink comes into contact with the glottis (the airway through the larynx) because the epiglottis has not covered it in time, we "swallow the wrong way" and start to cough fitfully. Because this has occurred in restaurants to people who have unwisely tried to eat and talk simultaneously, the heart attack brought on by suffocation has commonly been referred to as a "restaurant coronary."

Ah-Choo!

The sneeze is another form of breathing in which air is exhaled violently through the nasal passages. It is usually a reflex action to irritation of the mucous membrane in the nose, but may be caused by other stimulation, such as bright light flashing into the eye.

Particles ejected in a forceful sneeze have been measured at 103.6 miles per hour (165.76 kilometers per hour).

The most chronic fit of sneezing ever recorded is that of an English girl who started sneezing after catching a cold and continued to sneeze for 194 days.

Adam's Legacy

Authors have frequently projected the comic image of the shy, nervous young man trying to get up his courage to talk to a pretty girl by including a reference to the bobbing structure that rides up and down in his throat as he swallows repeatedly to lubricate his dry throat.

The "bobbing apple" actually is a prominent part of the larynx. It is more visible in men because the male larynx is larger than the female larynx and because its prominent part in women is covered by fatty tissue.

The part of the larynx we see riding up and down is called the "Adam's apple" because of a folk legend which claims that the biblical Adam had difficulty getting his bite of the apple down and got it stuck partway. The trait, of course, has been passed down to his male descendents. The reminder doesn't seem to have deterred men from responding to the "temptations" of women, however.

A Childhood Guardian

Not so many years ago, many people had their tonsils and adenoids taken out as a matter of course, most often before entering first grade. Today, infections of the respiratory tract are treated with antibiotics and other powerful medicines, and doctors often advise waiting to see whether a child develops all of the signs of chronic tonsil and adenoid enlargement before considering their surgical removal.

Our bodies have been provided with extra filtering tissues to see us through our early years of life when we seem always to have a cold or sore throat. The tonsils are part of the body's defense system and are located at the back of the throat where the soft palate meets the pharynx, one tonsil on each side. They are each about 1 inch by 1/2 inch in size.

When bacteria enter through the mouth, nose, or throat, the tonsils filter them out and fight them with lymphocytes. If the battle is fierce, the tonsils swell up with the effort and become red and hot and painful, particularly when you swallow. It is these tonsils that are sometimes removed when repeated infections make surgery advisable.

At the back of the tongue, there are 35 to 100 nodes of additional tonsillar tissue. These are the lingual tonsils, which act in much the same way as the other tonsils.

What we commonly call "adenoids" are themselves tonsils. These are the pharyngeal tonsils located at the back of the nasal passage. Repeated infections in the upper respiratory tract can cause permanent enlargement and thickening of all of the tonsillar tissues and this can cause blockage of the air passages, especially when the pharyngeal tonsils (the adenoids) are involved.

Children with adenoid trouble tend to breathe through the mouth and to speak with a nasal tone because of blockage to the air passages that gives the voice its resonance. People with this problem may breathe noisily and snore heavily. Mental and physical retardation are said to be caused by severe cases of "adenoids" because of inefficient delivery of oxygen to the brain and the rest of the body's tissues.

Usually the tonsils diminish in size and virtually disappear by the end of childhood when we are presumed not to need them to survive.

Soft as a Whisper

Did you know that you can talk without using your vocal cords? When we wish to keep our conversation from being overheard—or we are trying to protect our voice when we have laryngitis by not using it—we do just that.

The faster and more forcefully air is exhaled past the vocal cords, the louder the sound made by the voice. To lower the voice, we unwittingly pass a column of air through the "false vocal cords" (tissue folds located just above the true vocal cords in the larynx), bypassing the resonating chamber formed by the nasal passages, the mouth, and the pharynx so that the sound is not amplified. In this way, our words are passed out on this softly exhaled air as a whisper.

Katie, Beautiful K-K-Katie . . .

One set of muscles in the larynx pulls the vocal cords apart, opening the airway, permitting you to take a deep breath. An opposing set of muscles closes the vocal cords so that you can swallow and also so that you can speak—but not at the same time. These are coordinated muscular actions in the average person. The laryngeal muscles of some stutterers, however, are poorly coordinated and sometimes contract simultaneously in opposite directions to prevent fluent speech. Because whispering does not involve the vocal cords, however, stutterers do not stutter when they whisper.

The Changing Voice

The pitch of the voice (how high or low it sounds) depends on the length, tension, and thickness of the vocal cords. These factors affect the frequency of vibrations in the vocal cords. The tighter the cords, the higher the pitch of the sound. Short vocal cords produce higher tones; longer cords produce lower tones. Because males have longer

Upward movement of the diaphragm forces air up through the windpipe, setting the vocal cords vibrating. Because whispering does not involve the vocal cords, however, stutterers do not stutter when they whisper. Courtesy National Institutes of Health.

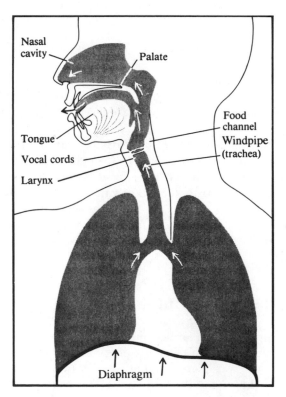

vocal cords (up to 1 inch in length), the male voice generally is deeper in pitch, while women and children with shorter cords have higher-pitched voices. The vocal cords of women average 1/6 of an inch in length.

Because the larynx, along with the rest of the body, grows rapidly during adolescence, young men often find they have difficulty controlling the tension of their vocal cords so that they swing from a tenor to a baritone in the course of a single sentence. We say that the voice "is changing."

The adult size of the larynx is not necessarily related to physical size, however. The baritone may be short, while the 7-foot basketball player is the tenor. It's the size of the vocal cords that counts.

The Sound of Your Voice

The qualities that make your voice "yours" and unlike any other are predetermined by the size and shape of the parts of your body involved in speech. Because no two people have vocal cords, mouths, noses, lips, or tongues shaped exactly alike, no two voices are identical. It is possible for each of us, however, to alter the timbre, intensity, and pitch of our voices through the voluntary control of the muscles of the respiratory organs, as when we sustain our breath when speaking or singing. Actors and singers study breath control and manipulation of the organs of speech to use the voice as an instrument. Impersonators develop this facility to a high degree.

Malformations in any of the parts of the body that we use to produce speech—a misshaped tongue, jaws, or cheeks, a cleft palate, missing teeth, a harelip, or enlarged adenoids, for example—can cause changes in the quality of the voice. An infection in the throat can irritate the vocal cords so they swell and the voice becomes hoarse. If the infection involves the larynx, laryngitis results and you may "lose" your voice. The attractive huskiness in the voice of some well-known popular singers is said to result from the growth of small, innocent tumors on their vocal cords. Removal of too many of these would destroy their "golden voice."

Words Exhaled

We project our voice by breathing. In normal respiration, muscles rotate the vocal cords in the larynx so that they move away from each other to permit air to pass up and down the throat without affecting the vocal cords. When we wish to project our voice in words or song, we take a breath and automatically rotate the vocal cords in the opposite direction so that they are close together and parallel to each other. At the same time, the vocal cords are tightened by muscles in the larynx.

When we exhale this breath, the air passes through the narrow opening between the cords and causes them to vibrate like the reeds of an oboe. The vibrating air is converted into an audible sound wave and a vocal tone. The faster and more forcefully air is exhaled past the vocal cords, the higher the pitch of the sound. This sound wave passes up into the resonating chamber formed by the nasal passages, the mouth, and the pharynx. There, it is amplified, changed, and refined in quality by the walls of these structures. The articulators (the lips, tongue, teeth, hard and soft palates, and the walls of the parts that make up the resonating chamber) then are used to form the sounds into recognizable, voiced speech which is projected into the atmosphere as we breathe out—exhaled words.

Artificial Speech

Man does not speak by voice box alone, and it's a good thing too. The larynx may be rendered useless in an accident, or may be removed surgically because of a cancerous growth. While not a common site for cancers to develop, cancer of the larynx accounts for 2 to 5 percent of all cancer cases. Each year at least 4,000 adults with this disease in the United States will undergo laryngectomy (removal of the larynx).

While scientists continue to study the ability of dolphins to communicate, no mammals speak as humans do. It is the human brain and nervous system that make it possible for us to verbalize our thoughts.

Speech requires storage in the brain of memories that associate sensations from our environment with certain words. For example, we learn as children that our furry playmate with the sharp claws is a "cat" and we remember that word ever after, barring damage to the memory centers in the brain.

Whether the larynx has been made useless by an accident or been removed because of a disease like cancer, the individual can still talk without a voice box, but must learn new ways to create sound waves and a vocal tone using vibrating air to project the sounds as voiced speech.

The most common way of teaching a person who has had a laryngectomy to speak is through a technique known as esophageal speech. This substitute speech is produced by expelling or belching swallowed air from the food tube, the esophagus. The articulators—

the tongue, lips, mouth, teeth, and the pharynx—then form the column of air into speech.

While the quality of this form of speech is quite good, it is difficult for some to master. Recent designs in biomedical engineering have resulted in the development of a number of manually operated speech synthesizers, and mechanical devices have been developed for insertion into the throat to aid in producing intelligible speech. Researchers at the National Institutes of Health (NIH) in the United States have refined surgical reconstruction techniques for laryngectomy patients that were first developed in Europe. These techniques allow patients to vocalize without learning esophageal speech or using a prosthetic device. In this technique, the upper part of the patient's trachea is reconstructed to provide a false glottis, the passageway for air through the throat that regulates air flow and pressure necessary for voice production. This technique cannot be used for all who need laryngectomies, but it is becoming more common in the United States.

STOMACH, LIVER, AND PANCREAS

Food Processing

The digestion and absorption of food take place in a muscular tube that runs for over 30 feet (about 9 meters) from the mouth to the anus. This is the digestive tract, sometimes referred to as the alimentary canal because we take our aliment (food) through it.

We eat food to nourish the cells of the body, but it is the intestinal tract that feeds the cells. For the nutrients in food to be delivered throughout the body, they must be reduced to a size small enough to enter the bloodstream. This is accomplished during the process of digestion in which large pieces of insoluble food are broken down into soluble chemical compounds that can pass through the walls of a long, convoluted tube, the intestines, or bowel, and into the blood for distribution to the cells.

Digestion of food begins in the mouth with the first bite. The teeth grind and tear the food apart into small pieces. These bits are mixed with fluid in the mouth from the salivary glands. Saliva contains an enzyme (a chemical substance that speeds up digestion) that acts on starch to convert it into sugar. Other enzymes will be added as the food makes its way through the digestive tract.

After chewing, the food is moved to the back of the mouth by the tongue. The tongue rises in the middle, gives the food a shove, and sends it on its way down the esophagus, the food tube.

When food enters the esophagus, the tube contracts in wavelike movements that carry the food along to the stomach. A valve at the mouth of the stomach lets food in gradually to prevent indigestion. The stomach holds a little under 2 quarts (1.9 liters) of semidigested food that stays in the stomach for 3 to 5 hours.

The elastic walls of the stomach release food slowly to the rest of the digestive tract. This storage facility makes it possible for us to get by with 3 meals a day instead of needing a continuous supply like grazing animals.

The stomach is lined with 35 million glands that produce about 3 quarts (2.85 liters) of gastric juices daily. Hydrochloric acid makes up roughly 5 percent of these juices and, together with other acids and various enzymes, continues to digest the food. Contractions in the stomach every 20 seconds churn the food and gastric juices into a pulpy, creamy fluid called chyme. The chyme is gradually squeezed into the small intestines (duodenum) where digestion is completed and most of the absorption into the bloodstream takes place.

While the food is in the small intestines, bile, manufactured in the liver and stored in the gall bladder, and juices from the pancreas mix with the chyme before the nutrients pass into the bloodstream through the walls of the small intestines.

The large intestine or colon (commonly referred to as the gut) receives undigested matter and continues the absorption of nutrients and, finally, of water. Once the water has been extracted, it is returned to the body to prevent the cells from becoming dehydrated. Nutrients absorbed through the walls of the small and large intestines are carried in the blood to the liver where they are processed and stored for release to the body, as needed, through the bloodstream.

Fifteen hours or more after that first bite started down the alimentary canal, the final residue of the food is passed along to the rectum and is excreted through the anus as feces.

By the time you eat your lunch today, last night's meal is just completing its trip.

Rude Noises

While contractions are churning food, gas can be trapped in the stomach and the churning of the food produces gurgling sounds. Most of

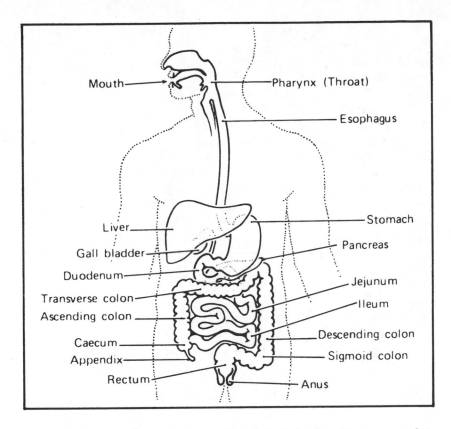

Mouth—
Pharynx (Throat)
Esophagus
Liver
Stomach
Gall bladder
Pancreas
Duodenum
Jejunum
Transverse colon
Ileum
Ascending colon
Caecum
Descending colon
Appendix
Sigmoid colon
Rectum
Anus

It takes 15 hours or more for food to go through the body's digestive process—a long count for down and out. Courtesy National Institutes of Health.

the time these are inaudible, but immediately after a meal—most often when one is seated in a quiet place such as a lecture hall or church—these churning noises may be heard as "stomach rumblings." On the other hand, when the stomach has been empty for some time, the contractions may start automatically again, particularly if the aroma of a good meal wafts your way. Contractions on an empty stomach can make the rumblings even louder. Gas in an empty stomach presses against the walls of the stomach to produce what we call "hunger pangs."

Air swallowed along with food or gulped nervously may be expelled up the esophagus as a "belch." The approaching belch (or burp) can usually be felt in time to allow for closing the mouth to prevent its escape with a loud, rude noise (although in some societies, a belch after a good meal is accepted as a compliment to the cook—and the louder the better).

Each day, 7 to 11 quarts (6.6 to 10.4 liters) of gas enter or are formed in the large intestines, or bowel. Some of this gas is expelled by belching, but some is passed from the stomach on through to the large bowel. Most of the gas is reabsorbed into the body as the stool makes its way to the anus so that only about ½ quart (0.5 liter) is expelled.

People with an overly active bowel that hurries the gas along, not giving it time for reabsorption, may have problems with passing excessive amounts of gas. The activity of bacteria in the large intestines adds small amounts of volatile compounds to the gas which gives it the characteristic unpleasant odor. Because bile, added from the liver and gall bladder during digestion, deodorizes the stool to some extent, people with diseases of these organs may have stools that are particularly foul smelling. Certain foods such as a diet high in meats and fats, certain vegetable proteins like those of beans, and fermented drinks like beer and ale also add extra intestinal gas and their own peculiar aroma when expelled.

Because fear or anxiety speeds up the large intestines, you may find yourself with another problem in situations of high stress. When this happens in a social setting, the strain for control can be unbearable for the sensitive.

Bon Appetit!

The pain of indigestion we call "heartburn" has nothing in common with the heart except its location. Heartburn is usually described as a burning sensation in the chest behind the breastbone, frequently accompanied by a feeling of food coming back into the mouth along with an acid or bitter taste.

When food is swallowed, it travels down the esophagus, the food tube, with the aid of wavelike movements in the tube. At the bottom of the esophagus, a sphincter (valve) opens to admit food into the stomach and closes quickly afterward.

Without this valve, swallowed food and other matter would plummet down the esophagus into the stomach to produce an attack of indigestion the likes of which you could not imagine. This is because pressure inside the stomach is always greater than that in the esophagus.

Sometimes this valve relaxes accidentally, especially if food has been hurriedly eaten or the meal is unusually large. At other times, heartburn occurs because the valve is too weak to close properly. When the valve is open, some of the gastric juices leak back up the esophagus where they irritate the lining of the food tube and produce the burning sensation.

In the United States alone, 22 million people have an attack of heartburn every day. Drugstores in the U.S. grossed $242 million in 1980 from the sale of antacids, often taken for heartburn.

Butterflies in My Stomach

If you have ever experienced the crampy tension of "butterflies" in the abdomen—perhaps accompanied by mild nausea and sometimes diarrhea—just before delivering a speech or at examination time in school, you know what "irritable bowel syndrome" (IBS) feels like. Also called nervous stomach or spastic bowel, this reaction to stress can cause all of these symptoms plus swings between constipation and diarrhea.

Usually IBS is not serious, however inconvenient and uncomfortable, and does not lead to the development of ulcers or other gastrointestinal problems. Control of the emotional reaction to stress and perhaps some dietary adjustments are all that is needed.

A problem that leads to similar trouble in roughly 20 percent of the adults in the United States and 60 to 90 percent of the world's adults is lactose intolerance. That is, they cannot easily digest foods containing lactose (milk sugar) such as milk, cheeses made from milk, butter, whey, or lactose. Should a lactose-intolerant person eat some of these substances, he will experience mild to violent reactions including gas pains, diarrhea, nausea, and vomiting, much the same as the symptoms of IBS.

Vegetables such as the infamous bean, peas, cucumbers, and some fruits produce gas and may contribute to the symptoms of IBS. A deficiency of fiber in the diet such as bran also can contribute to an irritable bowel or upset stomach. Several small meals rather than one or two large ones have been recommended for people with IBS to spread the quantity of food delivered to the digestive tract for processing over a longer time frame.

If adjustments in your diet and eating habits do not clear up the problem, a physician should probably be consulted. There are drugs on the market today that can help control the nervous tension as well as the "irritable" reaction of the gastrointestinal tract.

A Hole in the Wall

During digestion, strong juices made in the lining of the stomach are added to the thick mixture of partially digested food to further divide the food substances into their basic chemical parts. One of these gastric juices is hydrochloric acid, a relatively powerful acid that, outside the body, is strong enough to burn holes in wood. Under normal conditions the stomach is protected from burning or digesting itself by its strong lining which is coated with thick mucus that keeps the gastric juices from the stomach's tissues while they do their work on food.

For reasons not clearly understood, however, a sore or ulcer can occur in the wall of the stomach or small intestines (duodenum) when there is an imbalance between the acids and enzymes secreted by the stomach and the capacity of the stomach and duodenum to resist these juices.

About 4 million people in the United States have ulcers.

The Chemistry Laboratory

The liver is the largest gland in the body and one of the largest organs. At 3 to 4 pounds (1.35 to 1.8 kilograms), the liver is 7 times larger than it needs to be to perform its estimated 500 functions, providing the body with a margin of safety for this vital organ.

Among the chemical activities of the liver are the breakdown and absorption of food, especially carbohydrates and fats; the storage of food nutrients such as iron and copper, and the fat-soluble vitamins A, D, and B_{12}; the formation of vitamin A; the conversion of dead red blood cells into bile—essential to digestion; the filtering and detoxification of poisonous materials from the bloodstream; the manufacture of plasma (blood) proteins and blood-clotting substances, as well as the factor that prevents anemia; the production of red blood cells in the unborn; and the formation of many antibodies. An incredible list for one organ!

The liver plays an important role in a number of bodily functions such as digestion. While food passes through the body by way of the esophagus, the stomach, and the intestines, it is the liver—with the gall bladder, pancreas, and the bloodstream—that helps to decompose and absorb food and thus nourish the body.

The liver plays a major role in the balance of blood sugar in the body by alternately withdrawing and adding sugar to the bloodstream in the amounts required. When a candy bar or other carbohydrate is consumed, it is changed into glucose (sugar) in the intestines and sent out into the bloodstream through the walls of the intestines. The concentration of glucose in the blood triggers the pancreas' beta cells in the endocrine part of the gland to secrete the hormone insulin to aid the decomposition of the glucose. Any glucose not required immediately by the body is sent to the liver for conversion to a starchy substance, glycogen, which is then stored in the liver and in muscle tissue. Liver glycogen is changed back to blood sugar—the principal source of energy for the brain—when blood sugar levels are low between meals, and is released into the bloodstream. The glycogen in a muscle remains in that muscle until it is oxidized, burned up, during activity. When this glycogen is consumed and more is needed, the liver's store of glycogen is tapped. The liver stores 3 ounces (84 grams) of glycogen at a time, enough to last the average sedentary person about 18 hours.

Another major function of the liver is the detoxification of poisonous substances in the bloodstream, including things that are potentially toxic to the body, such as drugs, alcohol, caffeine, and nicotine. Of course, the accidental intake of poisonous substances such as carbon tetrachloride, a volatile fluid used in dry cleaning, chloroform, arsenic, or household cleaning fluids can be fatal. All of these foreign substances that cannot be broken down and used by the body are sent to the liver through the bloodstream for removal or to have the poison neutralized. Most often the liver adds chemicals to the material to encourage it to dissolve and so speed its elimination from the body through the urine.

The liver usually heals itself quickly when it is damaged, but when the amount of a foreign substance is too great for it to handle, or the problem is one of chronic use of a toxic substance such as in alcoholism or drug abuse, there may be permanent liver damage. In response to such abuse, the liver replaces its active cells with fatty tissue which gives it a golden-yellow appearance instead of its normal one of reddish brown. The liver becomes hardened, shrinks in size, and is "cirrhotic." Cirrhosis of the liver leads to various health problems and even death when the liver is unable to perform its essential functions.

Successful liver transplants have been performed in the United States since 1963. The most dramatic of these have been in very young children with congenital abnormalities or functional diseases of the liver. This surgery can take up to 12 hours because of the intricacy of the liver and its connections. The network of tubes in the liver that must be hooked up during surgery, placed end to end, would stretch for 60 miles (96 kilometers).

Color Me Yellow

Bile is made by the liver from the recycling of broken-down red blood cells. On the way to the duodenum, part of the bile is stored in the gall bladder for later use, and moisture is absorbed by the walls of the gall bladder from the bile. Sometimes small particles in the bile settle out or precipitate to form masses called gallstones which may be passed easily to the intestines for elimination or may grow to a size that will obstruct passage of bile and cause severe pain.

A small amount of bile is added to the waste products of digestion. Its pigment gives the stool its characteristic color. Bile also helps to deodorize the stool by reducing fermentation and putrefaction in the intestines. A bit of bile pigment is absorbed into the bloodstream and gives the straw color to blood plasma and to urine. Symptoms of a problem with the production or distribution of bile in the body are often colorless urine and pale stools that have a foul odor. This may be caused by dysfunction in the gall bladder or in the liver.

In addition to its pigments, bile is made up of salts that emulsify food fats that are then stored in the walls of the intestines for later use. Another function of bile is to carry off the poisonous substances that the liver removes from the blood for elimination through the intestines or the kidneys and urine.

An obstruction of the bile duct that carries bile into the body prevents it from being eliminated in the usual manner and can cause it to spill into the bloodstream. Sometimes the conversion of old red blood cells is greater than normal and the amount of bile formed increases. Diseases such as hepatitis or liver damage from certain drugs such as alcohol, birth control pills, or isoniazid (used to treat tuberculosis) may cause bile to spill into the bloodstream. When there is an excessive amount of bile in the bloodstream, it appears in the skin, the whites of the eyes, and the mucous membranes, giving the unlucky person a yellowish cast. This condition is called jaundice, from the French word, *jaune,* meaning yellow.

About 1 pint (½ liter) of bile is produced daily by the liver.

The Sugar Factory

The pancreas actually has 2 functions: to produce and release pancreatic juices into the small intestines (duodenum) and to produce and release insulin into the bloodstream to regulate the amount of sugar in the blood.

Lying in a horizontal position behind the stomach, the pancreas is 6 inches (152.4 millimeters) in length and is the second largest gland in the body (the liver is the largest). Its slender head or right side rests in the curve of the duodenum. About 1 quart (.95 liter) of pancreatic juices is produced each day. These are carried through the pancreatic duct into the common bile duct where they join bile from the liver and gall bladder on their way to the intestines. Enzymes (chemical substances that speed up digestion) in the pancreatic juices break protein into amino acids for use in building body tissues; change starch into sugar; and fats into fatty acids and glycerin. As in the rest of digestion, everything we eat is transformed into another substance that is usable in performing some bodily function.

Insulin is produced in the endocrine part of the pancreas, in the beta cells of the islets of Langerhans which make up less than 1 percent of the total size of the gland. Between 200,000 and 2 million islet beta cells secrete insulin into the bloodstream when the concentration of glucose triggers it. The increase in blood sugar that occurs through the digestion of carbohydrates such as candy bars or cookies causes an increase in insulin production to aid in the decomposition of the glucose. When blood sugar levels go down between meals, insulin production decreases. Unlike the hormones secreted by other endocrine glands, insulin production is triggered by the concentration of glucose in the blood.

During digestion, carbohydrates are changed to glucose in the intestines. Excess glucose is sent to the liver for conversion to the starchy substance, glycogen, that is then stored in the muscles and liver for release as needed through the bloodstream. When needed, the liver converts glycogen back to blood sugar (glucose), the principal source of energy for the brain and the body cells. Other glycogen is stored in muscle tissue and is burned up (oxidized) during activity.

The amount of insulin needed at any given time varies widely depending on such factors as food intake that delivers fluctuating amounts of glucose, the amount of exercise a person does, and consequently the amount of energy needed by the cells. Any excess carbohydrates not converted to glycogen are stored, as we all know, as fat. Exercise, therefore, can reduce body fat by improving the body's capacity to handle sugar.

When the liver fails to store glycogen properly, the pancreas fails to produce sufficient insulin, or the body is incapable of utilizing existing insulin supplies, diabetes mellitus—sugar diabetes—develops. In diabetes, the unmetabolized sugar stays in the blood and is excreted in the urine, making tests for the condition an easy matter.

Measures to control blood sugar levels in the diabetic have centered around maintaining a stable diet and, since soon after its discovery in 1921, taking artificial insulin by injection or orally. In their efforts to find a more perfect way to control blood sugar metabolism and prevent the long-term serious effects of this condition, researchers have devised some exciting new methods including pancreas or pancreatic transplants from a person who has just died or from a live donor. Another form of transplant, not being performed on humans yet, involves the pancreas glands of aborted fetuses. Such transplants in humans may be only a few years away, according to researchers in Australia and the United States. New research is exploring the transplant of the islet beta cells themselves, involving about a thimbleful of tissue extracted from the donor pancreas. Other researchers have concentrated on refinement of implantable insulin pumps for automatic, controlled infusion of artificial insulin into the body of the diabetic. Recent research has produced human insulin using recombinant DNA techniques with bacteria as the source. This product was introduced in 1982 in the United Kingdom and in Ireland. It awaits approval for marketing in the United States.

As we grow older, the body tolerates glucose less well, increasing the chances of our developing diabetes. A researcher at Stanford University in California reported in 1981 that although calorie control and exercise may not completely protect against a decline in beta-cell function, they may help keep the beta cells functioning well. The moral would seem to be: "Keep walking, Grandma, and kick the candy bar habit."

KIDNEYS AND BELOW

Laundering Blood

The body is supplied with 2 kidneys, one on either side of the back wall of the upper abdomen, roughly behind the liver and stomach. The kidneys act as filters that clean the blood by removing waste products through the production of urine.

The chemical balance of blood is maintained by its circulation through the kidneys which eliminate the organic wastes of digestion, excess salts, water, and small protein molecules present in excessive amounts through the processes of filtration and absorption.

The basic filtering units of the kidneys are the nephrons, a tiny network of tubules that, at a magnification of 100 times, appear like a nexus of human brains. Together, both kidneys contain about 2 million of these tiny filters that clear the blood of unwanted waste products. It is possible to lose many of these nephrons through disease or even one whole kidney and still lead a normal life.

The kidneys play a major role in maintaining the balance of water in the body. The weight of the human body is 65 to 70 percent water. The balance between the intake and output of water keeps the composition of the body's fluids constant. The intake of water is regulated mostly by the sensation of thirst. Thirst may be felt when there is a reduction in body water because less has been consumed, or when there has been a

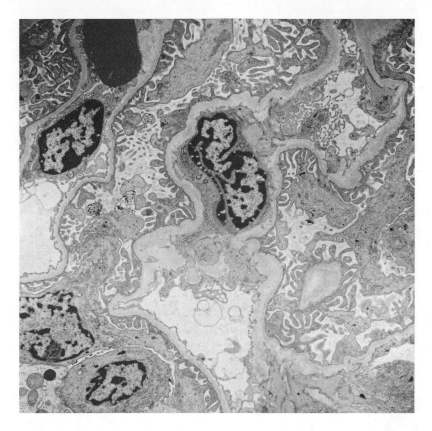

The human kidney, magnified 7,300 times, showing the complex microworld inside the nephron, the kidney's basic filtering unit. Both kidneys contain about 2 million of these tiny filters. Courtesy John M. Basgen, University of Minnesota.

loss of blood, or when extra water has been lost because of vomiting, diarrhea, sweating, increased salt intake—all those potato chips—or a physical condition that causes excessive urination. The strong urge for a drink of water seems to be prompted when there is a general dehydration of the tissues, or when less saliva is secreted and the membranes lining the mouth and pharynx become dry.

About 99 percent of the fluids removed from the blood by the kidneys are reabsorbed, together with glucose, salts, vitamins, and other substances needed by the body. In this way, the kidneys control the balance between the acid and alkaline conditions of the body's tissues and the balance between water and salt in the body's cells. The amount of fluid reabsorbed by the body is controlled by a hormone excreted by the pituitary gland located below the brain. This hormone controls the production of urine, preventing the kidneys from remov-

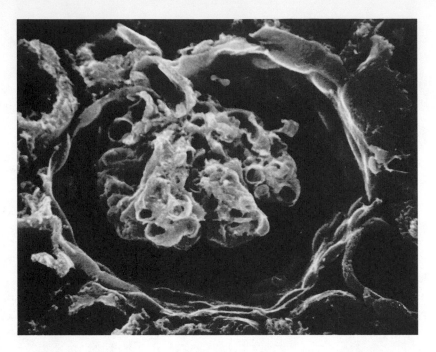

An electron microscope image, magnified 650 times, of one of the kidney's basic clusters of filtering capillaries—the glomerulus. The kidneys filter about 48 gallons (180 liters) of blood every 24 hours. Courtesy John M. Basgen and Tom Groppoli, University of Minnesota. Originally published in **Postgraduate Medicine,** *June 1981.*

ing too much water from the body's tissues and thus avoiding dehydration of the cells. When water intake is inadequate, the body draws on water stores in the tissues. If this should continue for too long, dehydration is the result. A water loss of from 5 to 10 percent of body weight is considered serious dehydration and a 20 percent loss is usually fatal. Under average conditions, a person may live for 12 to 20 days without water, but if exposed to heat simultaneously, as in a desert, may survive for only 2 or 3 days.

Without the removal of excess salts and fluid from the blood by the kidneys, fluids would collect in the blood and in the tissues to produce swelling (edema) of the face, feet, hands, ankles, and heart. This edema of the heart muscle forces the heart to pump harder and it becomes weaker and may stop. We get potassium from meats and fruit juices. Too little of this vital mineral and the muscles will weaken and fail, particularly the muscles involved in breathing. Too much potassium and the heart slows down and stops.

In removing excess fluids from the body, those from the glands are carried off into the urine as well, making possible the urological test for pregnancy and other conditions.

Each day the body excretes 1 1/2 to 2 quarts (1.4 to 1.9 liters) of urine containing the products of protein digestion, uric acid, urea, and creatinine. To do this, the kidneys filter about 48 gallons (182 liters) of blood every 24 hours—close to 4 times the body's liquid weight. This amounts to almost 1.3 million gallons filtered in a lifetime of 73 years, enough to fill a good-sized city water tank. At this moment, as much as one fourth of your blood is passing through your kidneys for laundering.

Kidney Abuse

The kidneys are subject to damage from many sources. Infection in the nephrons (filtering units) of the kidneys usually enters up the urinary tract from the outside. The urethra, the tube that leads from the bladder to the outside, passes through the penis in men and is 8 to 12 inches long (20 to 30 centimeters). In women, the urethra is only 1 to 2 inches (2.5 to 5 centimeters) in length, making the trip for bacteria from the outside shorter and infections in females more common.

Burns over a large part of the body may cause wastes from destroyed tissue to build up faster than the kidneys can get rid of them. Under these conditions, essential blood components seep from the wounds faster than they can be replaced by the kidneys.

Damage from a blow to the area over the kidneys—the "rabbit punch" of boxing—or a car accident can cause problems for the nephrons, as can many drugs and poisons.

The kidney usually can repair itself quickly, but the body's chemistry often must be adjusted medically when damage or infection is extensive.

It is possible to lead a normal life with only one kidney. However, when the remaining kidney tissue malfunctions or there is an intolerable loss of functioning tissue, life may be threatened.

Modern technology and surgery have made it possible for these people to survive as well. Kidney transplants have been successfully performed since 1954. An alternative to a transplant, however, or for use as a temporary measure while waiting for a donor kidney, is renal dialysis. This technique requires the patient to be attached to a mechanical kidney that simulates the laundering action of the natural kidney. Blood flows from a vein in the body into the dialysis machine where wastes are filtered out through a semipermeable membrane and washed away. The machine then returns the clean blood to the body through an artery.

In the past, the necessity for kidney dialysis meant a life restricted to close proximity to a hospital or other center where professionals could perform the dialysis. Refinements of these artificial kidneys have now reduced the size of the machine so that it is portable, making it possible for people who need this aid to do their own dialysis wherever they happen to be.

Nature's Call

Under normal conditions, the body produces 1½ to 2 quarts (1.4 to 1.9 liters) of urine daily. Chemical, nervous, or physical factors may, however, affect the quantity of urine produced on any given day and, therefore, the number of times it is necessary to answer nature's call.

The amount of urine may be affected by the volume of blood passing through the kidneys at any moment. When the body is chilled, for example, the blood supply to the skin is reduced to conserve internal heat. This causes an increase of blood to the body's organs, including the kidneys, and more urine is made.

Emotions such as fear or anxiety may raise the blood pressure and increase urine production. Excitement or anger can tighten the muscles of the bladder wall and, although the bladder may not be full, give the urge for relief. During pregnancy, when the growing fetus sits on top of the bladder for 9 months, the pressure gives the mother a frequent sense of urgency.

The caffeine in coffee, tea, some soft drinks, and other substances such as medicines are diuretics; that is, they stimulate the kidneys to remove more fluids from the body. Some drugs are prescribed in the treatment of high blood pressure and other conditions to act as diuretics in order to remove a larger amount of urine from the body's tissues. The nicotine in cigarettes has the opposite effect because it increases production of a hormone made in the pituitary gland located under the brain. This hormone controls the production of urine so that the kidneys do not remove too much water from the body's tissues and cause dehydration of the cells. Heavy smokers urinate less often, therefore, affording the smoker virtually the only physiological benefit from the habit.

Less urine is created at night (about one fourth the daytime production) because the body is less active at night, usually. Physical activity makes the heart beat faster and the blood to move more rapidly through the kidneys. This makes the kidneys work harder and produce more urine. Digestion of food and drink also causes more kidney activity because of the function of the circulatory system in that process.

Alcohol consumption causes the heart to beat faster and dilate the blood vessels stimulating the kidneys to manufacture more urine. Alcohol also slows production of the pituitary hormone that controls urine, so that it is produced more rapidly. Too much alcohol intake leads to mild dehydration and a craving for water. The dryness in the mouth and headache typical of a hangover are the aftereffects of dehydration from alcohol. The headache of a hangover is caused by dehydration of brain cells that literally hurt for water. If the amount of alcohol consumed was enough to cause vomiting, the dehydration would be worse—and so would the hangover. Pale, dilute urine is produced in large amounts when quantities of alcohol are consumed. To help avoid the unpleasant effects of a hangover, dilute your drinks with ice, use water as a mixer, and limit your intake by spacing the drinks out. If a hangover does occur, the only sure cure is time and rest —usually about 1 hour for every drink consumed. The dehydration cure is also slow. Liquids should be taken gradually, about 12 ounces every hour or so, depending on your body weight.

Training the Holding Tank

The bladder essentially is a holding tank, regularly filled and regularly emptied. There are 2 valves in the bladder (sphincters). One of these valves is at the base of the bladder and opens automatically when the bladder is filling. The second valve is farther down the exit tube from the bladder and is under voluntary control. Controlled opening of the second valve is learned in childhood.

The control pattern for relieving the bladder of urine is inherited. Children born of parents who had a bedwetting problem may have difficulties in being toilet trained. Conscious control of the bladder may be defective from birth and some diseases or spinal cord damage may prevent control of the bladder. In the aged, weakened muscles may cause valve control to be imperfect so that urine leaks from the bladder. Women who have had a number of pregnancies often develop urinary incontinence because of the persistent weakening of the valves from the pressure of the fetuses while in the womb.

Bladder training varies widely between cultures depending upon the importance placed by the society on the habit. Normally, bladder training is possible from about 15 months of age. Between the ages of 2 and 4, the capacity of the bladder to retain urine doubles to the adult maximum of more than a pint (more than 500 cubic centimeters) and toilet training is usually completed by this time in most Western societies. About 10 percent of all children will be late in developing control. Boys generally take longer to be trained than girls, although there is no difference between the male and female capacity to retain urine, popular mythology not withstanding.

The bladder is muscular and can stretch to hold urine without forcing us to empty it as long as the body is resting quietly. When the ureters (the tubes from the kidneys to the bladder) have delivered just under a pint of urine (about a half liter), the sensory signals in the bladder give the familiar feeling that emptying is required. When we are bouncing along in a car over a bumpy road, the signals send a more urgent message requiring concentrated control until a convenient stopping place is found.

The Smell of Urine

Urine has no odor when passed. Shortly after being passed, however, organisms in the environment attack one of the main waste products of urine, urea, which is manufactured in the liver as an end product of protein digestion. When urea is sent to the kidneys from the liver for processing, it is broken down into its chemical parts, one of which is ammonia. The decomposition of ammonia by organisms in our environment gives urine its "characteristic" odor and, if the urine or its decomposed ammonia remains in contact with the skin—in diapers or bedding, for example—it can irritate the skin and cause a serious rash. Urine that has an unusual odor may mean there is an infection or possibly some physical problem with the kidneys or bladder.

Over 1.4 ounces (40 grams) of urea are eliminated daily through the urinary tract. Ammonia is toxic to life. If only $1/1{,}000$ of a milligram of ammonia were to get into each 1.06 quarts (1 liter) of your blood, you would die. So let's hear it for the kidneys!

Urine Is Yellow—Most of the Time

The straw color of urine is provided by a bit of bile pigment from the gall bladder excreted into the bloodstream and extracted as the blood is filtered through the kidneys. The more concentrated the urine, the darker its color. Before you have had a chance to eat or drink in the morning, the first visit to the necessary produces urine that is golden to almost rust color. Drinking large volumes of alcohol produces quantities of pale, dilute urine.

Some people who are born with the inability to digest an amino acid called tyrosine properly excrete a substance called homogentisic acid

INS AND OUTS:

into the urine. When this occurs, and the urine stands for a while, it turns black.

Medicines such as levodopa used in the treatment of Parkinsonism (shaking palsy) can turn urine from a reddish color to black; others may turn urine pink to red, orange, or amber. The discoloration is seldom significant, but can be alarming if unexpected.

Male Labor

The basis of kidney action is the flushing of waste products from the body with a stream of water. It would be natural to assume that all of the wastes to be eliminated would be soluble in water. That assumption would be slightly inaccurate. For example, small amounts of uric acid are excreted in the urine and this compound is not soluble at all.

Microscopic crystals of solid substances are carried through in the urine without incident usually, but when excessive amounts of some substances are present, they can combine with others to form larger pieces of insoluble material called kidney stones.

Some of these are calcium stones made of calcium oxalate and calcium phosphate that form when there are excessive amounts of calcium, oxalate, or uric acid in the urine, or when the urine contains low levels of citrate. These stones can be passed through the ureters (the tubes that carry urine from the kidneys to the bladder) and then the urethra (the tube from the bladder to the outside) as long as the edges are smooth and they do not tear up the bladder wall or block the passage of urine. When they are rough and spiny, they cause excruciating pain that has been likened to the pain of childbirth.

Stones may be the result of excess calcium in the urine, or be brought about by a bowel disease or abnormality. People who have had intestinal bypass surgery often develop kidney stones. Another group involves those who have high levels of uric acid in the blood. This is common in people with the disease "gout," a painful condition in which uric acid is deposited in the joints of the extremities, particularly the big toe.

While kidney stone disease occurs in about 5 out of every 1,000 people in the United States, about 5 percent of these cases have no metabolic basis, but seem to occur often in people who do not like to drink water. While substantial amounts of water may be obtained from foodstuffs, following the old adage to "drink at least 8 glasses of water a day" may be sound advice to help keep the kidneys in proper water balance and free of stones.

Until recently, major surgery was one of the few options sufferers had to alleviate their pain. Now research is concentrating on a drug to prevent the formation of stones in susceptible people and new noninvasive techniques make it possible to dissolve, fish out, or disintegrate the stones. By inserting a tube into the kidney, the stone can be visualized through radiologic means and then ultrasound is applied and the stone is disintegrated. In another method, shock waves aid in removing the stone or destroying it.

The Dangling Worm

Hanging from the lowest loop of the large intestines, on the right side of the lower abdomen, is that useless appendage to the bowel, the appendix. Because it is shaped like an earth worm, its anatomical name is vermiform appendix.

The only time the appendix does anything is to give trouble. Occasionally, a small, hard, indigestible food particle can drop into this small outpouching of the large intestines and get stuck there. An irritation may develop over time and possibly an inflammation—appendicitis. If this inflammation is not brought under control with the use of antibiotics or other measures, surgery may be necessary to remove the offending tissue. If a seriously inflamed appendix is not removed in time, it can rupture and spill its infected contents into the abdominal cavity and cause peritonitis, a general inflammation within the peritoneum (the membrane that lines the abdominal cavity and surrounds the organs of the abdomen).

For a bit of flesh only 8.5 centimeters (3.3 inches) in length, a number of old wives' tales have grown up about the appendix and the causes of appendicitis, including the one about swallowed orange seeds—or sometimes, cherry pits—getting stuck in it.

As far as we now know, seeds and pits pass harmlessly through the digestive tract and are excreted.

Appendicitis has been treated surgically since the early eighteenth century when Claudius Amyand performed the first recorded appendectomy in 1736 in Great Britain. In the United States alone, in 1981, approximately 285,000 people lost their appendixes surgically.

Prostate Problems

The prostate gland surrounds the urethra, the tube that leads from the bladder to the outside of the body in men. This mass of gland tissue and muscle fibers produces seminal fluid which mixes with sperm to make semen, the liquid in which sperm may be transported.

In late middle age, despite a reduction of the amount of testicular hormone, the prostate can enlarge causing a painful obstruction to the urethra. This may be caused by hormonal changes, by venereal disease or other diseases, or by tumors in the tube or prostate. Because of pressure of the enlarged gland on the bladder's outlet, the individual has a constant urge to pass urine but may have difficulty in starting the flow and in emptying the bladder completely. Under these circumstances, urine that is left behind can become infected. A complete obstruction prevents passage of any urine and the urine can spill into the blood causing uremic poisoning, a slow death.

Treatment with female hormones seems to counteract this effect of the male hormones, but surgical removal of the part of the gland involved reduces the obstruction and does not affect the male's sex life.

The involvement of male hormones is an assumption, but it has been noted that the condition rarely happens in eunuchs.

The Undignified Malady

Hemorrhoids, many physicians now believe, are the result of humans walking on 2 feet. They are not caused by sedentary occupations, sitting on hard, cold surfaces, or worry, as some people used to think. They are not the first step to cancer of the bowel. They are harmless, but a considerable nuisance to those who have them.

The upright posture of humans makes it necessary for circulating blood to fight gravity to make its complete circuit in humans. This pull of gravity, combined with such factors as pregnancy, constipation, and straining, increases dilation of the blood vessels in the anal canal. When these vessels enlarge and fill with blood, either inside or outside the anal canal, a hemorrhoid is created.

Hemorrhoids that occur in the part of the anal canal covered by skin are external hemorrhoids, while those that appear in the part covered by mucous membrane are internal hemorrhoids or piles as they are commonly called.

Hemorrhoids are relatively painless but may be irritated when a hard stool is passed, causing some discomfort. Hemorrhoids produce itching and they can bleed when they break down, although some people may have them and never know it. Various medical treatments are possible to relieve the discomfort and even bleeding of hemorrhoids. Surgery is reserved for more severe cases, when other treatments have been ineffectual.

Dr. James Robinson, a retired British surgeon, speaking on the subject of hemorrhoids at the University of Texas Health Science

Center at Dallas in early 1983, mentioned the practice in medieval Europe of naming patron saints as protectors against dreaded diseases. The hemorrhoid was thought so undignified an ailment that a bona fide saint could not be assigned to it. Instead, prayers for hemorrhoids were to be directed to a gardener named Fiacre, because the condition resembled a bunch of grapes. This man became so famous that the French named an inn after him, the Inn of Saint Fiacre.

Chapter Seven

Coming into Play: Sex

THE SEXUAL CONTINUUM

A Half Century of Sexual Intercourse

People spend a great deal of time thinking about their own and others' bodies, but relatively little time participating in one of the body's greatest pleasures: sexual intercourse.

In the half century between the ages of 20 and 70, the average person spends 600 hours in the act; this comes to just 12 hours a year, 1 hour a month, 2 minutes out of each day. On the basis of time spent —less than 1/700 of a lifetime—intercourse is a very small part of sexuality.

The Energy of Intercourse

A Couple's Sexual Energy. During 10 minutes of sexual intercourse, a couple generates energy at the rate of almost 3 kilowatts, which is enough to run all household appliances, including the lights, refrigerator, stereo, and the bedroom air conditioner for those 10 minutes.

During a sexually active lifetime of 50 years, the couple would release enough energy to equal the energy in 1 ton of TNT. Convert this into fireworks and one great spectacular display could be put on to celebrate the sexual golden anniversary.

The World's Sexual Energy. If the lifetime sexual energy for the world's sexually active population of 3 billion were totaled, it would equal an energy release of 1.5 billion tons of TNT—a big bang with over 100,000 times the energy in the Hiroshima A-bomb.

For the 50 billion people in the earth's history who have ever lived to sexual maturity, the total sexual energy would come to 25,000 megatons, considerably more than either the United States or Soviet nuclear arsenals. This means that if humanity's total sexual energy were released all at once, planet earth would be rendered uninhabitable.

For a more hopeful future, the total sexual energy of humanity up to the present day (25,000 megatons) would be enough to launch and accelerate a 200-ton starship to one tenth the speed of light and send it off on a journey to the stars.

Those Special Spasms

Women have more sexual spasms, on the average, than men during orgasm. A male ejaculation lasts about 10 seconds, and most of the semen is expelled in 5 or 6 bursts, each contraction taking slightly less than 1 second. An average female orgasm lasts some 10 to 15 seconds, but can last up to a minute for some women. A young woman will have about 8 to 12 vaginal contractions for an intense orgasm and 3 to 5 for a mild one. The lower number of spasms also applies to older women.

Fourteen percent of women report regular multiple orgasms, whereas men rarely do. It is not uncommon for these women to have 6 or more orgasms during one sexual session. Only a few men (about 7 percent and usually very young) experience more than one orgasm during a single sexual act.

How do women and men differ when they're having more than one? Women's second and third orgasms are usually more intense and enjoyable than the first. But for those few young men who enjoy more than one, it's just the opposite—the first is almost always the best.

Finding the Grafenberg Spot

Women by the thousands are learning about their own Grafenberg spots for the first time—a very sexually sensitive area of the vagina that has been much neglected or overlooked because of all the attention the clitoris has received ever since Kinsey's research in the 1950s. Even most gynecologists have been ignorant of the "G" spot's existence. This is because its location in the vagina is outside the area of the normal pelvic examination.

Because there seemed to be real differences between what some women felt they actually experienced and the "objective" descriptions of sex research, researchers reexamined all the traditional questions about female orgasm in the early 1980s. Was the clitoris alone the major source for female sexual excitation? Were there really 2 types of female orgasm—one clitoral and one vaginal? Is there truly a female ejaculation as some women claim?

The new research centered on the Grafenberg spot—named after Ernest Grafenberg, a gynecologist who first described its sexual significance in an article that appeared in 1950, but whose findings were more or less buried under Kinsey's highly publicized research.

The Grafenberg spot is located in the upper wall of the vagina near the urethra, which is surrounded by unique erectile tissue, not quite one half of an inch beneath the surface of the vagina. Research has established that this area is the major source of stimulation for the so-called vaginal (uterine) orgasm, which many people have considered a sexual myth, mainly because of the prevailing belief in clitoral orgasms. These vaginal orgasms do not depend at all on clitoral stimulation, which means there are 2 different types of orgasm. And women report that the clitoral and vaginal orgasms are very different in intensity.

As the whereabouts of the "G" spot becomes better known by lovers everywhere, and as lovers learn what it can do for their sex lives, there'll be more happiness in the bedrooms. More and more women will experience intense vaginal orgasms for the first time and more of them will experience orgasm during intercourse, without the need for clitoral stimulation. The Grafenberg spot may become a common bedroom word.

Female Ejaculation?

Another sexual myth is about to be thrown out the bedroom window— that ejaculation is entirely a male sexual function. This is what the textbooks and experts have been telling us for the last 100 years.

The fact is that perhaps 10 percent of all women in the United States do ejaculate when they reach orgasm, and these women have identified the Grafenberg spot as the trigger for their ejaculations. More importantly, once the no-ejaculation myth is more generally exposed and the truth known, certain ill-founded inhibitions will be cast aside and millions more women may be able to let themselves go and experience ejaculations with "G"-spot-stimulated vaginal orgasms.

Regretfully, excessive wetness at orgasm has often been blamed on "urinary stress incontinence," and if a woman or her sexual partner wrongly interpreted her ejaculation as "peeing in bed," she would learn to control it, out of embarrassment, which would also stop her vaginal orgasms.

Researchers have proven that the female ejaculate is definitely not urine and is different from ordinary vaginal secretions. The fluid is, in fact, very similar to the chemical composition of the seminal fluid ejaculated from males who have been vasectomized.

Sexologists have discovered that women who ejaculate can produce contractions of the pubococcygeal (PC) muscle that are twice as strong as those in women who do not ejaculate. (The PC muscle stretches from the pubic bone in front, around the genitals on both sides, to the tailbone in the back.) It was also demonstrated that the uterine contractions are almost 3 times stronger for women who do ejaculate than for women who don't.

So ejaculation is a reality for many women, and it has a definite relationship to the strength of the PC muscle—a muscle similar to all muscles in that it can be exercised and made to perform better. (See the next entry, "The Sex Muscle.")

The amount of fluid ejaculated varies from woman to woman (just as it does from man to man), but the range is from a few drops to a full cup or more!

Sexercise: The Sex Muscle

The same muscle that wagged the tail of our ancient evolutionary ancestors has recently been shown to play an important role in women's sexual satisfaction. Both women and men have a pubococcygeal (PC) muscle, which runs on both sides of the genitals from the pubic bone to the tailbone. It is the support muscle of the pelvis and holds the internal organs such as the intestines in place.

A weak PC muscle is often responsible for many medical problems for women—urinary stress incontinence (when urine leaks during fright or physical exertion), prolapse (falling) of the bladder, prolapse of the rectum, and childbirth problems in general. Vaginal orgasms and female ejaculations almost never occur in women with a weak PC muscle, and that is why "sexercise" of the PC often becomes a major part of contemporary sexual therapy for women. A strong and healthy PC muscle usually means heightened sexual response and satisfaction.

A California gynecologist, Arnold Kegel, knew the importance of the PC muscle with respect to gynecological as well as sexual problems. His ideas, however, went against the status quo of the medical profession in the early 1950s, which tended to solve everything surgically.

Kegel had the impressive record of eliminating the need for surgery in 2,550 patients out of 3,000—an 85 percent cure rate—by putting them through his PC exercises. But Kegel's flex-it program for strengthening a weak PC muscle (or relaxing one that is too tense) would have to wait 30 years to get the attention it deserved.

Exercise, not surgery, is now almost always recommended. Three hundred sustained contractions each day for 90 days are often prescribed to build up the PC muscle. And what woman would refuse such a program when she knows that women with the strongest muscles are also those who have orgasms during intercourse? That plus this added bonus: These "sexercises" are almost impossible to do without becoming sexually aroused!

Pleasurable Wrinkles

The walls of the vagina are composed of fibrous and elastic tissue, which is usually a flattened, closed canal when there is no sexual response. Beneath this fibrous coat is a layer of smooth muscle, and beneath this is the mucosa layer with many blood vessels. The entire mucosa layer of the vagina has an intricate network of erectile tissue. Under magnification, the folds in the mucosa layer give the vagina a wrinkled appearance. These are the wrinkles that no one worries about.

The Womb's Walls

An amazing nexus of blood vessels and capillaries supply the uterus with copious amounts of blood. This hollow, muscular organ—which holds the developing embryo and fetus—has thick walls, about 1 inch thick, and they are even thicker during pregnancy. The complex interlacing muscles of the womb that are responsible for labor contractions must be well supplied with blood.

The uterus does contract several times during female orgasm, and these contractions are quite similar to those of the first stage of labor.

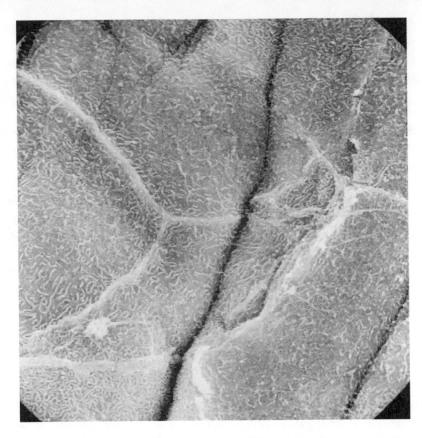

Two magnifications (above and on facing page) of the human vagina surface—4,400X and 10,200X. The walls of the vagina are composed of fibrous and elastic tissue, and they change throughout the menstrual cycle because of hormonal variations. The highly flattened outer cells are continuously shed and replaced. The microridges in the high magnification give the vagina its firm but elastic surface. Courtesy E. S. E. Hafez, Wayne State University School of Medicine.

The Smooth Hormone

Estrogens are the hormones responsible for the female shape—the breasts, the hips, the buttocks, all the extra curves. They keep a woman's skin and breasts soft and generally make her attractive to the opposite sex. But estrogens do more than advertise and attract. They also help out in the home stretch by lubricating the vagina and making good sex a smooth delight.

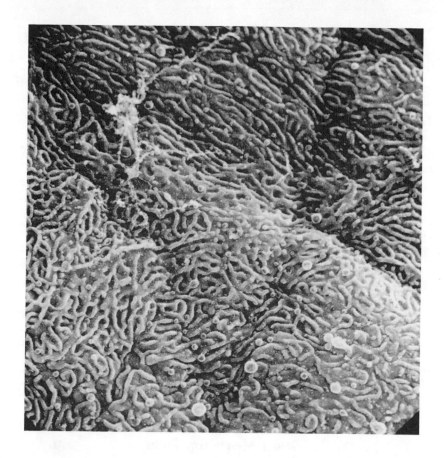

During and after a woman's menopause, however, the body produces less estrogen and the vagina often becomes dry, making sexual pleasure more difficult. But just as some men are prescribed a testosterone boost, so too can women replace their lost estrogen by taking pills.* There are over 35 different brand name prescriptions on the market for pill-form estrogen, and more than 60 million prescriptions are written each year—enough to keep things moving smoothly for the wiser and more experienced lovers.

---

* Estrogen therapy carries risks for some patients. Pregnant women should never take estrogen. Other patient groups—for example, those who have had a stroke, heart attack, angina, cancer of the breast or uterus—should not be prescribed estrogen. Consult your physician and be sure he or she knows your medical history.

The Male Hormone in Women

Testosterone, the principal male sex hormone, has greater influence on sexual drive of men *and* women than any other hormone. A woman's desire was once thought to be controlled by estrogen, a female hormone, but this is now known not to be true. If a woman loses her sexual drive after having had a normal one in the past, testosterone treatment can restore her sexual appetite. Women who have taken synthetic testosterone experience a tremendous surge in their sexual appetite.

The hormone's level is highest in women around the middle of their menstrual cycle, and this is why women are more sexually responsive at this time and why couples tend to be more sexually active during mid-cycle.

Some women produce 10 times more testosterone than others, and these women, according to one study, make love more often and enjoy it more. Researchers also suspect, and hope to prove, that women with higher levels of testosterone may have stronger bonding instincts and form more enduring relationships.

Good Morning, Dear

A man's normal potency is maintained by the male hormone testosterone, most of which is secreted by special cells (neighbors to the sperm-producing cells) in the testicles.

Men, like women, have sexual cycles, even if they are often less apparent. Testosterone levels in men are known to have seasonal and daily cycles. A scientific study in France showed that the yearly peak for testosterone is in October—the month ruled by Venus in astrological myth. The daily cycle for the male hormone—and this should surprise none of us because it *is* apparent—peaks in the early morning, and lovers have many Good Mornings to thank for it!

Building Up an Erection

The top side of the penis (corpus cavernosum) is responsible for a man's erection. But because there is no increase of blood flow to this area of the penis, how does the organ become engorged and erect with 7 times the normal blood flow?

Until recently, it was believed that there were separate blood flows to the top and bottom of the penis, but researchers have now found that this is not true. An erection, it turns out, is formed by blood that would normally flow to the bottom side of the penis. Researchers at the University of Copenhagen have discovered shunt-type arteries that connect the top side and bottom side of the penis. During sexual arousal, nerve impulses constrict these arteries, and this redirects what is usually bottom-side blood flow to the erectile tissue of the top side— Presto! Erection!

Uncoiling the Testicle Tubes

There are thousands of coiled tubes (seminiferous tubules) in the male testicles, where the sperm are constantly formed. If all of these tiny tubes were stretched out and placed end to end, they would span a distance of 800 feet (244 meters)—the height of the Pan Am Building in New York City.

Zippity at 60

When a man is 60 years old, every part of his body has slowed down— from his brain (which often experiences a slight loss of memory) to his heart (which pumps less blood) to his testicles (which produce less male hormone). At this age, a man's body produces about the same amount of testosterone that a 9- or 10-year-old boy does.

Gentlemen, don't panic. There is hope for us, as the following example will prove. A man had been totally impotent for 10 years, ever since the age of 50. Then he was treated with testosterone and . . . bang! He began having erections again. This lucky man also began having sexual dreams at night and erotic daydreams. He became a very happy 60-year-old.

Hormone therapy will not work for everyone, of course. Physical impotence can also be caused by neurological and vascular problems that testosterone therapy will not cure. However, as this man's case demonstrates, some impotent men can be helped. If that sexual decline is getting you down, talk to your urologist about putting some zippity-doodah into your golden years.

Some Help from Mr. Piggy

Pheromones are substances used by animals and certain insects to send chemical messages, messages that are received through the sense of smell. If animals send and receive pheromones that act for the most part as mating signals, why not people?

Some scientists remain skeptical about the existence of human pheromones, but the search continues to prove that these biochemical scents draw women and men together in unknown ways. The cosmetic industry is certainly not waiting for conclusive proof—they're competing hard and investing in research and development to get pheromones or their synthetic equivalents into their products. One perfume manufacturer, in fact, has already added the pheromone androsterone to its perfume formula.

This pheromone-spiked product may well get mixed reviews when spread on human faces. One U.S. study of 200 volunteers showed 3 different responses to the scent. About half the volunteers could not smell it at all. Another third could smell it at low concentrations, but did not like it (it reminded them of toilets!). And about 30 of the 200 people tested could smell it at higher concentrations and liked it. The response may have been very different, however, had the volunteers known the source of androsterone. The extract is derived from the hormone testosterone taken from inside boar's testicles!

Sex Scents

A group of British researchers got more positive results when they isolated a pheromone called alpha androstenol from male perspiration. The substance, after it was purified, smelled like sandalwood to most of the women tested, and the researchers claimed that the scent was a definite turn-on for these women.

It may be that pheromone messages are received by only a minority of people today, that most have lost this primitive ability to send or receive chemical messages. With the sense-distorting bombardment of stimuli experienced in contemporary industrialized societies, it should not surprise any of us to learn that this ability may be in rapid decline— that our eyes and brains have repressed our sense of smell because of the additional demands of late-twentieth-century living.

If, on the other hand, research offers definite proof of human pheromones, this knowledge could affect our lives in many unexpected ways. One researcher has gone so far to suggest that pheromones derived from the vaginal secretions of young women could be given to postmenopausal women as sexual attractants to enhance and increase the longevity of their sex lives. With longer lives for both men and women, and with better health for older people constantly on the increase, most of us would vote for extending sexual longevity as an alternative to the rocking chair.

Sexual Calories

How many calories do you burn up when you enjoy the ultimate sexual pleasure, sexual intercourse? About 200 calories, on the average, for each partner.

Sex/Drug Tidbits

• If you love sex, men, take it easy on the booze. A study showed that, on the average, it took longer to attain an erection after 3 drinks. But even worse, just one drink can decrease the size of an erection by about 50 percent!

• Heavy drinking reduces the amount of the male hormone, testosterone, in men. One of the results, eventually, is that their breasts get larger.

• Women who smoke marijuana agree that the drug increases sexual desire and intensifies sexual pleasure—if the right feelings about making love are already there.

• Men report that women on pot spend a lot more time giving fellatio than when they are not high.

• Users of cocaine often compare its "rush" to a sexual high or orgasm. An injection of cocaine can produce a spontaneous erection. But, for that matter, so can a few or several days of sexual abstinence—without the risk.

• Erection pills? Men who have occasional impotency or staying-power problems often fall into a vicious psychological cycle and compound the problem. One doctor tells his patients to take 2 chelated magnesium tablets 20 minutes before intercourse. It was good advice —it worked. Why? No one is sure, but magnesium is known to be involved in hundreds of metabolic reactions in the soft tissues of the body, and because of today's processed foods, many of us are deficient in magnesium. Drinking also depletes the body's magnesium supply. So if that physical and emotional letdown is not allowing you to be your best in bed, try 2 with water and find something else to do for 20 minutes.

Sexual Allergy

A few unfortunate women have extreme allergic reactions to male ejaculate, so extreme that some have almost died after sexual intercourse. Shock, inability to breathe, and severe asthma attacks are common in these cases, and for some of these women emergency adrenaline injections were needed to save their lives.

The allergen is not the sperm cells in the semen, but the concentrated protein layer that coats the cells. While the precise mechanism that triggers such severe reactions is not understood, doctors hope they can desensitize the allergic women by injecting the irritant in very small quantities and thus build up their tolerance.

The only choice these women now have is to avoid sexual intercourse or make sure their man uses a reliable condom. But this can hardly be considered normal sex—not when there's fear attached to it, not when catching your breath afterward means literally fighting for your life.

The PMS Complex

What have you got if you experience aches and pains, irritability, insomnia, depression, lethargy, fatigue, nervousness, dizziness, fainting, headaches? Not sure yet? Well, try adding constipation, cramps, fluid retention and the resultant weight gain of 3 to 10 pounds, abdominal bloating, swollen ankles, enlarged and sore breasts.

Depending on the severity and number of these symptoms, you've got premenstrual syndrome (PMS), which affects 60 percent of all women. No particular woman will have all these symptoms, of course, and those she does have may vary in intensity from month to month; but every woman has experienced some of them during her monthly cycle. It is the severity of them that determines whether a woman experiences mild discomfort as a result of the complex bodily changes taking place because of menstruation or whether she is a victim of PMS.

Poor Queen Victoria had premenstrual syndrome, and poor husband Albert was an abused husband because of it. Once a month she would rant at him, shouting unwarranted accusations and throwing any close-at-hand objects across the room. Albert no doubt got hit a few times. It's hard enough trying to argue with a queen during the best of times, but it must have been damn near impossible when the queen had PMS. And that goes for any woman with extreme PMS symptoms. At its worst, PMS makes the woman completely irrational and out of control—a situation that very few women experience. No amount of understanding, tender loving care, or placation is capable of snapping the woman out of it. In the past, every woman had to get through it the best way she could.

Today PMS is getting the serious attention and research it deserves, long overdue after centuries of neglect and misunderstanding. No doubt, some of the witches who were burned at the stake suffered premenstrual syndrome. When the tens of millions of people it affects are considered—not just the woman but the husband, children, friends, and colleagues around her—PMS becomes a major medical problem, one that deserves even more funding than it is currently getting.

Why all this suffering? Most researchers blame an imbalance of hormones as the basic cause, the same hormones that play such a major part in conception, pregnancy, and the birth of babies (which gives such joy to humankind).

During the second half of the menstrual cycle after ovulation, there are elevated levels of estrogen and progesterone in the female body. But researchers have not been able to arrive at a consensus as to which hormone or combination of hormones is responsible for PMS. Besides estrogen and progesterone, aldosterone (secreted by the adrenal cortex) and prolactin (the hormone that triggers lactation) may figure in the cyclical hormonal fluctuations that result in PMS symptoms.

All in all, PMS is very complex—a manifestation of the complex female reproduction system—and eludes easy definition or cure. There is no single treatment that seems to work for all women. This suggests that there are probably several distinct types of PMS, each with its own symptoms and potential treatment. But the answers are slowly forthcoming, medications are being tested and developed. None too soon! Even basic vitamin B_6 therapy has been found to help some women.

PMS begins 7 to 14 days prior to menstruation—that's a big portion of every month of a woman's reproductive years, and there are tens of millions of women who suffer the symptoms. If a woman bears the burden of PMS for 10 days each month for 20 years, that amounts to almost 7 years of her life—and of the lives of those closest to her. The equivalent of a human lifetime is lived under its influence for every 10 women who endure PMS for this amount of time.

Think of the pain and heartache, the lost potential that results. Think of the historical injustices it may have spawned. If you're a woman, think of yourself. If you have the PMS syndrome, you can do something about it today that you couldn't just a decade ago. What? Read on and think of flowers.

The Primrose Solution

The 1982 Nobel Prize in Medicine was given to a group of doctors for their research into prostaglandins. Prostaglandins are a group of fatty-acid derivatives that occur in all tissues of the human body and affect all organs. They are biologically active and are synthesized in the body from unsaturated fatty acids.

What do prostaglandins do for us? Well, they are known to affect the circulatory system, reducing blood pressure in very low concentrations. They also stimulate smooth-muscle contractions, including those of the uterus, and have other critical functions in the male and female reproductive processes.

While there are a great number of prostaglandins in the body, there is one in particular that the Nobel Prize team linked to premenstrual syndrome—prostaglandin E_1 (PGE_1, for short). The symptoms of PMS occur when there are low levels of prostaglandin E_1, and scientists have learned that these low levels can be caused by a deficiency of the essential fatty acid, gamma-linoleic acid (GLA). The GLA deficiency, in turn, is brought on by the stress and hormonal changes present before a woman's period begins. Without sufficient GLA building blocks, prostaglandin E_1 cannot be synthesized, and it therefore falls to low levels—the low levels that are scientifically linked to PMS symptoms.

Researchers in Massachusetts have claimed a 60 to 80 percent success rate in treating hundreds of women with premenstrual syndrome. What was the prescription? The women adhered to a nutritional program that included swallowing primrose-oil capsules twice a day for 2 to 3 months. Research is continuing to determine long-term dosage and possible side effects.

Primrose oil works because it is the only natural source (besides breast milk) that is rich in gamma-linoleic acid from which prostaglandin E_1 is synthesized. By drinking the nectar of the perennial herb, the primrose, some suffering PMS women may find relief from this monthly pain and distress. Primrose-oil capsules are available in many health food stores.

The Bloated Blahs

Fluid retention in body tissues is one of the most common symptoms of premenstrual syndrome, and it's responsible for a host of problems, from swollen ankles to headaches. This extra water weight is probably caused by increased levels of the hormone, aldosterone, which regulates the metabolism of sodium, chloride, and potassium in the human body. An increase in this hormone causes the retention of sodium and water by the kidneys and a woman experiences weight gain, bloating, and swelling.

But that's not the half of it. The same fluid retention in brain tissues may be the culprit behind many or most of the mental and behavioral problems associated with premenstrual syndrome—depression, insomnia, lethargy, fainting, nervousness, and tantrums, to name a few. That pressure in the head naturally changes the way a woman perceives the world.

There are several ways to lessen, if not completely alleviate, the effects of fluid retention. Here are some of the tried and true methods that may work for you:

1. Carefully limit fluid consumption for 12 to 14 days before the menstrual period to no more than a quart daily.
2. Discipline yourself to a salt-free diet.
3. Have your doctor prescribe a diuretic that will increase the flow of urine. The pharmaceutical industry offers many to choose from.

As for the symptoms of fatigue and irritability, frequent but small protein meals will keep blood sugar levels high. It is the drop in blood sugar levels that contributes to these symptoms.

The Impotence Complex

"It's all in your head." That was the gist of the traditional answer given to most men suffering from impotence. But there has been a dramatic medical about-face in recent years, and new diagnostic techniques and methods of treatment hold promise for many of the estimated 10 million impotent men in the United States. Doctors now recognize that many cases of chronic impotence are due to physical causes. As a result, fewer men are quickly sent off to the psychiatrist's office for a solution to their problem—a trip that could create a psychological problem that was not there in the first place.

The physical causes, if found, are usually hormonal imbalances or vascular problems. In a Boston study of 255 men with chronic impotence, no fewer than one third of them were diagnosed as having hormonal imbalances, most of which were treated and corrected with hormone therapy—especially testosterone.

Because erections depend on blood flow to the erectile tissue of the penis, any number of vascular problems (arterial disease, for example) that impede this blood flow can cause impotence. Some impotent patients are able to get erections while lying on their backs, but often lose them in the missionary position or when they begin pelvic thrusting. This problem is known as the "pelvic steal"—when blood is diverted from the penis and redirected to the thigh muscles by a mechanism that is not fully understood.

Because vascular problems may be the cause of up to 60 percent of all chronic impotency cases—and even a higher percentage in the older male group—doctors believe it is very important to measure the blood pressure and circulation of the patient's penis. A Doppler ultrasound technique is used to get a reading on circulation, and the blood pressure is taken by a special cuff that is wrapped around the penis.

The final option in treating impotency caused by blood-flow obstructions is microsurgery, and there are a few cases where potency has been successfully restored by replacing blocked arteries in the penis with synthetic arteries. An impotency expert at the Baylor College of Medicine says another surgical approach will be to replace the blocked arteries of the penis with the patient's own veins. Where will the veins come from? From the feet! From the ground up, so to speak.

The Aging Penis

Blood pressure in a man's penis, all-important for firm erections, declines year by year, decade by decade. So too does the up-angle of his erection, the amount and force of ejaculate, and often the length of the orgasm.

Most studies indicate that impotence in older men is due mainly to vascular problems. More thickening and hardening of the arterial walls (arteriosclerosis) has been measured in the penis than in other parts of the body. In this respect, a man's most pleasure-giving organ ages faster than the rest of his body, but a good woman will continue to make him believe it's ageless.

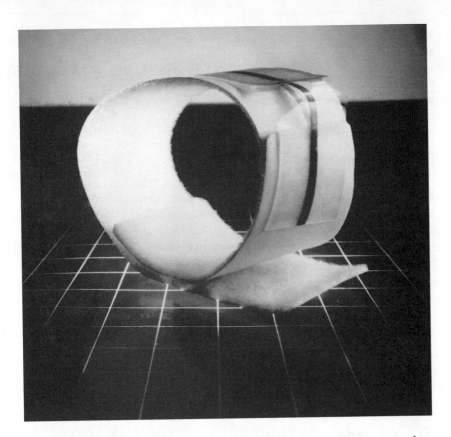

The Dacomed Snap-Gauge™ impotence testing device allows patients to test them-selves for physical impotence. Worn around the penis during sleep, it measures nocturnal erections that naturally occur in normally potent males. If the device does not snap open, there can be a serious impotence problem. Courtesy Dacomed Corpo-ration.

Monitoring Impotence

Severe impotence that is organic and not psychological in nature can be established by measuring erections during sleep. The standard test measures the patient's penis circumference—"nocturnal penile tumes-cence". If the circumference increases by 0.2 inch (5 millimeters) or less, the man is considered to have severe impotence.

The test is not foolproof, however, because some men have erec-tions of penile length with little or no increase in girth. Recently, however, take-home devices have been developed that measure both dimensions.

Some 60 to 70 percent of a full erection is needed for good penetration and intercourse. An attempted insertion with less will just produce negative reinforcement and jolt the male ego's most fragile territory.

Erection Pacemakers?

By some estimates, more than 100 million men worldwide may be experiencing some form of impotence. Total impotence caused by physical problems such as circulatory disease or nerve damage from radical prostatectomies has often been untreatable in the past, but new research suggests that it too can be corrected in the future.

Researchers have recently found bundles of nerves near the prostate that trigger erections in monkeys when electrically stimulated. By surgically implanting electrodes that can be activated by radio signals, the researchers induced and maintained the erections in the animals for periods of up to several hours.

Totally impotent men may therefore merely push a button someday to experience an instant, long-lasting erection! A Philadelphia-based firm, Biosonics, Inc., already has such a device under development. Its name: Male Electronic Genital Stimulator—MEGS, for short.

The Artificial Erection

When all else fails for the chronic impotent male, there is one last resort—the artificial erection. Known to medicine as the penile prosthesis, this device is implanted in the top side of the penis where the blood usually fills up and expands the erectile tissue.

There are several different designs currently available. One device consists of 2 silicone rods that are semirigid, but the drawback is that the penis is always semierect and must be forced into low profile by tight underwear or an athletic supporter for those who want to avoid social embarrassment. Another design, developed in West Germany, avoids this problem with flexible implants that have cores of coiled wire surrounded by silicone rubber. Its advantage is that the penis can be moved to rest or moved to act.

A more complicated penile implant consists of 2 inflatable cylinders, a reservoir with tubing, and a small pump. More surgery is involved for implantation and the device is therefore more expensive. Once implanted, the owner can squeeze the pump in his scrotum and fill up the

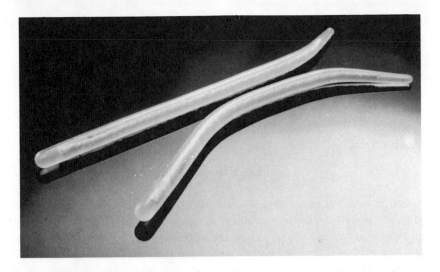

The artificial erection, known as the penile prosthesis, is implanted in the top side of the penis to correct severe physical impotence. One such device, the Jonas malleable prosthesis, has helped thousands of men restore their potency. Courtesy Dacomed Corporation.

cylinders with salt water. This results in an erection. After intercourse, he presses a release valve in his scrotum and the erection solution flows back into the reservoir which is implanted near the bladder. The main disadvantage of this implant is that leaks, always correctable, sometimes occur in the inflatable cylinders or the tubing. But the advantages are a more natural erection and superior penetration during intercourse.

Another decade will probably bring forth the near-perfect artificial erection; hand pumps will be obsolete and a flex of a muscle in the genital area will electrically begin the fluid transfer that creates the erection needed for joyful sex.

BEYOND THE PILL

The Pill Route

About 3 billion oral contraceptive pills are consumed in the United States each year by about 9 million women. If these 3 billion pills were laid out in a row, pill to pill, they could stretch from Fairbanks, Alaska, to Grand Forks, North Dakota, to Independence, Kansas, and then south to Hitchcock, Texas. From there, with more than 1 billion pills left, they could be put down all the way to Muscle Shoals, Alabama, onward to Intercourse, Pennsylvania, and then span eastward across the Atlantic to Gateshead, England. Finally, the pills would run out around Motherwell, Scotland—after a total distance of about 8,000 miles (12,800 kilometers).

Pill Mill

Ever since the first oral contraceptive pill, Enovid, was approved and marketed in 1960, there have been continuing concern and debate over the medical risks. Recent research findings, the result of data collected over many years from millions of women, have allayed many of the fears and clearly demonstrated certain health benefits.

A trio of reports in the *Journal of the American Medical Association* offered reassurance about the long-term use of oral contraceptives. Their findings indicated that women using the pill have a 50 percent lower risk of contracting ovarian cancer, a 50 percent lower risk of contracting cancer of the uterine lining (endometrial cancer), and a 50 percent lower risk of noncancerous breast tumors and other benign breast disorders. They also noted fewer cases of iron-deficiency anemia among pill users, fewer cases of pregnancy outside the uterus, and much less monthly discomfort from cramps.

Perhaps most important, there were far fewer cases of pelvic inflammatory disease (PID) among women. A common bacterial infection, PID affects some 850,000 women in the United States alone; it can lead to infertility, blockage of the fallopian tubes, and, in rare cases, death.

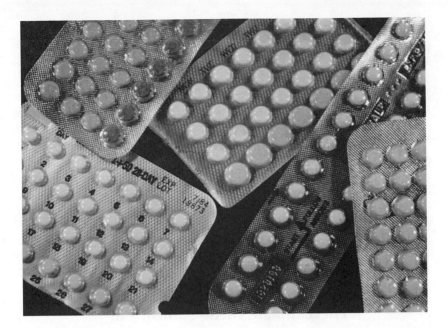

Over 3 billion oral contraceptive pills are consumed in North America each year by about 9 million women. If placed end to end, these pills could stretch a total distance of about 8,000 miles (12,800 kilometers). Courtesy National Institutes of Health.

In addition, the study did *not* find a higher rate of breast cancer, even among long-term pill users. The researchers estimated that, because of the pill, 65,000 women are spared hospitalization, surgery, or other treatment for these medical problems.

A few months later, British and California researchers countered these earlier reports with different findings on the risks of cervical and breast cancer, claiming that pill users have a *higher* risk of developing such cancers. Many factors may explain the different conclusions, but the most likely is the incidence of high-dose progestogen- and estrogen-formula pills used over long periods of time.

None of the researchers recommended giving up the pill, but suggested that women under the age of 25 not take pills with a high progestogen content. The pill is by no means without hazards: It has been linked to strokes, heart attacks, infertility, and blood clots. Because the circulatory risks are heightened in smokers and women over 35, most physicians recommend other forms of contraception for these groups.

Although research continues, and the pill has not been given a clean bill of health, the 9 million American women taking the pill should feel encouraged by the newly found benefits, while also being prudent about long-term use by having regular exams and remaining alert to problems.

Today's pill, the so-called new pill, has been drastically cut in hormonal content, which may lower the risks *and* reduce the benefits. Breakthrough bleeding is a common disadvantage of these pills. At least 5 years' research will be needed to collect sufficient data on the new pill before any valid findings can be published.

One disquieting report by a British doctor said that patients who had given up the low-dose pill to become pregnant had difficulty conceiving. Several cases that he treated with fertility drugs resulted in conception of twins and triplets. What an ironic twist of fate if many women who have been delaying motherhood find themselves the mothers of several children at once!

The Ultimate Birth-Control Pill?

Development of a new hormone contraceptive for women, expected to be safer than the steroid-containing pills now on the market, is in its clinical-trial phase. Eventually it may be available in pill form and will only have to be taken on 3 consecutive days each month rather than the usual 21 days.

Medical researchers have developed a synthesized version of the brain's natural luteinizing hormone-releasing hormone (LHRH), which regulates reproductive processes in both men and women and is essential for fertility. As a contraceptive for women, the synthetic version (about 140 times more powerful than natural LHRH) is taken on each of the first 3 days of the menstrual cycle. This changes the timing of a woman's cycle and extends its first half from 14 days to about 23 days, and shortens the second half (the luteal phase) from 14 to about 9 days. By shortening the second half of the cycle, the egg (possibly fertilized) journeys to the uterus lining, but the lining is not physically ready to accept a fertilized egg. No implantation of a fertilized egg can therefore take place—an engineered infertility.

If and when the LHRH-tailored pill is available, the fact that it will need only be taken after the start of each menstrual cycle will be a real benefit. This point in the female cycle is a natural reminder that few women could forget. The world has been waiting for the ultimate safe and effective birth-control pill. This may turn out to be the one. Stay tuned.

RU-486: A Secret Formula

A drug that blocks the action of progesterone on the lining of the uterus, with the result that the lining is sloughed off and no implantation of a fertilized egg can occur, is the basis for another future birth-control pill that holds great promise. Developed by a French research team over a period of 17 years, the drug's composition is still held secret; it has been designated RU-486.

If large-scale testing over time proves that RU-486 is ready for certification and mass distribution, it will have definite advantages over birth-control pills that prevent ovulation by hormonally influencing the pituitary gland. These hormonal pills may put the whole body at risk for 3 out of 4 weeks, and they are notorious for their many side effects. But RU-486 acts directly on the uterus by filling the progesterone receptors—cell proteins on the uterus lining—and blocking the hormone that makes implantation possible.

Another important advantage: An RU-486 pill is taken only 4 days a month—at the end of each monthly cycle—rather than the usual 21 days a month. And more important, testing so far has found no side effects. Researchers on both sides of the Atlantic are hoping that this new, more targeted, less risky approach to contraception will dominate the state-of-the-art, birth-control drugs.

Vaginal Rings

The future of contraception lies in new ways of influencing human hormones—the postpill era. This very active research area promises many new developments and breakthroughs in the next few decades.

One new approach to hormonal contraception is the vaginal ring, which contains and slowly releases a progestin hormone that prevents pregnancy. A synthetic plastic (Silastic) ring is inserted by the woman high into her vagina after each menstruation. She wears it 3 weeks, removes it, has her period, and inserts it again.

The major advantage of the vaginal ring over the pill is that it gives a month's protection with one insertion—no pill-popping (or possibly forgetting to take the pill) for 21 days every month. And unlike certain hormonal implants on the horizon, the ring is controlled by the woman herself!

The Vaginal Sponge

An ancient contraceptive method, used by Egyptian women more than 3,000 years ago, was redesigned and redeveloped by modern science, tested for 5 years, and finally approved by the Federal Food and Drug Administration in 1983. It is the contraceptive sponge, and it challenges other barrier-type contraceptives—the condom, the diaphragm, and foam—because it is 85 percent effective for 24 hours, is easy to insert, does not need individual fitting (one size fits all women), is disposable, and is available over the counter. All this for a modest $8-million research price tag.

The small ovalshaped sponge, made of polyurethane, is 2 inches in diameter, 1 inch thick, and weighs about 1/4 of an ounce. When inserted into the vagina (much easier to do than with a diaphragm), it fits snugly over the cervix and prevents the sperm from passing into the uterus. The sponge is also permeated with a spermicide, Nonoxynol 9. Once in, a woman can relax for 24 hours.

The contraceptive sponges that Egyptian women used were natural sponges gathered from the sea and then soaked in citric juice—a natural spermicide because of its high acidity (how effective it was is anyone's guess). So sexual history repeats itself—this time with FDA approval.

A Male Pill

There has been much talk about an oral contraceptive for men, but it will be some years, perhaps another decade, before tested and certified drugs will be behind the counter at your local drugstore. Current research offers no final answers, but it does indicate how sperm production eventually will be inhibited in the male testes—by some method of enzyme or hormone regulation.

One promising male contraceptive under active study is an import from China—the drug, gossypol. In the 1950s, Chinese scientists wanted to know why there were extremely low birth rates in a particular region of China. Eventually they found out that the people of the region used only crude cottonseed oil for cooking. They further discovered that the active compound in the oil was gossypol, and that it was causing the male infertility.

Recent research has discovered that gossypol selectively inhibits an important enzyme (lactate dehydrogenase-x) which plays a critical role in the metabolism of sperm cells and sperm-generating cells. The best aspect of gossypol is that it is selective and has a minimal effect on a man's sex hormone levels or his sex drive.

Chinese testing of thousands of men has demonstrated that the drug has a 99 percent success rate in causing male infertility, but it sometimes produces side effects of fatigue, loss of appetite, and lower potassium levels. Further research into the drug's biochemical mechanism will determine its long-term effects on men and whether or not it is safe. The fact that gossypol occurs naturally in the plentiful cotton plant would give this drug a real economic advantage over high-tech synthesized hormones.

Another promising agent for male (as well as female) contraception is a synthesized brain hormone called LHRH-A. This hormone imitator is a modified version of the brain's natural luteinizing hormone-releasing hormone that has major control over reproductive events in men and women. Natural LHRH causes the pituitary gland to secrete hormones (called gonadotropins) that flow through the bloodstream to the testes in men and the ovaries in women.

For men these hormones regulate the production of sperm and the sex hormones, especially testosterone. Researchers have found that the synthesized hormone (which regulates the release of these other hormones) acts as an antifertility agent when administered in amounts 100 times more potent than the natural form. In other words, in large amounts LHRH-A does the opposite of what it usually does: It inhibits sperm production, reduces sperm vigor and movement, and lowers testosterone levels in the blood.

Before this form of male contraception is viable, however, there are some problems that must be solved. Some men experienced a reduced sex drive and others became impotent as a result of taking the synthetic hormone—the result of lowered testosterone levels. A few men even had hot flashes like those women experience after menopause. Some researchers think that a combination of LHRH-A with testosterone might avoid these side effects, but further research is needed and the results cannot be predicted.

There may be no definite answers for several years. Indeed, the final form of the male contraceptive is open to question. It may not be a pill at all, but instead come in nasal spray form so that the nasal passages could readily absorb the drug into the bloodstream. Or it may be in the form of a lozenge that would be placed under the tongue and absorbed.

The time will no doubt come when women *and* men share the risks of contraception. *His* or *her* month of responsibility for taking the pill (or the nasal spray or the lozenge) may be the future reality. Or it may be all the man's responsibility. Better choices can be made based on the man's or the woman's medical history. There will be more freedom of choice for men and women once the male pill (or its equivalent) becomes available.

THE NEW FERTILITY

Fallopian Detour

Babies conceived outside the human body in a laboratory dish (in vitro fertilization—IVF for short) now number in the hundreds and in the next few decades will number in the thousands and tens of thousands. The medical techniques and know-how for this out-of-body, glass-dish fertilization, along with all the related medical preparations of the mother-to-be, are constantly being refined and the success rate is increasing.

Eventually IVF will make pregnancy possible for several hundred thousand infertile couples—especially in cases where the woman has blocked, diseased, or removed fallopian tubes, which prevent the ovum from traveling down its usual passageway and rendezvousing with the sperm.

Medical technology has set up a fallopian detour that takes the egg from the ovary through a hollow suction needle, then into a laboratory dish for a few days (where it meets the sperm, becomes fertilized, and divides a few times), and finally through the vagina into the uterus, via a catheter, where it will attach itself to the uterine wall and begin a very much desired pregnancy. The real beauty about successful out-of-body conception is that there are never any unwanted babies.

Gathering Eggs

Gathering tiny human egg cells (ova are about 1/25 of an inch in diameter) for out-of-body fertilization is a delicate process that requires precise timing and the use of high-tech medical instruments. If the eggs are taken too early from the follicles on the ovary surface, they will be immature and cannot be fertilized. If, however, they are fully ripe before the doctors attempt to gather them, spontaneous ovulation

---

230

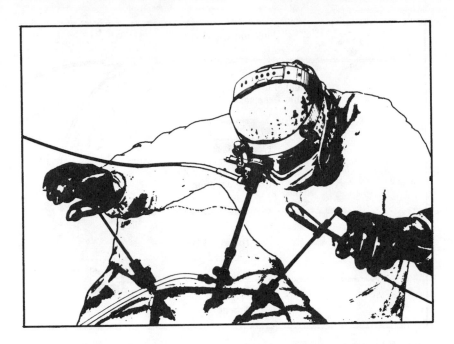

A surgeon removes a human egg from the ovary of a patient—the first procedure necessary for in vitro fertilization. The instrument in his left hand manipulates the ovary; the middle instrument is the eyepiece and light source; and the right hand holds the aspirator that removes the ova. Courtesy Richard Wolf Medical Instruments Corporation.

occurs—the eggs burst from their follicle nests, and are lost in the fallopian tubes.

It was Dr. Patrick Steptoe, the English gynecologist, who developed the egg-removal techniques that led to the world's first out-of-body-conceived baby, Louise Brown. He and his colleague, physiologist Robert Edwards, still prefer that a woman ovulate naturally, without the use of Pergonal (a combination of synthesized hormones), which other reproductive clinics are using to control ovulation—the maturity time *and* the number of eggs.

This controlled ovulation method was responsible for the first in vitro fertilized baby in the United States, Elizabeth Jordan Carr, under the medical care of Howard and Georgeanna Jones at Eastern Virginia Medical School, in Norfolk. After more than 40 failures at pregnancy with the natural ovulation method before egg extraction, they decided to use Pergonal, which led to the first full-term pregnancy in the United States. This process eventually led to a 22 percent pregnancy success rate for externally fertilized eggs, and this compares with a 25 percent chance of normal fertility during any one cycle.

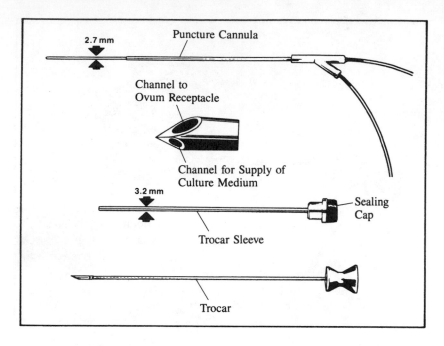

Human egg-gathering tools designed by Dr. Patrick Steptoe, the English gynecologist who delivered Louise Brown, the firstborn in vitro baby. The tiny ovum (about 1/25 of an inch in diameter) is drawn up through a hollow needle (center) by delicate suction. Courtesy Richard Wolf Medical Instruments Corporation.

How do doctors gather these human eggs that are smaller than the period under the question mark at the end of this sentence? Most important, they need enhanced eyes and hands to carry out this microsurgery, and sophisticated optical-fiber instruments which make human egg gathering possible.

Just before ovulation, a small incision is made in the abdomen near the navel and a laparoscope (a thin, flexible, magnifying tube with its own fiber-optic lighting system and a viewing eyepiece for the physician) is inserted and used to examine the ovaries and determine if the ripe eggs are about ready to burst from the ovarian walls. If they are, a hollow suction needle (1/29 of an inch in diameter) is guided into the ovarian follicle where the egg is about to burst forth, and the egg is sucked up inside and held until it is released and placed in the laboratory dish filled with a special culture—a temporary artificial womb. The suction of the hollow needle is so delicate that it could not even lift a feather.

Out-of-Body Wombs

True "test-tube" babies do not exist. The laboratory-fertilized egg that is implanted in the uterus spends less than 3 days in the glass dish— less than one hundredth of its full gestation time. Artificial wombs that could sustain and nurture human embryos and fetuses from fertilization to full term are possible in the future, but they are probably several decades away. The easiest part of the whole process, out-of-the-body fertilization and embryo implantation, has been accomplished over the last several years, but it has *not* been easy. The world's first baby conceived outside the human body was the first success out of more than 80 unsuccessful attempts by English Drs. Patrick Steptoe and Robert Edwards.

Before an out-of-body womb can be constructed, a tremendous amount of knowledge must be learned about the uterus, the placenta, and the complex hormonal system that helps these organs support and nurture human gestation.

Why create out-of-the-body wombs when nature does an adequate job most of the time, and with new prenatal medical techniques, more of the time?

If and when the technology for out-of-body wombs exists, it may offer a safer gestation and birth for certain mothers and their babies. It would make prenatal medical care, in which there have been several breakthroughs of late, even safer, more effective, and able to treat prenatal problems that are untreatable today.

Certain controlled prenatal diets could make the fetal brain develop at a faster rate. After all, growth in the uterus is in large part controlled by the mother's body size, and this limitation could be removed with artificial wombs. Advanced prenatal technologies could help procreate a larger number of high-intelligence individuals that would be equal to the ever-more-difficult challenges the future will bring.

We should not close this door, even though the many ethical questions must be confronted, for it may lead to no less than the survival of humankind.

Embryo Banks

Techniques for freezing, storing, and thawing unfertilized and fertilized human eggs are steadily improving, and there is little doubt that ova banks and embryo banks will join sperm banks within the next few

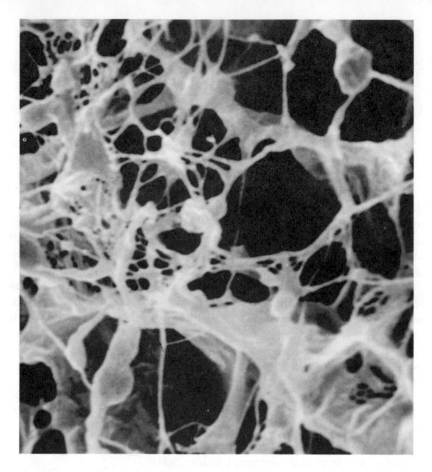

Cervical mucus (above) constantly changes during a woman's cycle because of hormonal variations. The success of sperm penetration and conception is dependent on the composition of the mucus. The degree of ferning of a dried mucus sample (facing page) can help indicate the best time for artificial insemination. Courtesy Ronald G. Cohn, Syntex Research; Dr. Lourens J. D. Zaneveld, University of Illinois.

decades. In fact, London's Royal Free Hospital, among others, has been freezing embryos with the hope of preserving them until such time as reliable techniques are available to thaw, revive, and implant them in a hormonally receptive uterus—and not necessarily the biological mother's; any healthy uterus will do. A breakthrough came in 1983, when Australian doctors successfully implanted an in vitro fertilized embryo that had been frozen for 4 months. In 1984, two healthy babies were born from in vitro fertilized, frozen embryos.

These embryo banks could provide deep-freeze "savings accounts"

COMING INTO PLAY:

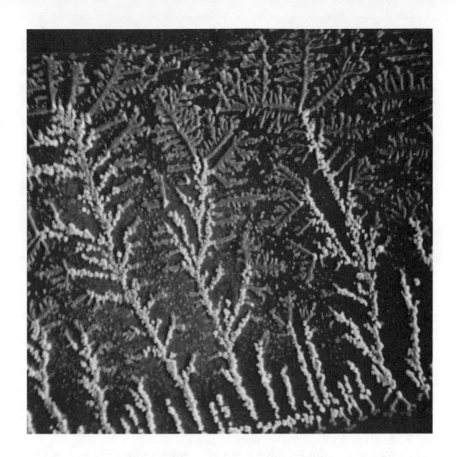

for couples and broaden their reproductive options. What kind of options? A couple could opt to store an embryo (we're talking about just a few cell divisions, about 8 cells) as a hedge against the time either of them might be sterilized. Career women who might want their children later in life could be helped by such banks, and the high-risk factor of late conceptions would be lowered. Also, such embryonic storage might someday allow genetic-health screening, depending on the couple's hereditary history, thus helping to insure the unborn's quality of life.

The ethical considerations are complex and controversial. For example, what if the parents of a frozen embryo were killed in an automobile accident and their only child, a 21-year-old daughter, decided to give "birth" to her own parents' baby, her own brother or sister!

Despite these controversial issues, any medical technology that promises new reproductive choices and less suffering for the parents or their offspring must be vigorously and thoroughly discussed. Embryo banks may provide future solutions to problems that do not yet exist.

The 1984 case of Mario and Elsa Rios, parents of two frozen embryos preserved by Australian doctors at the Queen Victoria Medical Center in Melbourne, demonstrates what kind of bizarre, real-life dilemmas can result from the new technology. The couple died in a plane crash, leaving no instructions in their wills about the fate of the frozen embryos they left behind. The world press covered the story, and a public debate followed. The fact that the frozen embryos had little chance of surviving the thawing process, which was a pioneering technique at the time, was given little attention.

Freezing Sperm . . . and Time

Sperm banks proliferated in the 1960s, partly because men wanted a hedge against vasectomy. Today there are some 25 sperm banks in the United States that hold frozen sperm samples from thousands of donors. The most famous sperm bank, in California, has exclusively as its donors Nobel Prize winners.

The semen sample is carefully screened, analyzed, and prepared before freezing. It is mixed with part of an egg yolk, gylcerol, and antibiotics—a sort of antifreeze for protecting the sperm. Then it is put in a glass ampule and stored in liquid nitrogen at a temperature as cold as −384 degrees F for later use.

Frozen sperm samples have been known to retain their potency for as long as 10 years, but this time varies greatly from one sample to another. Usually, however, frozen sperm retain some 60 percent of their potency for about 5 years.

When sperm is frozen, so too, in a sense, is time. Dead men have been known to father children with their frozen sperm.

Sperm Assist

Artificial insemination (AI) in humans has been going on for about 200 years, and more than 1 million people have been conceived this way worldwide. Some 10,000 to 20,000 babies are born each year in the United States as a result of this conception method. Most often couples choose artificial insemination because the male either has a low sperm count or is sterile. If he has a low count, his more hearty sperm can be separated from the less active and introduced into the vagina. If the male is sterile, a donor's sperm is collected in a syringe and introduced into the woman's cervix through the vagina for 3 or 4 days around the time of ovulation. Another technique often used is to place the donor ejaculate in a cervical cap—a small plastic cup—put it in the cervix and leave it there for about 24 hours. Donor sperm is also used in AI if the male partner carries some hereditary disorder which the couple do not wish to pass on to their children.

The chances of a healthy, fertile woman becoming pregnant from the artificial insemination of donor sperm are very good—most women become pregnant within 3 to 6 months. If the cervical cap technique is used, the odds are even better—about equal to those for a fertile couple. Pregnancy via this method is all but assured for the fertile female; it just may take some women a few more months to conceive.

And what are the results of these sperm assists that lead to conception? Usually proud, happy parents of boys, not girls. Probably this is because the male Y chromosome is lighter than the female X chromosome. When semen is stored in a container, the top third contains 80 percent male Y chromosomes; the middle third about 50 percent Y and 50 percent X; and the bottom third about 80 percent X, female chromosomes. But the girls, it appears, are catching up. Their sex is dominating the out-of-body fertilizations that are increasing in number.

Sowing the Earth and Beyond

The human seeds—ova and spermatozoa—necessary for the next generation could be held in the palm of your hand; or, for that matter, within a microscopic ark that could be sent just about anywhere in the solar system.

The Slow Journey

The fallopian tubes (oviducts) transport the ovum into the uterus each month. Estrogen secretion just before the mense causes the hairlike cilia to proliferate and increase their beating action, which sweeps the egg toward the uterus, a journey that takes about 3 days at a speed of 1/16 of an inch per hour.

Safety in Numbers

There are about 2 million human female eggs (ova) in both ovaries at birth and about 300,000 survive to puberty, but only 450 or so of these mature and are expelled during a woman's reproductive years.

The ovum is the largest cell that the human body produces. Even so, it is only about 1 millimeter (1/25 of an inch) in diameter, about the size of the period at the end of this sentence, just visible to the human eye.

When 200 Million Are Too Few

Two hundred million sperm would seem to be enough to keep the birth rate of the United States going (at 1980 rates) for over 60 years if every one of them found and penetrated an ovum.

If a man's ejaculate from orgasm held that many sperm, however, it would be considered a low sperm count and probably too few to

Two hundred million sperm in a man's ejaculate indicate a low sperm count; at least 400 million are usually necessary to impregnate a fertile woman. Courtesy Ronald G. Cohn, Syntex Research.

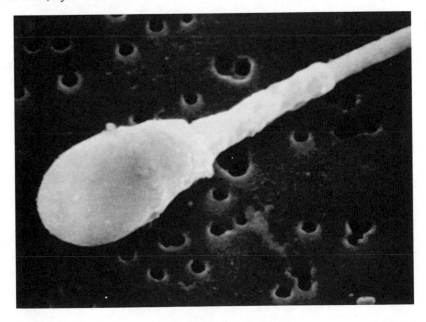

COMING INTO PLAY:

impregnate a fertile woman. Add another 200 million healthy sperm and you're likely to have offspring.

The Semen Solution

Semen coagulates during or just after ejaculation, and then liquifies 5 to 20 minutes after it is in the vagina. This protects and immobilizes the spermatozoa for a short time, which may help conserve their energy for the migration to the ovum, or perhaps allows them to enter the cervix without coming into contact with the vaginal fluid that can adversely affect sperm mobility if it is too acid.

Over 90 percent of semen is water and less than 2 percent is sperm. The average amount of ejaculate is a little less than a teaspoonful, which totals some 4.5 gallons in a man's lifetime—about 1,040 cubic inches of the stuff.

A Slow Swim

Sperm cells are the smallest cells of the human body—only 1/500 of an inch in length. Each spermatozoan has a head, neck, and tail as distinct parts, and it is the head—only 1/10 of the total length—that carries the male's genetic message in 23 chromosomes and determines the sex of the child.

When male orgasm occurs during female ovulation, spermatozoa travel in a straight, rotating line through the cervix into the uterus, and then through the uterus into the fallopian tubes where they may rendezvous with an egg (ovum)—a distance of about 6 or 7 inches, not counting the vagina.

The fastest sperm, under ideal conditions, can swim 8 to 9 inches every hour; the slowest about 2 to 3 inches. The most likely time for conception would therefore be about 1 hour after ejaculation. At an average of the 2 speeds, it would take a sperm 4,163 years to swim the Atlantic Ocean, from New York to London.

The Good Race

Some 10 to 30 billion sperm cells are formed in the male testes each month, but most of them never have a chance to swim the good race. Every ejaculation contains an average of 400 *million* and some may be

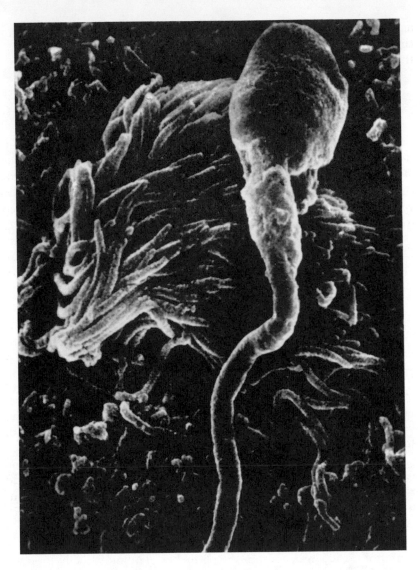

A sperm swimming up the fallopian tube toward its rendezvous with an ovum. Its average speed is about 5 inches (12.7 centimeters) an hour. If a sperm could swim the Atlantic Ocean at this speed, from New York to London, it would take more than 4,100 years. Courtesy NOVA and National Institutes of Health, Research Resources Information Center.

as high as 600 million. If a young man and woman have intercourse 3 times a week, every month at least 4.8 billion spermatozoa are given their freedom—more than the human population of the earth.

What Lethargic Sperm Lack

In 1982 scientists at the National Institute of Child Health and Human Development discovered the first known biochemical cause of male infertility—an enzyme deficiency that causes motionless or sluggish sperm. Without an adequate amount of this enzyme (protein-carboxyl methylase—PCM, for short), sperm never get off the starting line to compete in the great race to the egg.

Researchers discovered that infertile men had only one fourth the PCM enzyme activity that fertile men had, and that this lower PCM level was similar to that of vasectomized men.

The testes have one of the highest concentrations of PCM in the human body, but the enzyme is also known to be involved in controlling the movement of white blood cells and bacteria. A complex series of biochemical reactions controls all cell movement in the human body, and PCM activity is just one component. But if PCM is out of balance, so too are other components of the body's complex biochemistry.

Molecular-level research has great promise for infertility disorders. Apparent defects in sperm—for example, a flaw in the tail of sperm—account for a very small number of male infertility cases, and so this discovery can lead to a treatment for male infertility as well as to a breakthrough male contraceptive.

Think of it: "Darling," says Marsha to John. "Don't forget your pill tonight!"

Computer-Designed Sperm

Besides the research on why some sperm can't swim, other studies are concentrating on computer analyses of sperm—the complex interrelationships between their shape, motion, and speed. Sperm that swim in a corkscrew motion, for example, are fastest if they also have flat heads. What will any of this prove? For one, possible knowledge for improving techniques and conception rates for artificial insemination. What else? Better sperm "sprung" from the human mind. Better sperm for better babies.

INSIDE THE WOMB

First Swim

Our first swim is a submerged float rather than an Australian crawl. We all float, turn, move our limbs while suspended in the amniotic fluid of our mothers' wombs before birth. This first swim lasts many months, during all but the early weeks of pregnancy. No wonder most young babies take so well to the bathtub and swimming pool waters.

The amniotic swimming pool is contained in a transparent sac composed of the inner fetal membrane, the amnion. Together they are commonly known as the "bag of waters" and form an in utero vessel that is the unborn's entire world. This vessel provides: shock absorption and protection from injury; regulation of temperature; a barrier against infection; room to grow, move about, and exercise; a reservoir for fetal waste products, mostly urine; and a two-way route for exchange of fluids and hormones through the membrane wall—normally all the comforts a womb has to afford. About the fourth month of pregnancy, the unborn begins to taste the waters that form its liquid world by swallowing the amniotic fluid. Result: the smallest hiccups known to human life.

The Amniotic Ambiance

What is the recipe for amniotic fluid besides its transparent and almost colorless water? Some shedded skin cells, a few white blood cells, a small quantity of albumin (a simple protein), small amounts of hormones, organic and inorganic salts, a pinch of calcium, fetal urine, and other liquids secreted through the unborn's skin.

The amount of amniotic fluid increases during the pregnancy and is, on the average, a bit more than 1 quart (1 liter) at full term, although up to 2 quarts (1.9 liters) is not unusual.

Much of the fluid is formed and absorbed directly through the amniotic membranes. The total volume is probably also regulated by the membranes, so that when volume increases, pressure rises, resulting in an increase in fluid absorption, which returns the volume to normal.

As the fetus grows, the amount of fluid increases, and it is also continually absorbed and renewed. The fluid is therefore completely replaced every 3 hours. For the near-term baby, this amounts to slightly over 1 quart every 3 hours and almost 8½ quarts each day of replaced fluid. How much does this add up to over the last 7 months of pregnancy? Almost 1,800 quarts (about 450 U.S. gallons) of amniotic fluid are replaced, an amount that would weigh 3,600 pounds—some 528 times the baby's birth weight.

Womb Hearts

No heart beats for the first 4 weeks of human life. Then, about 1 month after conception—when the embryo is about ¼ of an inch in size—a simple one-chambered heart beats its first beat—the first of about 3 billion in its lifetime. This early embryonic heart thumps about 65 beats each minute, compared to 72 for the average adult at rest and to its own high 140 beats just before birth. Sixty-five beats each minute is some 9 times faster than the heartbeat of a giant whale.

During the third week of human gestation, the silent heart is just 2 tiny tubes sheathed by muscle cells. Toward the end of this week, these tubes begin to fuse into a single chamber. In another 7 days, this tiny heart will pump blood through the few rudimentary arteries and veins.

This tiny human heart is found next to the developing brain, but it is gradually pushed lower toward its final position in the body as the mouth grows between it and the brain. The new heart, after all, will eventually have to beat on its own and depend on the mouth to sustain it. During these early weeks of pregnancy, our hearts are *almost* in our mouths!

What size are our newly beating hearts? About ¹⁄₄₀ of an inch, not much larger than a visible speck of dust, but still 5 times larger than the fertilized human egg from which it grew. Even a hummingbird's heart is larger.

Beyond the Genital Ridge

During the first 6 weeks of pregnancy, there are no distinguishing male or female characteristics in the embryo. Even though the baby's sex has been genetically determined at time of conception, the sexes are physically alike at this time and have the same sex glands and organs. Embryos have both male and female genital ducts.

About the seventh week of development, the genital ridge (genital tubercle) begins to secrete testosterone in the male and estrogen in the female. Sexual differentiation begins and becomes readily apparent about the tenth week. The clitoris and penis develop from this genital ridge.

The male and female hormones are critical in normal prenatal sexual development. Experiments have shown that large-dose injections of the male hormone in female animals produce male sexual organs even though the fetus is female. If the testes are removed in a male fetus, female sexual organs will develop.

In humans, such sex errors are the result of genetic abnormalities. It is the genetic message, after all—male (XY) or female (XX)—that determines whether testosterone or estrogen will be secreted from the genital ridge and begin sexual differentiation just before the second month of pregnancy. But it is possible for a fertilized egg to carry the wrong combination of sex chromosomes. Such genetic errors can result in XXY males—sterile males with small penises and testicles who also have girlish breasts and often exhibit psychosexual behavior disorders. This affliction is known as Klinefelter's syndrome.

Another sexual error involves a missing chromosome; it is known as Turner's syndrome. In this condition, the female's ovaries are missing and she is sterile. Also, she is sexually infantile in appearance. The infantile appearance resulting from this syndrome, however, can be successfully treated with female sex hormones.

When the hormones start to flow from the genital ridge, we hope the genetic message is heard loud and clear. Otherwise there can be real sexual problems—such as boys with uteruses and girls with clitorises as large as small penises.

Prenatal Sex

By the sixteenth week of gestation, the unborn's male or female organs are basically formed and sex determination is visually possible. Hair also appears on the head. Four weeks later, the legs lengthen appreciably and the distance from the umbilical cord to the pubic region increases. From the thirty-sixth week to the fortieth week, the male's small smooth scrotum grows larger, becoming wrinkled and pendulous, and the testes descend into it from the inguinal canals. The female's labia majora also become well developed during this month. From a physical neuter to unborn boy or girl in just 24 weeks.

This is prenatal sex—genetically set, and for the most part beyond everyone's control, including the doctor's.

Early I.D.

Two months after conception—when the fetus is 1.4 inches (3.5 centimeters) long and weighs only 1/15 of an ounce (2 grams)—the eyes, ears, nose, and mouth become recognizable. At this point in gestation, fingers and toes are also formed—the unborn has fingerprints, but the fingernails will not appear for another 4 months.

These tiny fingerprints are unique and will remain so for the rest of the individual's life. Their whorls are different than those of the other 4.6 billion people living on earth.

Womb Weight Boom

A newborn baby weighing in at 7 pounds (3.17 kilograms) has increased its weight about 10,000 times since conception. This is the largest weight gain in human life. Even after 4 weeks of gestation, the embryo weighs slightly less than 1/70 of an ounce (0.4 gram).

Imaging the Unborn

The idea of seeing into the human womb and watching the fetus develop (and in later stages kick, hiccup, or suck a thumb) may have been the fantasy of some pregnant women over the centuries, but in the last decade it has become a medical reality.

Ultrasound (also called ultrasonography) is one of the most important recent breakthroughs in diagnosing the unborn—and is much safer than X rays. This high technology is based on beaming high-frequency sound waves (20,000 to millions of vibrations a second, above the range of the human ear) through the mother's body to the fetus, where they bounce off as echoes, reflected whenever they meet body matter of different densities. They return to a receiver, recorded, and translated into an image on a TV screen. Finally, doctors interpret the fuzzy, hardly prime-time images.

Ultrasound was first used in the 1950s to estimate the gestation age of the fetus and to confirm the suspicion that there might be a multiple birth. Today the technology of ultrasonography has advanced to a remarkable degree and, along with amniocentesis and into-the-uterus fiber-optic fetoscopy, accounts for the prenatal diagnosis of some 200 defects and other problem conditions in the unborn, not including chromosomal disorders.

Through the use of ultrasound technology, it is now possible to detect such fetal abnormalities as limb defects, enlarged heart, fallopian-tube pregnancies, too much or too little amniotic fluid, an obstructed urethra, obstructed kidneys, abnormally small or large heads, or a complete absence of a brain and a spinal cord.

In addition, ultrasonic imaging—which generates multiple-pulse echo systems that are activated in sequence—creates an ultrasonic motion picture. Doctors can see pulsations in the umbilical vessels, the placenta, or the fetal heart.

About midterm in pregnancy, the 4 chambers of the fetal heart can be observed, often down to the detail of imaging cardiac valve function. Even the unborn's heart rate can be measured. Respiratory movements can be seen, fingers counted (important because extra digits usually signify a serious birth-defect syndrome), and eye movements recorded. Changes in fetal eye movements can indicate whether or not the unborn is neurologically normal.

Contemporary ultrasound does have its limits of resolution—it can image nothing smaller than about 1/13 of an inch (2 millimeters). This therefore excludes early embryonic imaging. After all, at 6 weeks, the embryo is only 0.5 of an inch (1.25 centimeters) long, so the earliest useful imaging and diagnosis can be accomplished is at about 10 weeks, when the fetus is a bit over 2 inches in length. No doubt better resolution and accuracy of diagnosis at even earlier stages of gestation will come about in the next few decades. It is likely that most fetuses with physical malformations will be diagnosed by the twentieth week of pregnancy. And there may come a day when mom and dad can see their unborn baby's first heartbeat, first wince, first smile!

Womb Zoom

Ultrasound gives an overall view of the gestating uterus without actually entering the body. Fetoscopy, however, zooms in for close-up portraits of the fetus and its surroundings, but to do this doctors actually enter the uterus with a fiber-optic endoscope through a small incision (about 1/8 of an inch, 3 millimeters) in the abdomen. Doctors carefully guide the endoscope by watching the ultrasonic big picture, so fetoscopy depends on ultrasound. Because this is a surgically invasive procedure, it is more risky than ultrasound, but the images are clear and detailed, and fetoscopy can actually obtain fetal blood or skin

COMING INTO PLAY:

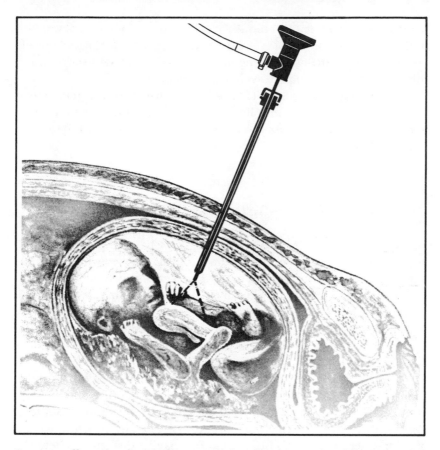

Fetoscopy allows the physician to zoom in for closeup portraits of the fetus and its environment, inspecting a field of view less than a square inch. Blood and skin samples can also be obtained for laboratory study. This is a GieBen Model. Courtesy Richard Wolf Medical Instruments Corporation.

samples for thorough laboratory analysis. By entering the womb with this well-lit, zoom-lens probe, smaller areas of the fetus—eyes, ears, mouth, joints, genitalia—can be examined. Because of the optical system, the area examined is usually limited to 4 square centimeters—less than a square inch.

The blood and skin sampling capability of fetoscopy is of great importance to prenatal medicine. Blood diseases, including hemophilia, have been diagnosed in the unborn. A blood sample is obtained by guiding the probe to the umbilical vein on the inside surface of the placenta, and a very thin blood-sampling needle (less than 1/60 of an inch in diameter) is inserted to collect the blood.

Fetoscopy is a recent technique that is performed in only a few major medical centers, but it holds great promise beyond its diagnostic role because it can actually enter the uterus. In the not-too-distant future, this technology will be performing fetal medicine. Medications can be directly administered, and eventually cell transplants and genetic material can be introduced into fetal tissues or the bloodstream to treat genetic or acquired diseases of the unborn. The womb will become a mini operating room.

Before-Birth Brain Surgery

Brain surgery in the womb? Yes. Surgeons have implanted runoff, stainless steel valves (shunts) in the skulls of fetuses with abnormal amounts of cerebrospinal fluid in the 4 spaces between the brain lobes (a condition known as hydrocephalus). This is a life-threatening condition for the fetus because the engorged spaces swell and press on the brain, halting its growth. More than half of all such fetuses are still-born, and those that survive have serious brain damage and medical problems for life.

Now, by diagnosing and treating the problem before birth, severe brain damage and facial disfigurement in the unborn may be prevented. The first 3 unborn patients benefited from this brain surgery. One of them has a normal appearance as a result, even though his growth is delayed and his brain anatomy may be distorted. There is a gestation time limit for such in-the-uterus surgery. Midterm, about 4 months, is the earliest that such surgery can be performed, and so the damage done up to that point is beyond treatment for now.

The surgery—which requires the surgeon to push a needle through the muscles of the abdominal wall into the amniotic cavity and then through the fetal skull—requires about 20 minutes. The fetus's head, however, is a small target—smaller than a tennis ball, about 2 inches (5 centimeters) in diameter. And the ultrasound imaging system is not your usual-quality TV image. The unborn baby is also a moving target, even though sedation can help diminish this problem somewhat. Still, doctors have always come within 1/5 of an inch (0.5 centimeter) of their target in the fetal brain.

The next 2 decades will see even more dramatic advances in treating the unborn patient, and even earlier treatment will be possible. The more distant future promises a rebuilding of the fetally damaged brains of infants, with brain tissue transplants and even some minicomputer implants.

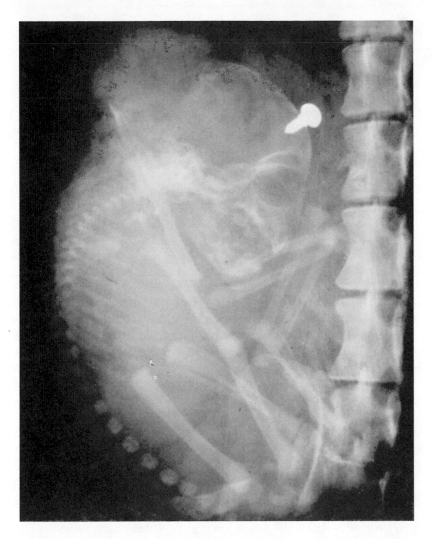

An X ray of a fetal monkey shows the implanted shunt valve used to drain off abnormal amounts of cerebrospinal fluid that cause brain damage before birth. This prenatal surgery has been successfully performed on the brains of unborns still in the womb. Courtesy National Institute of Child Health and Human Development.

The Half-Born Patient

Other in-the-womb surgery on the unborn includes treatment of a blocked urethra in a fetus by inserting a 4.7-inch-long catheter through the woman's abdomen into the fetus's bladder. The catheter draws off the dangerous buildup of urine that can permanently damage kidneys and cause death. Anchor-shaped to keep it in place, the catheter extends from the fetal bladder through the abdominal wall and out to the amniotic fluid.

One unborn patient with a blocked urinary tract was treated in a different—indeed, a historic—way. In this case, the urine buildup was too far advanced to be treated with the insertion of a catheter, so the surgeons made incisions in the abdomen and uterus, drew the lower half of the fetus from the uterus, and surgically extended and rerouted the tubes that carry urine from the kidneys to the bladder. The tubes were brought to the outside of the body, and the urine therefore avoided the blockage and flowed harmlessly into the amniotic fluid.

This was the first open-womb surgery ever performed. The pregnancy continued normally after the operation on the "half-born" patient in the twenty-first week, and the baby was *fully* born in the thirty-fifth week of pregnancy. Shortly after birth, it became apparent that the baby's lungs had been irreversibly damaged as a result of the blockage before the surgery was performed. The baby's lungs could not support life, and it died 9 hours after birth. Despite the afterbirth death of the patient, the state-of-the-art prenatal surgery was successful in correcting the diagnosed problem. It was just diagnosed and corrected too late.

Successful surgery on a fetus—whether wholly inside the uterus or partly outside—points the way for surgical treatment of many life-threatening prenatal conditions. Those whose tiny bodies experience the operating room's air will be a special group of babies that were born one and a half times.

MOMS AND NEWBORNS

Mom's Monitoring

Mothers-to-be who want to find out how their unborn baby is doing, from the twenty-eighth week of pregnancy on, now have a "measuring stick." A study at the University of Pennsylvania showed that the unborn's general state of health can usually be determined by the number of fetal movements in any 12-hour period each day. If there are 10 or more movements during this period, mom can be fairly certain that baby is healthy. The results of the study of 150 women show that fewer than 10 movements strongly indicate some kind of prenatal complication or the possibility of stillbirth.

Pregnant women can therefore monitor their unborn's health by making and using a simple chart. If there is little movement for 2 or more days, get to an obstetrician.

Hypnosis for Moms-to-Be

It has been more than 25 years since the American Medical Association went on record to say that hypnosis "has a recognized place in medicine." Much has happened in that quarter century. In the area of obstetrics alone, hypnosis is commonly used to relieve some of the side effects of pregnancy (for example, metallic taste in mouth, crawly skin sensation, or a general feeling of invasion), and for making labor and delivery less painful and healthier experiences.

Doctor advocates urge even wider use of hypnosis in obstetrics because clinical experience has demonstrated it provides real comfort to expectant mothers in all phases of pregnancy and childbirth. Most of the women who go through the training sessions during the last half of their pregnancies can stand up and walk about during the initial stages of labor, and then can walk into the delivery room for the birth. After delivery, they walk out of the delivery OR with the new baby in their arms.

Only a few patients (about 5 percent) can be treated by hypnosis alone, but even for those women who need something more, the training can reduce the amount of drugs they need to about one quarter of the normal dosage.

The training sessions teach patients the techniques of self-hypnosis. By learning progressive relaxation techniques, women can induce a trance that puts their minds in a beautiful place or previous enjoyable experience.

In most cases, this is not done at actual delivery because doctors believe women should be fully aware of their birth experience. But hypnosis can be used for the incision made during an episiotomy (enlargement of the vulvar orifice for obstetrical purposes). For this procedure, the patient is given a choice between a local anesthetic and a mental trip to her own "pleasant place." Most women decide to take the mental vacation.

The power and benefit of hypnosis is no better demonstrated than by the fact that many women have had successful cesarean-section surgery without any anesthesia whatsoever. Would that all of us could find such a "pleasant place" during stressful times!

A Measured Labor

The frequent pelvic examinations during labor, to determine the degree of cervical dilation, have several drawbacks. They are often uncomfortable for the expectant mother; they can cause infections; and they keep busy medical personnel scurrying between patients, wasting valuable time traveling up and down the corridors.

These manual pelvic exams, however, may soon be a part of medical history. A new device has been developed by researchers at Case Western Reserve University that records cervical dilation during labor. This tiny, lightweight, ultrasonic device is called a cervimeter sensor, and it measures only 1/25 inch × 1/25 inch × 1/5 inch. It is attached by clips to opposite sides of the cervix during the early stage of labor and gives data on the changes of cervical dilation through all stages of labor. Its measurements of cervical dilation are more exact than manual examinations, and it will be especially useful in high-risk pregnancies, along with other measuring devices (for example, one to measure the fetal heart rate), to help doctors evaluate the progress of labor and prepare for a possible high-risk delivery. During testing of the cervimeter, it was found that only one recording each second was necessary for adequate information, although it is capable of continuous measurements. Even if just the one measurement per second is recorded, an impressive total of cervical soundings is chalked up during labor. If a first-pregnancy labor lasts 16 hours (not at all unusual), the medical record will show almost 58,000 cervical measurements!

Blondes Wait Longer

Blondes definitely do not have more fun when it comes to childbirth. Why? Because, on the average, brunettes deliver their babies slightly sooner than do blondes.

Boys in a Hurry

Boys are born sooner than girls, on the average. That's what a Scottish study from the University of Aberdeen concluded after studying some 52,000 births over a period of 28 years—from 1961 to 1979. The reasons are not clear, but doctors suggest that the higher weight of male babies may trigger earlier birth. Or could it be that males are often more impatient than females, even before birth?

Early Arrivals

About 7 percent of all babies born in the United States each year are premature low-birth-weight infants. This means that out of just over 4 million babies born, almost a quarter of a million are "preemies"—a birth weight of 5.5 pounds or less. Sadly, these low-weight babies account for 75 percent of all newborn deaths and 50 percent of all brain-damaged infants. But there is cause for optimism. Infant deaths have declined rapidly since the mid-1960s. Intensive neonatal care (and the accompanying technological advances during the last 20 years) has resulted in greatly improved survival rates for these babies, and prospects are very bright for additional breakthroughs during the next decade.

A baby that arrives early is a high risk because it is still a fetus—a fetus outside the womb—not a full-term baby. About half of all premature babies have a serious, life-threatening heart defect, where a small temporary artery that bypasses the inactive lungs of the unborn child does not close because of early birth.

Half of the preemies weighing under 3.3 pounds suffer from brain hemorrhaging, and many die. Blindness often results if the minute blood vessels of the eyes receive just a bit too much oxygen from life-support systems. Other common threats to these tiny newborns are: deficiency of sugar in the blood (hypoglycemia); jaundice caused by an underdeveloped liver; accumulation of acids because of immature kidneys; and a host of infections that prey on the newborn's susceptibility.

Considering all this, it's better to be born too late than to be born too early. Still, the new treatments are saving the lives of 10,000 early arrivals each year.

The Smallest Survivor

The smallest premature baby ever born was a female—Marion Chapman, born in South Shields, England, on June 5, 1938. She was just over 1 foot long and weighed in at 10 ounces (283 grams).

That she survived at all is amazing. It's all the more amazing when you learn that a low-weight group of premature babies born at the Harvard neonatology clinic some 4 decades later still had only a 44 percent chance of survival! Add to that the fact that the Harvard-born group of prematures weighed between 26 ounces (1.6 pounds) and 35 ounces (2.2 pounds), more than 2½ to 3½ times the English baby's birth weight, and Marion Chapman's unique birth record is even more impressive. But that's not all. The Harvard babies had the best care that medical knowledge and technology could offer in the 1970s; Marion Chapman was born unattended by a doctor. Later a doctor nursed her and fed her with a fountain pen filler.

Even with high technology, intensive care centers for premature babies, Marion's 10 ounces continues to hold the record. To better comprehend the birth weight of this English wonder baby, go pick up a can of Campbell's tomato soup—that's about what little Marion weighed.

Catching the First Breath

The most serious threat to premature babies—the one that literally takes their tiny breaths away—is respiratory distress syndrome (RDS, for short). This disease is a major killer and threatens some 50,000 newborn babies in the United States each year. It was fatal for about 25,000 of them until the mid-1960s.

A study at the University of California at San Francisco showed that, 20 years ago, only 10 percent of the babies who weighed 3¼ pounds (52 ounces) or less survived. By 1979, however, the survival rate for RDS babies dramatically increased to 80 percent.

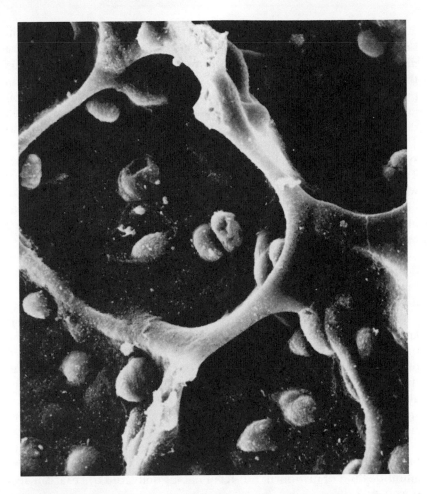

The air sacs (alveoli) of healthy premature lungs, magnified 2,600 times. The round cells normally secrete an oil-like liquid coating that prevents lung collapse in newborns. The lack of this in many premature infants causes respiratory distress syndrome (RDS), which threatens more than 50,000 newborn babies each year. New prenatal tests and treatments are saving tens of thousands of babies each year. Courtesy National Institutes of Health.

Respiratory distress syndrome used to be known as Hyaline membrane disease (hyalin from the Greek word *hyalos,* meaning glass). The disease afflicts the newborn by forming a glassy membrane that covers the air sacs and ducts in the lungs. As a result, the lungs can't expand properly because the air spaces within the underdeveloped lungs collapse when the newborn's first breath is exhaled. Severe breathing difficulties often develop, which can lead to asphyxiation and death.

In 1983 a new test was developed to detect respiratory distress syndrome. Called the Beckman Lumadex-FSI Fetal Lung Maturity Test, it is a 10-minute test on an amniotic fluid sample that determines whether or not the unborn's lungs have enough surfactant (an oil-like liquid) coating to prevent lung collapse at birth. An earlier test was involved and complex, had to be done in large laboratories, and took 2 to 3 hours.

Once RDS is diagnosed in the unborn, several options are open to doctors: They can administer drugs to speed development of the fetal lungs; delay delivery with drugs so that the fetal lungs develop; or be prepared at time of birth to use life-sustaining respiratory equipment.

One such device that prevents lung collapse in RDS newborns is known as a Gregory box—a small pressure chamber that fits over the infant's head and constantly feeds high-oxygen air, at slightly elevated pressures, into the premature lungs. The lungs are thus held open and the newborn's struggle for breath is ended. Normal breathing is usually developed within 7 days. This treatment, developed at the University of California Medical School at San Francisco, yields a 90 percent survival rate.

The near future also holds promise for donated lung surfactant to help RDS preemies. Where will this breath elixir come from? From the amniotic fluid of just-born, full-term babies delivered by cesarean section.

Today, even with the dramatic progress of the last 2 decades, some 12,000 babies die each year in the U.S. from respiratory distress. These recent breakthroughs will save thousands of lives by strengthening these smallest of lungs and filling them with life-giving air.

Death Before Birth

"How old was my mother when I was born?"

Most of us would reflect and answer an age: 18, 23, 30. The rare few would think or say, "She was dead."

Today's medical high technology makes it possible to mechanically maintain a pregnant woman's heart and respiratory functions when her brain is dead—legally death. These life-support systems can keep her unborn baby alive and growing until such time as delivery can be performed by cesarean section. Unborn babies have been kept alive for more than 2 months in prenatal intensive care. When these babies grow up, they may say, "I was born 2 months after my mother died."

Musical Legacy

About 200 cases of birth after the mother's death (most often brain death) have been recorded, but the number will dramatically increase in the next few decades because of available life-support technology and in utero diagnostic techniques, which include: monitoring the fetus's heartbeat, ultrasound imaging, amniotic-fluid analysis, and measurement of placental hormone levels. Doctors generally agree that there is little chance of saving the unborn if the pregnancy has not progressed for at least 28 weeks (about 7 months).

How the mother died is also an all-important factor in the chances for the unborn's survival. Death by asphyxia, such as in drowning or smoke inhalation, reduces the oxygen to the fetus to such a degree that a healthy birth is all but impossible.

The medical problems of keeping the fetus alive in such cases are profound, time-consuming, and costly. Frequent adjustments to the respirator are often necessary to keep adequate oxygen in the fetus's blood. Intravenous injections of protein, sugar, and fat are given through the mother for nourishment. Hormones to compensate for the mother's damaged or nonfunctioning pituitary gland must also be given. It amounts to round-the-clock intensive care that rescues an innocent baby from its own mother's death.

The medical staff also acts to compensate for the lack of movement and sound stimulation that a normal pregnancy provides the fetus through the pregnant woman's everyday activities. Nurses stroke the mother's abdomen and speak to the unborn with soothing words.

In a 1983 California case, where the mother's heartbeat and respiration were mechanically sustained for more than 2 months so that the baby could develop to a survivable stage, a tape recorder was placed at bedside and played the mother's favorite music. The sound of music reached the unborn boy floating within the amniotic ocean, and his heartbeat increased in response. He was soon delivered, all 3.3 pounds (1.5 kilograms) of him, in excellent condition, no doubt forever bonded to his dead mother's favorite music.

Newborn Heavies

The largest baby? There's some disagreement as to who can claim the title. Even if we discount the heaviest deformed babies who do not survive for long—for example, a baby born in 1939 in Illinois who only lived for 2 hours and who weighed in at 29¼ pounds—there is still reason for dispute.

The Middle East dominates the records, but are the weights accurate, was something lost in translation? A Turkish baby, born in 1961, reportedly weighed 24 pounds, 4 ounces, but the report was questioned many years after the fact and is no longer considered reliable. A more reliable claim, at least not disputed so far, comes from Iran: A baby was born in February 1972 that weighed in at 26½ pounds.

It is the Canadians, however, who can claim the certain heavy baby, based on parentage, not on medical scales and possibly tired and mistake-prone medical assistants. Anna Swan, of Nova Scotia, was almost 7½ feet tall. She married Martin van Buren Bates, shorter by about 3 inches, but still over 7 feet, and they became the tallest married couple on record, a record that still stands.

This tall woman produced a baby weighing 23 pounds, 12 ounces, and the fact has the authority of the *New York Medical Record* (March 22, 1879) behind it.

The world's largest babies at birth compare to normal babies at 1½ years old (their average weight is about 25 pounds). A 24-pound newborn has increased its weight over 33,000 times since conception.

Chapter Eight

Testings and Tamperings: Body-Brain Responses

DRUGS

A Drug by Any Other Name . . .

All medicines are drugs, but not all drugs are medicines. Alcohol is a drug, for example, and so are aspirin, cocaine, and caffeine.

Drugs taken *as* medicines, even though they have no actual medicinal properties, have one powerful effect in common—the placebo effect. The word "placebo" comes from the Latin word meaning "to please." A placebo, in the medical sense, refers to a substance taken in the belief that it is a medicine that goes on to have an observable effect on the user.

Placebos are inactive substances used often in comparative studies conducted on experimental drugs. One group of patients is given the "real thing" while another group gets the placebo, which may actually be a sugar pill. Neither group knows what they are taking. When the study is completed, researchers evaluate the degree of genuine effect from the drug.

Doctors who prescribe a medicine for a patient knowing that it will have little effect on the patient's problem may do so in the belief that the placebo effect will function—as it often does.

So strong is the effect on the mind of those who choose to believe, it is even possible to become addicted to placebos. The *Merck Manual* reports "at least 2 patients . . . were addicted to placebos. One consumed 10,000 placebos in one year."

Passing Through

When a drug enters the body, the response is the same as for any other foreign substance: The body attempts to metabolize or break down the substance, use what is beneficial to the body, and excrete the rest.

The first step in this process is for the drug to pass through the lining of the intestinal tract and enter the bloodstream. (Injected drugs, of course, go directly into the bloodstream). Because the walls of the intestinal tract are lined with fatty cells, drug molecules, among other chemicals, that dissolve in fat will pass through with relative ease. Other drugs that are water soluble may have difficulty getting through the tiny pores of these membranes and may be excreted as waste without ever reaching the bloodstream. Drugs that remain in the intestinal tract for a period of time may alter the normal bacterial growth in the bowel to produce digestive problems, including diarrhea as in the case of some of the early forms of antibiotics.

When a drug begins to circulate in the bloodstream, it is distributed to all parts of the body, where it is absorbed. At the same time, the process of elimination begins. The kidneys filter out water-soluble molecules of the drug and excrete them unchanged in the urine. As the drug passes through the liver, fat-soluble molecules are converted by the liver's chemical-processing function into compounds that are more water soluble and which can then be excreted in the urine as well.

The way a drug acts in the body is called its pharmacokinetics and includes its absorption into the bloodstream, its distribution to the cells, its metabolism into other forms in the liver, and its excretion, usually through the kidneys.

Drug Delivery

New forms of drugs make it possible for medicines to be delivered to their targets with greater accuracy, at controlled rates, with fewer side effects and less damage to tissues and organs not intended for treatment.

• Enteric-coated tablets have a wax matrix that prevents them from dissolving until they reach the small intestines.

• Sustained-release preparations also are contained in a wax coating. When the tablet dissolves, the wax slowly releases the medicine and controls the absorption rate of the active ingredient.

• Transdermal patches are bandaidlike patches impregnated with medicine that can be applied to the skin for continuous, rate-controlled absorption of drugs. These are being used to treat such problems as motion sickness and heart problems.

• A tiny disk of medicine placed under the eyelid administers a steady flow of the drug pilocarpine, used to treat glaucoma.

• Another patch placed on the mucous membrane in the mouth delivers a rate-controlled dose of nitroglycerin to treat heart problems.

• Implantable drug pumps deliver insulin to the diabetic as needed; other drug pumps deliver chemicals directly to the site of a tumor without affecting surrounding tissues. Research studies are in progress for the development of transdermal and vaginal products for female-hormone-replacement therapy during menopause and for a direct-contact product to treat hay fever and other allergies.

Hitting the Target

To produce its desired effect, a drug must reach its target and remain at the target long enough to do its job. Some medicines are specifically targeted and act only on certain types of tissue. For example, iodine is absorbed by thyroid tissue and is used for that reason to test for disease in that organ; fluoride is absorbed by bony tissue, especially teeth, and digitalis is absorbed by the heart.

Other medicines are targeted to a specific constituent of body fluids. Heparin, a drug used to prevent blood clots, produces its effect by combining with and deactivating proteins in the blood's plasma that are essential for clotting. Antidotes for some poisons such as lead work by attaching themselves to the molecules of the poison, drawing the poison into their own molecules, and then transforming the result into a soluble compound which then can be excreted. Many drugs, however, cause more than one effect, producing "side effects."

Drugs that are not targeted to specific tissues or other substances in the body may never reach their destination if they dissolve before they get there and can have unpleasant effects when they do; for example, the laxative Bisacodyl, if dissolved in the stomach, can cause nausea

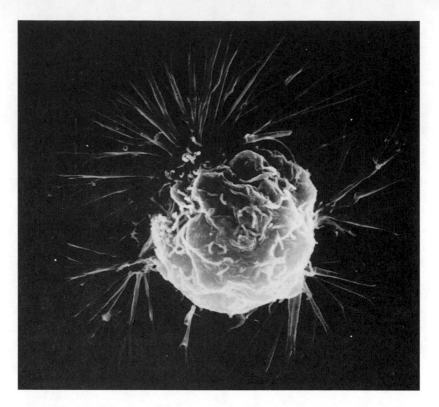

An electron micrograph of a cell cultured from breast-cancer tissue. The dramatic-looking tentacles result from specimen preparation and are not unique to cancer cells. New drug-delivery systems such as implantable drug pumps will deliver chemicals directly to the site of the tumor without affecting surrounding tissue. Courtesy National Institutes of Health.

and vomiting and would not be effective against the constipation for which it was taken.

Drug-Drug Interactions

Two or more drugs in the body at the same time may have no effect on each other. There are a number, however, that can interact and affect the way one or the other or both behave in the body. Some of these interactions create a combined effect that is greater than the effect of each alone. This is called potentiation. For example, an antihistamine can increase the sedative effects of anesthetics, barbiturates, tranquilizers, and some painkillers because they are central-nervous-system depressants like the antihistamine.

Other drugs taken together can cancel each other out or act against each other. This is known as antagonism. People with a tendency to form blood clots may be prescribed an anticoagulant drug such as warfarin. If the person also has arthritis and is taking a drug like phenylbutazone, the result can be severe bleeding in various parts of the body.

An antacid can cause an anticoagulant drug to be absorbed slowly and prevent it from working properly. Aspirin increases the blood-thinning effects of anticoagulants and can lead to severe bleeding if taken in combination.

Taking Your Medicine

Taking some medicines with carbonated soft drinks, acid fruit or vegetable juices causes the drug to dissolve quickly in the stomach. When this happens, the drug is prevented from reaching the intestines where it can be readily absorbed into the bloodstream.

Drugs swallowed with a full glass of water—at least one—will be absorbed twice as rapidly as one swallowed with a sip. Water speeds emptying of the stomach and dilutes the medicine, spreading it over a larger absorptive area in the intestine.

Take Before, With, After Meals

If you are taking drugs, the food you eat and what you use to wash it down can make the drugs work faster or slower or prevent medicines from working at all. Eating certain foods while taking drugs can be dangerous and even fatal. For these reasons, some medicines often are prescribed to be taken on an empty stomach, some just before meals, others between or with meals.

Food may affect drugs by enhancing or slowing down absorption of the drug into the bloodstream. A few drugs may speed up absorption. For example, fat-soluble drugs, such as the antifungal griseofulvin, are absorbed better when taken with a fatty meal rather than alone or with a high-protein meal (this also helps prevent or reduce the side effect of an upset stomach).

More often, however, food and drink interfere with absorption. Both penicillamine, used to treat rheumatoid arthritis and some other conditions, and the antibiotic tetracycline are absorbed half as well if taken with food. For tetracycline, it is the calcium in dairy products such as milk, cheese, and yogurt that interferes with absorption.

Because most drugs are tested on fasting subjects, recommended dosages may not take the potential for food interaction into account, leading to unfortunate experiences and later adjustments in instructions for taking the medicine.

Drugs and Food Nutrients

Just as some foods can affect the way certain drugs act in the body, so drugs can affect the body's use of food. The elimination of some food nutrients may be speeded up, there may be interference with the body's ability to change food nutrients into usable forms, or the body's absorption of nutrients may be hindered. Nutrient depletion of the body occurs gradually, but for those taking drugs over long periods of time, these interactions can lead to deficiencies of certain vitamins and minerals, especially in children, the elderly, those with poor diets, and the chronically ill.

Some drugs inhibit nutrient absorption by their effect on the bowel wall. One of these is mineral oil, the venerable old laxative still widely used by the elderly and in nursing homes. It has been reported that as little as 4 teaspoons (about 20 milliliters) of mineral oil taken twice a day on a regular basis can interfere with absorption of vitamin D, K, and carotene, a substance the body converts to vitamin A.

Birth-control pills are known to lower blood levels of certain vitamins such as folic acid, B_6, and vitamin C. Aspirin and other salicylates may produce deficiencies of vitamins B_6, B_{12}, C, E, K, folic acid, and iron.

The Dangerous Palate

Because foods and beverages contain natural and occasionally artificial chemicals, they can not only interact with drugs you take and affect the way the medicines work, but can cause other medical problems and, in some rare instances, may threaten your life.

One of the most dramatic of these rare occasions is the interaction that occurs between monoamine oxidase (MAO) inhibitors—drugs sometimes prescribed for depression and for high blood pressure—and foods high in a substance called tyramine, found in foods aged to increase their flavor.

Foods high in tyramine include cheeses, pickled herring, sour cream, yogurt, chicken livers, raisins, bananas, avocados, soy sauce, broad bean pods (fava beans), yeast extracts, meats prepared with a meat tenderizer, chianti-type wines and beer, and food or drink containing caffeine.

An MAO inhibitor in combination with any one of these foods will suppress the enzyme that breaks down the tyramine so that it is acceptable to the body. When this enzyme is prevented from doing its work, the chemicals from these foods build up and the blood pressure is elevated, sometimes to crisis levels that lead to brain hemorrhage and even death.

Drugs and Alcohol

As a drug itself, alcohol can cause serious interactions with other drugs and have damaging effects on the body, particularly the liver.

Alcohol is a central nervous system (CNS) depressant. If taken with another CNS depressant, alertness, judgment, and performance skills can be affected. The result can be fatal, particularly if the person is operating machinery or driving a vehicle while under the influence. An increase in the combined effect of the 2 drugs also can occur and be lethal, for example, when barbiturates are mixed with alcohol.

Among the drugs that alcohol interacts with are prescription pain medicines or sleeping pills; appetite suppressants (diet pills) used in some weight-reduction programs; tranquilizers; theophylline (medicine for asthma); tricyclic antidepressants and MAO inhibitors; medicine for seizures; oral antidiabetic medicines and insulin; antihistamines; and aspirin and other agents used for the pain and inflammation of arthritis. Heavy alcohol consumption also may decrease the body's ability to absorb thiamin, vitamin B_1, vitamin B_6, and folic acid from foods.

People who develop a tolerance to the sedative effects of alcohol may find they need larger doses of sleeping pills or tranquilizers to get the desired effect. This can lead to an accidental overdose.

For similar reasons, alcoholics and patients with alcohol in their system need larger quantities of anesthetics to induce sleep. Once these patients are "under," the sleep is deeper and lasts longer.

Over time, the excess use of alcohol or drugs leads to the destruction of liver cells and cirrhosis or hardening of the liver. The liver cannot function properly in that condition and deadly toxins build up in the body. Various illnesses follow and death is the usual outcome.

Drugs and Smoking

About 1 in 3 adults in the United States regularly smokes cigarettes. The nicotine in the body of the smoker can increase the metabolism of drugs by the liver and decrease the efficacy of specific drugs or make reactions to drug therapy more unpredictable. For some drugs, the smoker may need to take a larger dose and may have to take the drug more often than nonsmokers. Smoking also may result in increased risks of drug use, may affect an individual's response to certain diagnostic tests, and may interact with some substances in food.

Among women who smoke and also use oral birth-control pills, the risk of heart attack, stroke, and circulatory diseases is increased. This risk is even higher in women older than 37 and in heavy smokers. There is some evidence that women between the ages of 39 and 45 may have an increased risk of heart attack if they smoke and take noncontraceptive estrogen medications.

The dominant effect of smoking on drug metabolism comes from the ability of nicotine and other tobacco constituents to speed the process by which the body uses and eliminates a drug. This means not only that the drug may be less effective, but that the duration of its effect may be shortened. Under these circumstances, the drug will not be able to do its job and the patient and the doctor may erroneously conclude that the drug is ineffective and stop using it.

Smoking appears to interact with a number of drugs including theophylline, a bronchodilator used to treat asthma; pentazocine used in combination with other drugs to induce anesthesia; imipramine, an antidepressant; gluthetamide, a sedative; furosemide, a diuretic; and propanolol, a beta-blocker used to treat cardiac conditions. A recent study of diabetics reveals that smokers who are diabetic require a 15 to 20 percent higher dose of insulin than diabetic nonsmokers and the heavy smokers need an even higher dose.

It is possible that smokers may have increased needs for vitamin C, vitamin B_{12}, and vitamin B_6, although the reason for this is unknown. These smoking interactions may be a key to the fact that smoking mothers tend to have smaller babies who, because of their low birth weights, have an increased risk of dying early in life.

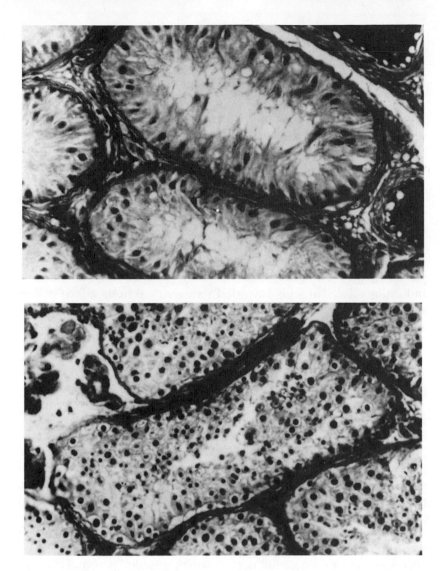

Excessive alcohol use destroys the liver cells—cirrhosis of the liver. The cells are altered, fill up with fat, and eventually die, allowing deadly toxins to build up in the body. Alcohol abuse also damages the germ cells in the male testes. The cells become smeared and misshapen (top) compared to the normal testes cells (bottom). Courtesy National Institutes of Health.

Mary Jane

While marijuana is beginning to gain wider acceptance in medical circles for the treatment of glaucoma and the nausea and dizziness associated with chemotherapeutic drugs used to treat some forms of cancer, physicians and scientists do not consider it a safe drug for recreational use.

The known or suspected chronic effects of marijuana use were reported in August 1982 in the *Morbidity and Mortality Weekly Report* published at the Centers for Disease Control from a study by the National Academy of Science's Institute of Medicine. These effects include short-term memory impairment and slowness of learning and impaired lung functioning similar to that found in cigarette smokers. Indications are that with extended use, more serious effects follow, such as cancer and other lung diseases, decreased sperm count and sperm mobility in the male, and interference with ovulation and prenatal development of the fetus in the female. Women who are users are 5 times more likely than nonusers to deliver low-birth-weight infants.

Heavy users also may experience an impairment of the immune response and there may be adverse effects on heart function.

The by-products of marijuana remain in the body fat for several weeks after use, with unknown consequences. Their storage in the body increases the possibility for chronic as well as residual effects on physical and mental performance, even after the reaction to the drug has worn off. The effect of marijuana on reaction time, motor coordination, and visual perception makes it dangerous to drive, operate machinery, or fly an airplane for up to 8 hours after the high disappears.

Prolonged marijuana use by young people seems to be associated with the "amotivational syndrome," characterized by a pattern of energy loss, diminished school performance, troubled parental relationships, and other behavioral disruptions. Although more research is needed to substantiate these findings, recent national surveys report that 40 percent of heavy marijuana users experience some or all of these symptoms of "amotivational syndrome."

That Competitive Edge

The use of anabolic steroids by athletes has a long history. Anabolic steroids are synthetic forms of testosterone, the male hormone. They

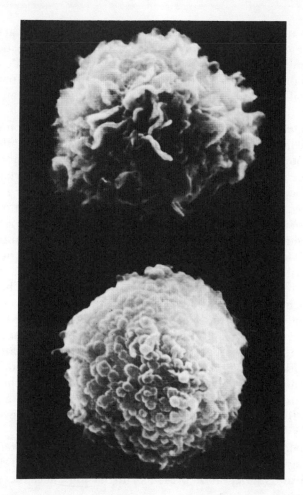

A striking contrast between lung cells of a nonsmoker (top) and a smoker (bottom). The clear lung cell of the nonsmoker appears open and fluffy—like a flower opening to the light—in contrast to the closed and cobbled-appearing cell of the smoker. Courtesy National Institutes of Health.

have been used by athletes for many years in the belief that they help heal tissue damage faster after exercise, build muscle tissue, and increase aggressiveness that gives a competitive edge. While there is a good deal of controversy in medical circles about their actual benefits, it is generally felt that what little the steroids may do for an athlete is not worth the risks to future health.

Natural testosterone helps the body store nitrogen, a component of all proteins, which promotes the growth of muscle and other tissue. Anabolic steroids are taken on the assumption that they add to nitrogen storage and so increase muscle buildup. This may work for female athletes, but they must endure the masculinizing effects of the hormone: acne, a deeper voice, and facial and body hair. The normal male athlete who already has substantial muscular development is storing all the nitrogen he can possibly use. Additional muscle buildup is not possible. Moreover, the effect on nitrogen storage of the anabolic steroids lasts for only about 1 month.

For the male, the risks of taking steroids are many. The pituitary gland which stimulates the testicles to produce testosterone stops its stimulation when it detects adequate (or excessive) levels of the hormone in the bloodstream. This causes the testicles to shrink in size and to decrease the amount of sperm produced. The prostate gland, a frequent site of cancer in males, enlarges because of the added testosterone and may stimulate a tumor already present in the gland to become cancerous. If the body converts the steroids into a substance similar to the female hormone estrogen, the male may develop additional breast tissue.

Both males and females who take anabolic steroids may experience liver damage, bleeding from the gastrointestinal tract, increased fat in the blood, and higher blood pressure, increasing the chances of future heart attacks.

Anabolic steroids cause the epiphyses of bones (the ends where growth occurs) to close prematurely. Because many people do not stop growing until after their teens, athletes given steroids at a tender age will stop growing.

Until recently, there were no accurate tests to detect steroids in an athlete. In fact, it was possible and a common practice to give other drugs that masked the presence of steroids in the urine. New testing methods, which were used in the recent Pan American games, can detect even 1 billionth of a gram of this illegal drug.

The Sober Truth

Drinking coffee will not counteract the effects of intoxication. The caffeine in coffee does nothing to lower the blood levels of alcohol, nor does it counteract the effects of alcohol on the central nervous system. Drinking large amounts of coffee—or anything else—will not sober someone who is drunk. The only prescription for sobering a drunk is time and a healthy liver that can remove the poisonous alcohol from the bloodstream. Pouring coffee into a drunk only produces a drunk full of coffee.

The Caffeine Habit

Caffeine is a drug found in coffee, tea, cocoa, cola drinks and some other soft drinks, and chocolate. It also is contained in many drugs you can buy without a prescription, such as headache, allergy, and stay-awake pills. Some prescription medicines also include caffeine.

Caffeine acts as a stimulant to the central nervous system. People react differently, but in general it can cause insomnia, nervousness, irritability, anxiety, and disturbances in the heart rate and rhythm. People who consume large quantities of caffeine-containing drinks and also take medicines that include caffeine may experience any or all of these symptoms to a heightened degree.

Because caffeine crosses the placental barrier—the connection between the mother and the developing fetus—and has been found in breast milk as well, concerns have been raised about the need for pregnant women to limit or stop their caffeine consumption during pregnancy.

The most recent evidence indicates that drinking moderate amounts of coffee during pregnancy is not associated with poorer pregnancy results. This Harvard study, reported in *The New England Journal of Medicine,* questioned more than 12,000 women at the time of delivery about their coffee consumption during the first 12 weeks of pregnancy, the time when most birth defects occur. They learned that 57 percent of those questioned drank no coffee and that only 5 percent drank more than 4 cups of coffee a day.

The researchers also found that over 22 percent of the women in their study were smokers at the time of delivery. In that 22 percent, the frequency of smoking was over 3 times greater among heavy coffee drinkers than among nondrinkers. When birth defects were correlated with coffee-drinking habits, no significant link was found; however, the association between coffee drinking and low birth weight which they did find disappeared when the data was corrected for smoking. This led the researchers to conclude that smoking is the real culprit. They recommended, however, the moderation of caffeine use—as with all drugs—during pregnancy.

As many as 22.5 million adult Americans consume an amount of caffeine from food and drugs equal to at least 10 cups of coffee every day.

VITAMINS

What Are Vitamins?

Vitamins are organic substances essential in very small quantities for the body to maintain normal growth and metabolism. Most vitamins are not made in the body and must be obtained from outside sources, principally from the foods we eat.

There are a few exceptions. The skin makes vitamin D when it is exposed to sunlight. Niacin may be produced in the body from an amino acid found in protein, tryptophan. Bacteria in the intestines manufacture vitamin K by acting on consumed foods. Vitamin A is made in the body from plant foods containing carotene found in green, leafy vegetables and carrots and in some other yellow and red vegetables and fruits.

Vitamins play a role in the body's defense and repair mechanisms. They do not themselves provide energy or serve as building units in the body, but act as coenzymes in tissue cells to cause certain metabolic reactions. They may help in forming genetic material, hormones, blood cells, or chemicals necessary to the nervous system. They also help the body to process other major nutrients such as proteins, carbohydrates, and fats. The specific ways in which vitamins function in the body are unknown.

Most scientists agree that a substance is a vitamin if a lack of the compound in the body produces specific deficiency symptoms and supplying the vitamin cures those symptoms. The Food and Drug Administration requires submission of studies showing that a deficiency of the substance in the body will produce a specific disease condition for the substance to be labeled a "vitamin."

In 1982, Americans spent $2.2 billion on vitamin supplements. Roughly 40 percent of the United States population takes a supplement regularly.

Natural Vitamins

There is no difference between vitamins naturally present in or extracted from foods and those that are manufactured from chemicals. The molecules of a "synthetic" vitamin look exactly the same to tissue cells as those of a "natural" vitamin—or else they wouldn't be able to function as vitamins in the body—so vitamins present in food, those added, and those taken as supplements have the same effect. Those who succumb to the advertising blandishments of promoters of natural vitamins are wasting their money on an often-much-more-expensive product. In addition, if people consume many vitamins, they may be risking harmful effects on the supply of the truly natural vitamins in the body, as well as interactions between excessive amounts of these vitamins and other medicines they may be taking.

A recent survey at the Yale-New Haven Clinical Research Center of 41 over-the-counter multivitamins revealed that the majority contained vitamin levels that were more than 200 percent higher than the U.S. Recommended Daily Allowance (RDA) listed on some food labeling. In some of the supplements, particularly those for pregnant women, there was an inadequate amount of some vitamins and minerals.

Getting Your Vitamins

All of the vitamins needed by the body can be obtained by eating a balanced diet, a variety of foods from each of the 4 food groups: milk, meat (or protein substitutes), vegetables and fruits, breads and cereals. A balanced diet also gives the body proteins, minerals, carbohydrates, and fats necessary to good health. In fact, vitamins often cannot work without the presence of other foods. Vitamins A, D, and E, the fat-soluble vitamins, for example, need fats for absorption by the body.

The total amount of each vitamin that you take in each day includes what you get from the foods you eat and what you may take as supplements. This total amount should not exceed the Recommended Daily

Allowances (RDA) unless you are taking vitamin supplements under the supervision of your doctor.

The Recommended Daily Allowances for vitamins represent the intakes of vitamins that should prevent the development of symptoms of deficiency disease and help maintain long-term health in the average body. A substantial safety margin is built into the RDA tables to allow for individual physical differences and the body's capacity to absorb vitamins.

Set by a panel of experts, RDAs are not precise numbers, but give a general idea of how much you need. They do not cover amounts needed for problems caused by a serious lack of vitamins. They are guidelines only, not minimum daily requirements. In other words, you do not need to consume the listed RDAs for a given vitamin—from all sources—every day to stay healthy. If you are a senior citizen, in fact, the RDA listings may not be helpful at all since everyone from age 50 on up is lumped together in one category.

Too Much of a Good Thing

Taking a little over the Recommended Daily Allowance (RDA) of a particular vitamin in food or vitamin supplements usually will have an insignificant effect on the body. However, megadosing, taking doses of at least 10 times the RDA for the vitamin over a long period of time, can lead to a harmful overdose and serious side effects or interactions with other chemicals—including medicines—present in your body. In fact some people have died because of vitamin megadosing.

Excess quantities of fat-soluble vitamins such as vitamin A are stored in the liver for long periods of time and may produce diarrhea, double vision, loss of hair, headaches, and a drying or cracking of the lips or skin, among other symptoms.

Vitamin C (ascorbic acid) taken in megadoses can raise the level of urine acid and cause an attack of gout in people with that condition. Megadoses of vitamin C may cause kidney stones. Infants born to mothers taking megadoses of vitamin C have been reported to develop scurvy, the condition prevented by small doses of the vitamin. Diabetics may get false urine test results from megadoses of vitamin C. The anti-blood-clotting effects of anticoagulants may be counteracted by megadoses of vitamin C.

The risks of taking megadoses of vitamin D include calcium deposits throughout the body, deafness, nausea, kidney stones, high blood pressure, high blood cholesterol, fragile bones, and loss of appetite.

With long-term use of large doses of vitamin E, you may feel as though you are coming down with the flu, develop pain in the stomach, nausea, tiredness, and weakness.

Excessive doses of vitamin K given to laboratory animals have produced anemia.

Drugs and Vitamins

Because they also are chemicals, vitamin supplements you buy without a prescription—even in normal dosages—can interact with other chemicals (drugs) you may be taking.

For example, the effects of the anti-Parkinsonism drug, levodopa, may be negated by a dose of as little as 10 milligrams of pyridoxine, vitamin B_6. The effects of anticoagulant drugs such as warfarin may be counteracted by megadoses (doses at least 10 times the Recommended Daily Allowances taken over a period of time) of vitamin C or by large doses of retinol (a vitamin A derivative). The seizure control of the drug phenytoin may be reduced by taking too much folic acid.

Deficiencies in vitamins C, D, B_{12}, riboflavin, and folic acid may be caused by use of oral diabetes medicine and muscle relaxers, among others. Antibiotics can cause deficiencies of iron and potassium, and vitamins A, B_{12}, C, and E.

Long-term use of diuretics to treat such conditions as congestive heart failure can lead to serious potassium depletion. If the potassium is not replaced in heart patients taking digitalis, the heart may develope an irregular or weak beat, undermining the benefits of the drug.

Chronic use of antacids can cause phosphate depletion that leads to mild muscle weakness, and to vitamin D deficiency in its more severe forms. Despite this, or perhaps in ignorance of it, $741 million was spent in the United States in 1982 on antacids sold without a prescription, over the counter.

DIET

The Battle of the Bulge

The overweight person has never lacked for advice: The bookstore shelves overflow with volumes on the latest diet fad, magazine articles appear regularly on the subject, and friends and doctors offer their version of the "right approach." Basically, they all say the same thing, take in fewer calories and exercise regularly by pushing away from the table and engaging in a sport you like. You are what you eat is the implication.

The findings of researchers at Boston's Beth Israel Hospital help to explain why some people can indulge their culinary preferences without gaining weight, while others gain on even a low-caloric intake.

The Boston researchers found that the levels of an enzyme called sodium-potassium ATPase was at least 20 percent below normal in the blood of the obese people they tested. ATPase regulates the body's sodium and potassium levels using energy and burning up calories in the process. Reduced ATPase levels in some overweight people may indicate that calories are not being burned and are instead stored as fat. The researchers indicated that the thermostatic control provided by the enzyme seems to malfunction in some obese people.

Another mechanism that helps keep weight stable is a substance called "brown fat," a kind of dark, fatty tissue found around the adrenal glands, the aorta, and the kidneys. Such tissue is said to diffuse excess calories as heat. Brown fat is said to decrease with age and may explain the tendency of the elderly to gain weight.

The Spice of Life

Salt, sodium chloride, has long been recognized as an essential ingredient of the normal diet. Sodium is necessary to maintain the body's blood volume and to control the movement of fluids in and out of cells. Sodium plays a crucial part in transmitting nerve impulses and in the metabolism of proteins and carbohydrates to produce energy. The chloride part of the salt molecule aids in maintaining the acid balance in the body and is necessary for some enzymes to do their jobs.

While all of these bodily activities can be kept going with an intake of less than 1/10 of a teaspoon of salt, the average American adult has been estimated to consume 2 1/2 to 3 teaspoons (10 to 12 grams) of salt each day. The healthy kidney disposes of excess salt, but some people who seem predisposed to develop high blood pressure may find excessive sodium intake a contributing factor. Although the evidence linking excessive sodium intake to the development of high blood pressure is not clearcut, doctors generally recommend reduction of salt intake as a wise move.

Athletes and others who do hard physical work in high temperatures must watch their salt intake more closely because of the amount lost in sweat. However, those who take salt tablets to make up this difference may develop a form of heat exhaustion from an overdose of salt. Too much salt in the bloodstream can lead to the formation of clots that can cause kidney failure, heart attacks, or a stroke. An overdose of salt is more dangerous than too little salt because it can be fatal.

During hot weather, the addition of more salt to food at the table and consumption of larger amounts of fluids, especially water, will make up for the salt lost in sweat.

Adult Americans consume 912 to 1,095 teaspoons (3,650 to 4,380 grams) of salt annually.

The (Im)Perfect Food

Milk is the original "natural food." Because of its association with motherhood, it has acquired an almost unassailable position as the "perfect" food. However, people who cannot drink milk or eat dairy products made from milk without suffering crampy abdominal pains, gassiness, and diarrhea would argue the point.

The most common cause of milk intolerance is a deficiency of the enzyme lactase which breaks down the principal sugar in milk and milk products, lactose. As many as 50 million adults in the United States and 2 to 4 billion people in the world are unable to digest lactose adequately.

Lactose is a large molecule, a double sugar or disaccharide, that must be split into its 2 component sugars, glucose and galactose, so its components can be absorbed through the walls of the intestines and converted to energy in the body. Lactase is made by cells that line the walls of the small intestines. If the amount of lactase produced is insufficient to digest the lactose consumed, some of the lactose will remain in the small intestines. The undigested lactose sits in the bowel where it draws fluid from the body's tissues. The 1¾ ounces (50 grams) of lactose in 1 quart (0.95 liter) of milk brings in at least 1 quart of water from outside the intestines. This increased water raises the volume and number of stools produced. At the same time, the bacteria normal to the intestines use the undigested lactose as food, forming lactic acid and hydrogen gas as by-products. The result is painful abdominal distention and cramps that transport the lactose to the large intestines where gas and diarrhea ensue.

The amount of lactase in the body is at its highest immediately after birth. Levels taper off after weaning from a diet of milk to other forms of nourishment. The degree of this decline appears to vary in different ethnic groups. Studies have indicated that by adulthood, at least one half to three fourths of African and American Blacks, Arabs, Israelis, and Asians are lactase deficient. Even among Caucasian populations of northern European ancestry, lactose intolerance occurs in 5 to 20 percent of young adults. Although figures are lacking, the condition appears frequently in people over the age of 40.

Playing on Fruit Fuel

Mothers of little-leaguers or young soccer league players have been supplying oranges for the pregame or half-time quick energy session since the beginning of these contests. A recent study at Tufts University indicates that, once again, mother knows best. According to the Tufts researchers there is solid evidence that fruit sugar (fructose) is a better source of energy than the glucose you would get from eating candy.

When you eat candy, you get an almost instantaneous surge of glucose into the bloodstream, and the body's response is to send a large amount of insulin into the bloodstream to metabolize the glucose. This drops the glucose blood level back down to where it was before you ate the candy, and sometimes even lower. With less glucose in the blood, your muscles burn more glycogen, the carbohydrate fuel supply from the liver, and you feel fatigued.

Fruit sugar, on the other hand, enters the bloodstream at a slower rate and does not need insulin to start its metabolism. The buildup of energy is slower in the body, and there is no rush of insulin either. Blood levels of glucose are kept relatively constant, you feel better, and your loss of glycogen slows down.

AGING

Why the Body Ages

While the human life span limit for most people has been set at 70 to 85 years for roughly the last 100,000 years, mankind continues its search for a "fountain of youth," something that will prolong life. The quest is for the key to longevity.

Some scientists believe that aging is genetically programmed, pointing to the graying of hair, menopause, and the fixed life span of humans. Laboratory tests with human cells, moreover, have demonstrated patterns of division and reproduction, growth, and healing mechanisms that closely parallel those of natural changes in the body's cells as they age, leading to the conclusion that these changes in humans are preprogrammed.

Other scientists suggest that aging occurs when cells are damaged faster than the body can repair them, producing errors that cause genetic damage. As these errors in DNA structure accumulate over time, the tissues and organs of which they are a part begin to malfunction and eventually break down.

One of the more recent theories of aging is that proposed by George Sacher, the late biologist. Sacher believed that aging was closely tied to evolution: Nature developed longevity genes to lengthen the life span and allow certain animals—those with large brains who produce small litters—sufficient time to produce several offspring and then live long enough to rear their young. At the same time, in order to keep a species fit, aging patterns evolved to prevent the older animals from reproducing the species because they are more likely to have defective young. Hence women experience menopause, and men in general experience reduced potency.

Old Dogs and New Tricks

The old adage, "You can't teach an old dog new tricks," has generally been extended to apply to humans as well. Even those who study human development have held that the intelligence of the human mind levels off and eventually declines throughout the adult years. A recently completed 21-year study of the intellectual performance of aging adults refutes this universal assessment.

The study by K. Warner Schaie, Director of the Gerontology Research Institute at the University of Southern California, in Los Angeles, demonstrated that at all ages the majority of people studied maintained their levels of intellectual capability—or improved it—as they grew older. Even between the ages of 74 and 81, almost 10 percent of the people tested performed better than they had at younger ages.

While the Schaie study found no single uniform pattern across the adult life span, factors discovered that affect individual variations include some physical conditions such as heart and circulatory problems, socioeconomic level, including education, and adaptability toward changing life-styles.

It would seem that educated people from a socially advantaged background who remain generally healthy and have a flexible attitude and life-style through their middle-aged years are likely to maintain their intellectual abilities in later life.

Sleeping Interruptus

A common myth about elderly people suggests that people need less sleep as they get older. Studies at the Stanford University Sleep Research Center, supported by the National Institute on Aging, indicate that it is the ability to sleep rather than the need that diminishes with age. In addition, the researchers have shown that older people awaken often during the night, even those who believe they are getting a good night's sleep.

In the Stanford studies, 35 percent of the elderly volunteers had periods of breathing difficulty while asleep. Many times in 1 hour these subjects stopped breathing, awakened briefly during the period of stopped breathing, and then began normal breathing without being aware of what had happened.

The findings of the researchers suggest that old people are often victims of this syndrome, sleep apnea (stopped breathing), and that it affects their daytime alertness and may result in their being erroneously labeled "senile." There also is some evidence that sleep apnea characterized by heavy snoring may be associated with heart disease. Additionally, the relatively common practice of prescribing sleeping pills for the elderly can lead to further depressed breathing and increase the risk of sudden death during sleep.

Old Before Their Time

Children with gray hair, cataracts, wrinkled skin, and diminished growth? Yes, it happens. Progeria and Werner's syndrome are 2 conditions that cause premature aging in children.

The first signs of progeria may appear in the first year of life when there is a failure to increase in size and weight. Children with this condition fail to mature sexually, have a delayed and abnormal growth of teeth, distortion of face and head size, and a loss of all body hair, among other signs. The skin appears old with patches that are tight and dry or dull and wrinkled. The "liver spots" of old age appear as they grow older—brown blotches of color on the skin. Hardening of the arteries may result in early death—at age 12 to 16—from heart attack or stroke.

Werner's syndrome does not become apparent until age 15 to 30, but there are many similarities with progeria and it has been suggested that it is a form of progeria. A short stature is characteristic, with premature graying of the hair and balding, cataracts, a change in skin texture, a loss of bone tissue (osteoporosis), and improper functioning of many glands, particularly the gonads (the testes and ovaries). People with this condition, unlike those with progeria, can survive to their forties or fifties and a few have lived to their sixties and seventies. Death is usually from cancer or from heart disease caused by hardening of the arteries.

Both of these conditions are extremely rare. Progeria occurs in the United States about 1 in every 250,000 live births. There are reported to have been only 73 cases of progeria worldwide since 1886 and 130 cases of Werner's syndrome since 1904.

A Ripe Old Age

The National Center of Health Statistics recently reported that "Americans born in 1982 can expect to live longer than those born in any previous year, to an average age of 74 years."

According to research findings presented in a 1981 paper at the American Association for the Advancement of Science Meeting in Washington, D.C., by Drs. James F. Fries and Lawrence M. Crapo, mankind reached its current maximum life span of 3 score and 10 (give or take a few years) about 100,000 years ago. Our present life span seems related, at least in part, to natural selection and the need for people to remain productive until their children no longer need their protection. Accordingly, human tissues and the organs of which they are a part deteriorate at a slow but constant rate from about age 30 and eventually fail fatally in all of us at about the same old age.

However, Fries and Crapo indicate it is possible to increase physical efficiency throughout your lifetime, even while organs are deteriorating. They explain that a serious runner free of disease, for example, can increase his body's performance for most of his lifetime because the organs seldom are used to their physical capacity, even by athletes.

Under ideal conditions, researchers state, the natural human life span's limit would be 85 years and 99 percent of the American people would die of old age between about 73 and 79.

Despite national and international claims about the record longevity of aged citizens—ranging from 120 to over 145 years—the greatest authenticated age to which a human has lived is 116, the age of a Japanese man living on Tokuno Shima Island who was born June 29, 1865.

Change of Life

People pass from childhood to puberty (which marks the start of adolescence) when their sex organs begin to be functional and the individuals become capable of reproducing themselves. For females, this event is marked by the start of menstruation usually at about age 13. Males generally begin puberty toward the end of their fourteenth year. At the onset of puberty secondary sex characteristics begin to appear—breast/beard development, deepening of the male voice. While physical adolescence comes to an end at around 19 with cessation of body growth, for some, emotional factors may last into their twenties.

After passing through early maturity (adolescence to about age 35) and the childbearing years, women face menopause in later maturity (35 to 55 or 60), after about age 50. At menopause, menstruation becomes irregular and gradually stops, ending the reproductive capability of the woman's body.

The female ovulation cycle that results in menstruation for the unimpregnated female is controlled by the release to the ovaries of the follicle-stimulating hormone (FSH) by the pituitary gland under the influence of the hypothalamus in the brain. FSH triggers the production of ova by the ovaries with the help of another hormone, estrogen. In menopause, there is a significant drop in the female hormones, particularly estrogen, resulting in an excess of FSH and hormonal imbalance.

If the reduction in hormones is relatively gradual, the woman may have few if any symptoms. Women who experience a sudden drop in hormone levels may experience more severe symptoms, including hot flashes, vaginal dryness, depression, itching skin, palpitations (an awareness of the heart's beating), and insomnia. The hormone changes of menopause result in a thinning of the walls of the vagina and the secretions of their mucous membranes, so that, while sexual drive may not change, intercourse may be painful and lead to anxieties that put a strain on a relationship.

Hormonal imbalance also is responsible for episodes of flushing experienced by roughly half the menopausal women. The reason for hot flashes is not known for certain, but it has been suggested that they are connected with a momentary alteration of the body's temperature control center in the brain, the hypothalamus. According to this theory, the body adjusts to the new thermostatic setting by causing perspiration and flushing to throw off the excess heat.

Connected with the reduced supply of estrogen is the development of osteoporosis, a thinning of bone tissue in postmenopausal women.

TESTINGS AND TAMPERINGS:

This condition leads to fractures and accounts for the high rate of bone fractures among women age 55 and older—10 times the risk for men the same age.

Estrogen-replacement therapy (ERT) to treat the symptoms of menopause and prevent osteoporosis is used cautiously these days by doctors because of the established link between ERT therapy and an increased risk of developing cancer of the uterus, high blood pressure, and gall-bladder problems.

Male Menopause

The notion of a male menopause is a contradiction in terms. Menopause means literally the end of menstrual periods. Since men do not menstruate, they cannot have a menopause. However, a mid-life climacteric is recognized as occurring in some males, with emotional effects similar to those experienced by women.

At this time, the male becomes aware of his aging body and may slip into depression. He becomes anxious about his ability to perform sexually and may become more sexually active to compensate for such feelings or lose the urge. Excessive concern about impending retirement, children growing up, and future options can lead to depression if these anxieties are not handled as they occur. A mature acceptance of the normal changes of life is necessary to successfully pass through this phase.

The Cutting Edge

Depending on the body's general physical condition, it reacts well to invasion for surgical procedures at virtually any age. The *Guinness Book of World Records* records that the most advanced age at which a person had surgery was 111 years, 105 days for a gentleman who had a hip operation in 1960. That record was surpassed in 1983 when a man born in 1871 underwent surgery to correct a cataract. He did so well, the doctor is reported to be planning surgical correction of the cataract in his other eye.

Drugs and the Aging Body

Aging affects the functions of the body and along with that, the pharmacokinetics of drugs—the way drugs behave in the body. A drug's pharmacokinetics include its absorption into the bloodstream, its distribution to the cells, its metabolism in the liver, and its excretion, usually through the kidneys and bladder. For example, the distribution of a number of drugs depends on their attachment to albumins in the blood. With aging, the concentration of serum albumin, a blood protein, declines. This lowered concentration of protein causes changes in drug binding, or attachment, and, as a consequence, in drug distribution. On top of that, the poor circulation of the blood experienced by many of the elderly and their slower absorption of medicines through the walls of the intestines may decrease the potential effectiveness of medicines. Malnutrition, a frequent problem in the elderly, also can affect the body's ability to absorb and use medicines.

Distribution also is affected by the higher proportion of fat to protein tissue in the elderly. More fat tissue means more room for fat-soluble drugs to be stored. These tissue changes can affect the amount of time a drug stays in the body, the amount of medicine absorbed by the body's tissues, and the action of the medicine in the body. The greater the percentage of fatty tissue, the more concentrated and powerful the effect of the drug—medicine, alcohol, caffeine, nicotine.

The filtering action of the kidneys and the ability of the liver to detoxify drugs such as barbiturates also decline with age, causing drugs to leave the body more slowly, a change even more important when 2 or more drugs are taken at the same time.

Because of the aging body's decreased ability to maintain the usual balance between all systems, the elderly may be more sensitive to the effects of some drugs. Unusual side effects also may be experienced because of aging changes that cause the body to retain larger concentrations of certain medicines. A dose that may cause nausea in a younger adult may lead to confusion or other side effects in the elderly. Senility has often been the diagnosis for a person only suffering from confusion and other conditions caused by too many drugs in the system.

To further complicate the problem for the elderly, research on drug therapy is conducted on young and middle-aged adults—mostly males —who are not over 50. Dosing and drug-reaction information are often inadequate or totally lacking for children and the elderly.

With all of the adverse effects that can afflict the elderly person because of consumption of drugs, it is distressing to note that 25 percent of prescription drugs in the United States are taken by 11 percent of the population—those over 65.

LIMITS TO SURVIVAL

Great Expectations

The relationship of dwarfism to impaired pituitary function has been recognized since 1908; however, only recently has it been possible to reverse the condition and enable the dwarf to attain a more normal height.

The human growth hormone is produced in the front portion of the pituitary gland and is essential for normal growth. A deficiency of the growth hormone (hGH), pituitary dwarfism affects twice as many boys as girls. It is most often diagnosed in children between the ages of 1 and 3 and sometimes older.

People afflicted with this deficiency are generally healthy and have normal mental development. The average person with this deficiency grows less than 1.5 inches (38 millimeters) a year. Maximum growth generally is 45 to 55 inches (1,143 to 1,397 millimeters).

Although a deficiency of the human growth hormone is the most common cause of pituitary dwarfism, other things can produce the same effect, such as kidney disease, heart or liver disease, malnutrition, or inherited short stature.

With early diagnosis, treatment of pituitary dwarfism is possible before the growth years have passed. The normal growth period ends at around age 18 or 19, while the growth of a hormone-deficient person may be extended to 20 or 25 years of age. More recent research has demonstrated that some short children also may respond to treatment with hGH therapy. With continued therapy, growth of about 3 inches (76.2 millimeters) each year can be expected until about 15 to 17 years of age.

Until recently, 30 to 50 pituitary glands had to be removed during autopsy to extract the growth hormone needed each year to treat one child—at a cost of about $5,000 per year. A synthetic growth hormone has been developed using recombinant DNA techniques that prevents some types of dwarfism in children and will be much less expensive than extracting hormones from human pituitary glands once it is approved for marketing.

No, I Don't Have a Cold . . .

Allergies are the result of a physical reaction to something in the environment. Allergic reactions range from an annoying skin rash, to nasal problems (a runny nose, blocked sinuses, sneezing), to an upset digestive tract, to violent reactions that swell the body's tissues, send the lungs into spasm, lower the blood pressure to dangerous levels, and cause sudden death.

The allergic reaction is a response from the body's immune system. Designed to fight off invading germs, the immune system reacts to ordinary substances in the environment in the same way. When a foreign protein, called an antigen, is encountered, the immune system produces 2 kinds of white blood cells. One attacks the foreign substance directly, while the other produces antibodies, immunoglobulins. Immunoglobulins are protein molecules that attach themselves to the surface of the invader to get it ready for destruction.

The antibodies continue to circulate in the body so that when an antigen is encountered again, up to 500,000 immunoglobulin E (IgE) molecules may attach themselves to the outside of the mast cells that lie on the surfaces of the antigen. The irritating substance enters the mast cells between the immunoglobulin molecules which causes the IgE molecules to react by pulling together. These molecules then stimulate the mast cell which causes it to release histamine and other chemicals that produce the symptoms of the allergic reaction in a form typical of the location of the affected mast cells.

Among the most common allergies are hay fever, asthma (reported to be related to allergy about 40 percent of the time), skin rashes or eczema, hives, animal dander, plant or chemical, penicillin and other medicines, and foods such as shellfish, nuts, eggs, and milk. Between 2 and 10 percent of all children in the United States under the age of 3 are allergic to milk, although breast milk does not seem to bother them.

About 35 million Americans suffer from allergies periodically or all of the time.

St. Bernard to the Rescue

When a skier winds up in a snowbank, the Swiss would tell us to send the St. Bernard with his trusty keg of brandy to revive the unfortunate victim—despite the fact that alcohol is one of the worst things you can give a person in a cold-stress situation.

Generally, the body's temperature is maintained through a number of mechanisms triggered when signals from nerve endings, mainly in the spinal cord and skin, are transmitted to the hypothalamus, the temperature control center in the brain. These signals set off an intense constriction of the blood vessels, which conserves body heat by reducing blood flow to the extremities. The body also stops sweating so that an additional bit of heat is saved. When we are cold, the normal reaction is to shiver. Shivering increases body heat by as much as 5 times the basal rate.

Alcohol is a drug which has strong vasodilator effects; that is, it dilates or widens the blood vessels causing increased loss of heat and sweating which adds to that loss. At the same time, alcohol interferes with the breakdown of carbohydrates from food which slows down heat production in the body. In addition, alcohol in combination with drugs such as antihistamines for hay fever or other allergies, cold medicines, sedatives, tranquilizers, sleep medicines, barbiturates, and medicines to treat depression produces a rapid decline in body temperature.

While the St. Bernard's brandy may have had positive benefits for the liquor industry, it is the last thing a victim of cold stress needs.

The Big Chill

Staying in a cold place for an extended period of time can cause problems for anyone. In its extreme form, exposure to cold temperatures can lead to hypothermia, a condition in which the body temperature goes below 95 degrees F (33 degrees C), rectally. When the body's rate of internal heat production cannot keep up with the rate of heat loss to a cool or cold environment, death usually follows.

Hypothermia may occur in anyone exposed to severe cold without enough protection. Skiers, mountain climbers, workers on offshore oil rigs, or victims of airplane or boating accidents have been victims of hypothermia. The cause of death in some "drownings at sea" has actually been from hypothermia. However, even mildly cool temperatures of 60 degrees F (15.5 degrees C) to 65 degrees F (18.3 degrees C) can trigger hypothermia, particularly in the elderly, infants under the age of 1 year, and some adults who do not shiver, react to cold normally, or take the usual steps to keep warm; or those who are unable to move around well, are ill, or cannot afford warm clothing, adequate heating fuel, or proper nutrition. Hikers or campers who are caught in the rain and can't find shelter sometimes develop hypothermia.

In addition, some medicines such as those used to treat high blood pressure, certain heart conditions, and migraine headaches can affect the loss of body heat or the body's ability to respond to cold temperatures.

Frozen Alive

The chances for recovery from hypothermia depend on the severity of the cold temperatures and how long the person was exposed, as well as the person's general condition before the accident. If body temperature did not fall below 90 degrees F (32.2 degrees C), chances for a normal recovery are good. If body temperature falls to between 80 degrees F (26.6 degrees C) and 90 degrees F (32.2 degrees C) most victims will recover, but may experience some lasting health damage. Most victims, especially the very old, will not survive a drop in body temperature below 80 degrees F (26.6 degrees C).

An exception to these norms was the case of 19-year-old Jean Hilliard in Minnesota in December 1980. In temperatures of 15 degrees below zero and with howling wind, Miss Hilliard had an accident with her car and had to leave it to find shelter. Walking a distance of 2 miles with only a short jacket for protection, she collapsed and was not found until the next morning.

Doctors reported her body was frozen as solid as "a cordwood stick." Her temperature did not even register on a medical thermometer, and was therefore below 88 degrees F (31.1 degrees C). Her heart rate was 6 to 8 beats a minute (the normal is 72 for a female), and she was breathing only 2 to 3 times a minute. Gradual thawing with moist electric heating pads brought her back to consciousness, and further treatment saw her to full recovery.

Each year brings reports of 10 to 15 similar cases of dramatic recovery following hypothermia, but they are the exceptions rather than the rule.

Frostbite

When body tissue is destroyed by freezing, the condition is called frostbite. Ice crystals actually form in the fluid around tissue cells and blood stops circulating as blood vessels freeze. Frostbite usually occurs in those people unable or unwilling to get in out of the cold, such as people lost in a snowstorm or skiers who stay too long on the slopes when it is very cold. It is particularly insidious since there is no sensation of pain at first.

When the skin temperature drops from the normal 98.6 degrees F (37 degrees C), the blood vessels in the skin constrict to conserve heat for the internal organs. Because it is cut off from its blood supply, the source of its heat, the skin cools quickly to 59 degrees F (15 degrees C). The body attempts at this point to save the skin by opening its blood vessels and bringing warm blood to it. The skin becomes red, feels warm, and a burning sensation starts, developing into severe pain. When the skin continues to cool, it becomes numb and the pain disappears. Circulation stops completely when the skin temperature drops below freezing. At this point, the tissues freeze and the skin takes on a white, waxy appearance that feels like a piece of frozen meat.

The skin, muscles, and blood vessels freeze first. As body temperature continues to drop, even the bones and tendons freeze.

The next time you go mountain climbing or backpacking in an icy, snowy place, be sure to dress properly, keep dry, and get back to your campsite before dark.

In the Heat of the Day

Heatstroke is the failure of all of the body's cooling mechanisms. Normally, the temperature control center in the brain maintains body temperature at about 98.6 degrees F. The brain's cells react principally to the temperature of the blood that passes through them. When the temperature of the blood rises, the nerves carry signals to all parts of the body. In response, the blood vessels near the surface of the skin are widened so that more heat is given off. At the same time, the metabolic processes in the internal organs are decreased so that less heat is produced. The point at which the brain's cells become so damaged by the rise in heat and lose their ability to function is heatstroke. Among the symptoms are faintness, dizziness, headache, nausea, a body temperature of 104 degrees F (40 degrees C) or higher, rapid pulse, very hot but dry skin, and loss of consciousness in rapid succession. Death may follow if the victim is not treated immediately.

Heat Exhaustion

Unlike heatstroke which can strike suddenly, heat exhaustion usually develops over several days. It is the most common form of illness due to hot weather. Heat exhaustion results from a loss of water and salt. The symptoms include weakness, heavy sweating, nausea, and light-headedness.

The average person is more susceptible to heat exhaustion when exercising. Athletes, on the other hand, seldom suffer heat exhaustion despite the fact that they lose great quantities of fluid during their exercise. This is because their hearts pump blood more efficiently and deliver it to vital areas at a more efficient rate. Their bodies, therefore, can function with lower levels of fluids. Moreover, athletes understand their need to take or replace fluids before, during, and after exercise, and regularly consume liquids when exercising.

Drunk on Water

Just as the headache of a hangover from too much alcohol consumption is caused by dehydration of the brain's cells, water intoxication can produce a very bad headache and even convulsions.

The body usually has the same concentration of minerals inside and outside each of its cells. Water contains few minerals. When you drink large amounts of water, the concentration of minerals outside the cells is diluted. Because the concentration of minerals inside the cells is still the same, the fluid with lower mineral concentration flows into the fluid with higher concentration inside the cell, causing the brain cells to swell and "cry out" with the pain we perceive as a headache. This situation also can cause convulsions.

If you notice that you get a headache when you drink large quantities of water, you may be among the people who are susceptible to water intoxication. The solution is to drink less water, unless you eat something at the same time. The alternative, if you cannot eat at the same time, is to quench your thirst with fruit juices high in mineral content.

How Dry I Am

The body can survive for weeks and even months without most of the nutrients we get from food—carbohydrates, fats, proteins, vitamins and minerals. Without water, however, the body will not last even a few days.

The body requires the equivalent of about 6 to 8 glasses of liquids a day. Some of this comes from the food we eat and drink. The principal component of tissue cells, urine, sweat, tears, and blood is water. Water also is a by-product of every energy-producing reaction that takes place in the body, such as the metabolism of carbohydrates into glucose. Lacking adequate water in the body, cells become dehydrated and the chemical reactions that occur in our cells are inhibited.

Under these conditions, cells cannot build new tissues and do not use energy supplied by food nutrients efficiently. Inadequate hydration prevents the formation of urine. The poisonous substances normally removed by the kidneys from the blood in forming urine then build up in the bloodstream creating an extremely hazardous and life-threatening situation.

Sweating helps the body dispose of excess heat and maintain a normal body temperature. If the body does not have enough water to produce sweat, body temperature rises to dangerous levels. With insufficient water, the body's blood volume is reduced, providing less blood to carry oxygen and food nutrients to all parts of the body. As a consequence of this dehydration, muscles become weak and a feeling of fatigue sets in. If you are unable to rehydrate yourself in time, you will die.

When you engage in sports, do heavy work, or do exercise that causes you to sweat, you need much more water than you usually drink to replace what is lost. A good general rule is to drink a glass of liquid with every meal and, of course, every time you feel thirsty. However, don't wait until you feel thirsty to replace lost fluids. It may be too late. Harvard Medical School studies have shown that healthy kidneys can process up to 80 glasses of fluid every day.

Losing Your Senses

A lack of taste or smell not only deprives us of the everyday pleasures of smelling freshly cut grass, the turkey roasting at Thanksgiving, or the flavor of other good meals, but can interfere with our sex life and may be dangerous.

The importance of smell in sex was rated in a national survey done by the Fragrance Foundation and reported in an article in *Parade* Magazine, April 10, 1983. On a scale of 1 to 10, the average score was 8. The same article reported that sexual desire diminishes in about one fourth of the people who have lost their sense of smell.

Lighting a match can be dangerous if you can't smell leaking gas. People who are unable to smell smoke may die because of their inability to receive this early-warning fire signal.

The sense of smell may be lost as a result of blocked nasal passages caused by years of sinus problems, or a bad attack of the flu or other infections may be the cause. Severe allergies, asthma, head injuries, or congenital abnormalities have all led to a loss of smell or taste. Some drugs such as captopril, used to treat high blood pressure, may cause a temporary loss of taste. Long-term use of potassium iodide may leave a metallic taste in the mouth. Strong chemotherapeutic agents taken by some cancer patients have resulted in changes in taste and smell. A tumor in the brain near the center for smell may cause the loss of this valuable sense.

People who have partially lost their sense of taste may still be able to distinguish between sweet, sour, salty, and bitter; but without smell, they cannot distinguish the flavor of foods. Flavor is the combination of smell, texture, and taste.

As many as 16 million people in the United States alone may suffer from disorders of taste or smell.

Hitting the Dreaded Wall

When an athlete "hits the wall," the result is not a bloody nose, but a loss of energy in the muscles. When carbohydrates from the food we eat are metabolized by the body, they are converted to sugar (glucose) in the intestine and sent through the walls of the bowel into the bloodstream. Any glucose not required as energy or fuel by the body immediately is sent to the liver for conversion to glycogen, which is then stored in the liver and in muscle tissue.

When there is inadequate glycogen to supply the needs of a muscle, the muscle begins to hurt and coordination of the muscle is lost. This is "hitting the wall," a common occurrence during endurance competition such as long-distance cycling, cross-country skiing, long-distance swimming, and marathon races. This happens most often, in fact, during marathons run in hot weather because exercise then uses up more glycogen than similar activity in cooler temperatures.

The glycogen stored in a muscle remains in that muscle until it is oxidized, burned up, during activity. The glycogen cannot move or be transferred to another muscle. This explains why the muscles that are being used the most in exercise will run out of glycogen first. A marathon runner's legs will run out of glycogen before his arms do, for example.

It is possible to keep going after "hitting the wall." If activity continues, the muscles are forced to burn fat, blood sugar, and then their own tissue. At that point, every move becomes excruciatingly painful.

Bonking

Athletes engaged in endurance sports—continuous competition for more than an hour—who lose liver glycogen during competition may experience "bonking." The symptoms of bonking include breaking into a cold sweat, shakiness, dizziness, and lack of muscle coordination.

It is possible to recover from bonking if you are able to eat immediately, thus restoring liver glycogen, the principal source of energy for the brain. Taking nourishment during an athletic event prevents bonking.

The major difference between "bonking" and "hitting the wall" is that in hitting the wall, you run out of muscle glycogen and cannot recover because it cannot be replaced instantaneously. In bonking, you run out of liver glycogen that can be replaced by eating and permits you to come back and continue the event.

It is possible to "bonk" and "hit the wall" during the same event. If you push on after hitting the wall when the muscle's store of glycogen has been used up, the muscles will burn liver glycogen in addition to fat, blood sugar, and their own tissues.

Radiation Sickness

Radiation takes 2 forms and affects the body in different ways. Ionizing radiation is what you can get from a nuclear blast, medical X rays, or fallout from a nuclear power reactor. Nonionizing radiation may come from high-voltage power lines, radar installations, or microwave towers.

The principal difference between the 2 forms of radiation is the energy they produce and what they do with it. Energy from ionizing radiation is strong enough to knock loose electrons in the molecules in cell tissue. These free electrons can break a chromosome, one of the chains of DNA molecules that contain the cell's genetic information. These chromosomes can repair themselves, but, according to one theory, may make incorrect repairs which may lead to uncontrolled, malignant reproduction of the cell, cancer. Nonionizing radiation lacks the energy to dislodge electrons, but can affect biological processes by heating tissues and by some nonthermal means.

Current research is reexamining the statistics on the 80,000 survivors of Hiroshima and Nagasaki. Studies of these groups over the years have examined the development of cancer and other diseases among the victims in relation to the estimated doses of radiation they received. It is now generally accepted that the original estimates of the number of people who would eventually develop cancer and other diseases from the fallout were too low. The horrible medical problems initially experienced by the survivors were therefore caused by even lower doses of ionizing radiation than originally estimated.

Living by the Clock

The internal rhythms of the body regulate our eating and sleeping habits and our daily activities as well as kidney and bowel function, body temperature, and hormone levels in the blood. These daily cycles are governed not by sunrise and sunset, but by internal cues or "clocks" as they are called by Dr. Martin C. Moore-Ede, Associate Professor of Physiology at Harvard Medical School and coauthor, with Frank Sulzman and Charles A. Fuller, of *The Clocks That Time Us.*

These internal time clocks, referred to by others as circadian rhythms, operate on about a 25-hour cycle and must be reset each day by stimuli outside the body, such as light and mealtimes. As long as these cues are not too much out of synchrony with the internal clock, the clock resets and the body's rhythms remain normal. However, if the time cues are shifted rapidly by more than an hour or so, the internal clock fails to catch up right away and resets itself by about an hour each day until it is once again in tune with the external cues.

Jet lag is the result of this disharmony between the internal time clock and external stimuli. People who work in industry, in hospitals, and public servants such as policemen and firemen who are required to work rotating shifts also may suffer from the effects of being out of phase with their internal clocks.

Dr. Moore-Ede and associates point out that there is more than one internal clock and that these various clocks do not react to external time changes in the same way. So, it is possible for an internal clock to be out of phase with the real world and out of phase with the other internal clocks.

The majority of people who experience a major change in time zones have periods of insomnia or they may fall asleep at the "wrong time." Fatigue is common. Digestive problems may result, along with constipation, a frequent occurrence in long-distance travel. Digestive juices excreted at the "regular" time for meals may have no food in the digestive tract to neutralize them. These juices may eat into the walls of the bowel and can cause peptic ulcers and other gastrointestinal problems.

All of these reactions may result in impaired judgment in a work situation or may ruin a vacation. Because our internal clocks are normally regulated for optimum performance during the day and a lower efficiency in the early hours of the morning, roughly between 3 and 5 A.M., a person shifted to work during these early morning hours may not be as alert as normal and can make errors in judgment. Accident statistics apparently support this assessment, and Dr. Moore-Ede notes that the Three Mile Island accident happened at four in the morning with a crew that had just started the night shift.

Hanging by Your Heels

The ancient form of crucifixion was in the inverted position for good reason—the observed effects led to a quick, if painful, death.

Today, fitness enthusiasts deliberately hang upside down in gravity boots to relieve stresses placed on joints in the body by the sedentary habits of modern living.

In the inverted position, body weight and gravity pull vertebrae in the spinal column apart and stretch muscles in the back. However, hanging upside down also raises the blood pressure and pulse rate, the pressure of fluids inside the eye, and pressure on arteries supplying the eye. The *New England Journal of Medicine* (November 25, 1982) reported that two people had awoken with black eyes after inversion in gravity boots.

The practice can be dangerous, especially for people not in perfect physical condition, those with high blood pressure, glaucoma, or the elderly. Researchers at the Chicago College of Osteopathic Medicine are now examining the effects of inversion on people with a high risk of having a stroke, those using aspirin regularly, and people with spinal problems and hernias. One can only speculate that a combination of 2 or several of these effects caused the death of victims of crucifixion.

Experiments by Soviet and American scientists on the effects of bed rest with the head tilted down—not a fully inverted position—reproduces some of the early effects on the body of weightlessness in space including rapid and pronounced shifts of body fluids along with related symptoms such as facial puffiness, nasal congestion, and a feeling of fullness in the head. Tests following the head-down tilt showed it took the heart some time to return to normal functioning—and these tests were on astronauts and cosmonauts in peak condition.

Which Way Is Up?

In outer space, without the gravitational pull of the earth, significant realignments occur in the structures of space travelers' inner ear. Coupled with interactions with other sensory systems, a variety of symptoms is produced, including space motion sickness, which has affected 30 to 40 percent of individuals flying in space.

Scientists believe that the problem of space motion sickness occurs when the body tries to adapt to the absence of gravity and shifts in its position that cause disorientation. Under these conditions, the brain receives conflicting signals from the inner ear—which registers pressure changes and affects the sense of balance—and the eye. The brain interprets these signals as incorrect because of the absence of directional markers in a weightless environment.

These abnormal signals, and reactions of the eyes and muscles to a moving environment, may combine to cause the release of a brain chemical into the fluid that bathes the brain and spinal cord, triggering vomiting, according to recent research by NASA scientists. This specific brain chemical has yet to be identified.

Because space motion sickness is accompanied by other physical reactions, NASA has named it space adaptation syndrome (SAS). Among the signs and symptoms reported are varying degrees of fatigue, excess salivation, gas or belching, loss of appetite, apathy, sleepiness, weakness, headaches, unusual sensitivity to repulsive odors or sights, excess discomfort to previously tolerated levels of heat or cold, and vomiting.

Some of the problems experienced, such as headaches, are thought to be caused by the shift of body fluids—1 to 2 quarts (0.95 to 1.9 liters)—from the lower to the upper half of the body that occurs because of the absence of gravity's downward pull.

Tests seem unable to predict who will develop SAS and who will not. Scientists indicate that people react differently in various gravitational environments and that it depends on basic susceptibility to the motion environment, and the rate and degree of adaptation. It has been demonstrated that previous participants are less likely to suffer with SAS than first-timers.

The symptoms of SAS usually appear soon after orbit and are aggravated by head and body movement, especially if the eyes are open. The

TESTINGS AND TAMPERINGS:

symptoms usually disappear within 2 to 4 days into the flight and do not recur. However, those who have experienced SAS on a flight—particularly those on longer flights—have sometimes had a recurrence of inner-ear effects after returning to earth.

Experiments on the recent *Spacelab 1* flight and others planned for the future were aimed at determining whether the SAS problem is with the otolith of the inner ear that controls information about gravity and linear motion, or with the semicircular canals that have to do with the angular motion of the head. Parallel to those studies are those that seek to learn whether it is gravity or light that is most important for humans in deciding which way is up.

Out of This World

Space travel demands the ultimate in adaptation from the human body. Space travelers must endure long periods of time in stationary positions, learn to move and work in a weightless environment, and live in close proximity with their fellow passengers. On top of all that, the space traveler must adapt to the physiological responses of the body to a weightless atmosphere which begin as soon as the body is in zero gravity.

Long-term space flight leaves muscles so weak that returning Russian cosmonauts—who have been on the longest space flights to date—have been barely able to stand and required many weeks of rehabilitation to recover. Bones lose 0.5 to 1 percent of their calcium content each month in a weightless environment. Some body fluids shift from the lower to the upper half of the body because of the absence of gravity's downward pull. While the heart and circulation seem to adapt efficiently within the first few hours of flight, there have been signs of heart abnormalities during the early stages of reentry to earth's gravity. The heart even loses some weight during space flight because some cardiac muscle is lost. The pulse rate on land after return from a long flight is higher than before the flight.

Red blood cells are depleted during flight, changing their ratio to white blood cells. Short astronauts and cosmonauts realize a fantasy during long-term flight by increasing 3 to 6 centimeters in height—but return to normal after reentry. Inflight weight losses average 4 to 5 percent during the first 5 days of a space flight and, after that, weight gradually declines for the rest of the mission. It is thought that early weight losses are due to a loss of fluids while the later losses are metabolic. Body composition changes include large losses of water, protein, and fat during the first month of a flight. Fat is probably regained while muscle mass is partially preserved depending on exercise regimens during flight.

Estimates have been made that humans can stay in space safely for periods of up to 4 months. While astronauts and cosmonauts are testing the limits of mankind's endurance, experiments continue on ways to improve the adaptation of the body to the changes imposed by weightlessness and to counteract the detrimental effects of space flight after reentry. Perhaps future space medicine can even find a way to avoid the puffed-up faces that astronauts experience because of the different distribution of blood in the body that occurs in zero gravity.

Chapter Nine

Glimpses from Now: Future Body, Future Brain

TRANSPLANTS AND ARTIFICIAL BODY PARTS

Restoring the Human Race

In the last 5 years, almost $1/1{,}000$ of 1 percent of the human race has been successfully rebuilt with new parts—tissue grafts (for example, kidney transplants), hip and knee replacements, heart pacemakers and artificial valves, breast implants, hydroencephalus shunts, penile implants, testicular prostheses (available for the replacement of the 30,000 testicles removed annually), artificial eyes, ears, noses, tongues, larynxes, and hearts, implanted nerve stimulation devices to relieve debilitating pain and to energize paralyzed bladders, implanted brain pacemakers for victims of cerebral palsy and epilepsy, artificial skin for burn victims, and synthetic blood. Not to mention an array of vein and arterial grafts.

Between 1978 and 1983, the number of people who have gained a more acceptable mode of existence, thanks to the spare body parts industry, is 4 million—more than the population of Chicago.

Beginning with a Bitch

At the beginning of this century, attempts to transplant kidneys were pioneered by two doctors, Dr. Alexis Carrel and Dr. C. C. Guthrie. In 1905, they published the nature and results of one of their experiments entitled "Transplantation of Both Kidneys From a Dog into a Bitch with Removal of Both Kidneys from the Latter."

Since then, the experiment has been a prototype for millions of modern kidney transplants.

Organ Pilot Team

The same Dr. Carrel later teamed up with a famous personality at the Rockefeller Institute in New York to develop other spare body parts. In 1928, the two men worked together in designing special kinds of blood pumps to keep organs alive in vitro. Dr. Carrel's collaborator was the pioneer aviator, Charles Lindbergh. Lindbergh, following his 1927 transatlantic flight, was seeking other challenges, this time much closer to home.

Kidneys and Sausages

The first artificial kidney machine was patented in 1943, and while it performed the same work of a real kidney (which fits in the palm of your hand), the artificial kidney's size was that of a baby carriage. Its tube, used to transport blood and waste in and out of the body, was made of sausage casing.

GLIMPSES FROM NOW:

Typing the Tissues

Thousands of cornea and bone-marrow transplants are performed each year, but only 600 liver transplants were performed in the 5-year period from 1978 to 1983. Why? One of the main reasons is that corneas and bone marrow do not require tissue matching, while livers do.

Matching tissues means making sure compatible antigens coexist between organ donor and organ recipient. Antigens are genetic, proteinlike chemical markers of the tissue's cells which, in the presence of genetically different antigens, alert the body to produce antibodies that fight and destroy the invasive material—foreign bacteria, viruses, or in the case of organ grafting, the donated liver. When the antigens of the donated liver fail to match the antigens of the recipient (patient), he dies. (The only backup system in liver-transplant operations is another transplant. In kidney-transplant operations, however, the patient may resort to temporary dialysis if rejection occurs.)

In identical twins, antigens are the same, and tissues from donor to recipient—twin to twin—are perfectly matched. In other siblings, the chances of having the same antigens are 1 in 4. But in 2 unrelated individuals, the chances of matching antigens effectively are 1 in 1,000.

Bone Marrow

Bone marrow is the main producer of blood and a key part of the body's immune system. Bone-marrow transplants are often necessary in people with leukemia or with diseases of the immune system known as "severe combined immunodeficiency" diseases. Ironically, transplanting of the new immunologically potent marrow would often stimulate the production of antibodies that would gradually kill the patient —host—in a disease known as graft-versus-host reaction. As a result, bone-marrow transplants had necessitated the perfect matching of tissues between donor and receiver up until 1983. This had meant that two thirds of all potential bone marrow recipients would not find an acceptable donor.

In 1983, scientists came up with a technique to "purify" the marrow by ridding it of T cells—white blood cells whose presence during grafting of the marrow brings on the dreaded graft-versus-host disease. The typical amount of bone marrow transplanted is about 1 ounce. This purifying technique could mean that a million sufferers of leukemia, blood disorders, severe aplastic anemia, thalassemia, rheumatoid arthritis, plus all kinds of allergies, could be cured with about 56,000 pounds of purified bone marrow.

Fetal Lifeline

Newborn babies have something valuable to contribute to medicine these days. It is the umbilical cord, exchange place for mom's nutrients and baby's wastes. The veins of umbilical cords have become replacement arteries implanted in 20,000 victims of arteriosclerosis and other arterial diseases. The cords are not throwaway items in the delivery room.

In the past, synthetic tubes made of materials like Dacron, along with blood vessels from cows, have been used as arterial implants—all with limited success. The synthetic tubes were found to promote clotting and bacterial growth, and the cattle-vessel grafts were prone to inflammation and eventual bursting.

But umbilical tubes are like Teflon-coated skillets. Both have a "surface energy" (SE) that prevents sticking or clotting.

In addition, the 3- to 5-foot vein of the umbilical cord is the only vein in nature with no valves or branches, making it a very ideal conduit.

When the umbilical cord is cut from a baby, it temporarily loses the SE factor. But this is immediately restored by "tanning" the vein—a process similar to tanning leather, and which uses the same tanning chemicals.

After tanning, the veins are checked for proper SE, tears, cholesterol deposits, and structural soundness. Only 20 percent of the veins pass inspection, but these are still more than enough to meet the demand for grafting in hearts, arms, and legs. If all the acceptable veins were tied together, they would form a gray-red lifeline long enough to stretch back and forth from New York to San Francisco 9 times.

Mysterious Virus

Whenever possible, the background of the organ donor is investigated. For example, if the potential donor had a neurological disease that could have been caused by a virus, that donor will probably be disqualified. The following story illustrates why.

In 1979, a 37-year-old woman underwent a corneal transplant, a procedure with a 90 percent success rate. It shouldn't have happened, but 50 days later the woman died.

The woman's transplanted cornea came from a forester who, apparently, had died from Guillain-Barré syndrome—a disease of the nervous system marked by progressive paralysis. Because the transplant victim exhibited these same symptoms, doctors attributed her death to Guillain-Barré syndrome as well.

However, looks can be deceiving, and the subsequent autopsy showed that a certain virus unrelated to Guillain-Barré had invaded the unfortunate woman's eyes and brain.

Suspecting that this virus may have been contributed along with the donated cornea, doctors reexamined the dead forester. Sure enough, the same virus was present. Why had doctors mistakenly concluded that Guillain-Barré syndrome was responsible for the 2 deaths instead of this virus? Because neither the forester nor the woman had a record of being bitten by an animal.

The virus, transmitted during the corneal transplant, was rabies.

Hitting Pay Dirt with Cyclosporine

In the soils of Wisconsin and Norway, 2 fungi were discovered in 1970 by Sandoz Corporation microbiologists. The fungi produced a certain weak antibiotic, which wasn't any big news in itself. What did become sensational was the follow-up discovery that this same antibiotic—cyclosporine—suppresses the self-destruct responses of the body's immune system and wards off infection during and after organ grafting.

Doctors immediately began to administer the immunosuppressant drug to patients of tissue grafts, and acceptance has become the rule rather than the exception. Kidney-transplant success jumped from 50 percent without cyclosporine to 80 percent with the drug, while the success of liver grafting shot up from 35 percent to 70 percent using cyclosporine. Heart transplants were no exception to this improved success rate. Cyclosporine-A was used in the famous Baby Fae transplant operation in 1984, when the 15-day-old girl received a baboon heart.

One year's supply presently costs $4,000 to $6,000, although this price will fall when cyclosporine becomes cheaper to make. Yearly sales could be in the neighborhood of $20 million, so the Sandoz microbiologists weren't kidding when they said they struck pay dirt upon finding those 2 fungi in soil samples.

Replaceable Man

The artificial body parts industry owes its feats of wonder largely to advances in biomechanics, electronics, and microsurgery.

Biomechanical engineers are combining their knowledge of torque, load, lift, stress, and drag with noncorrosive, infection- and clot-free metals and plastics to restore damaged or lost body organs, tissues, and limbs.

Tiny electronic minibrains—microcomputers—and equally minute motors work together to govern arm, leg, and hand movements.

Microsurgery, besides enabling the neurosurgeon to splice sheared nerves back together, is making possible the suturing of tiny blood vessels.

Listed below are spare body parts that have made it possible for millions of people around the world to overcome disabilities brought on by amputation, paralysis, birth defects, deformities, and disease; but, ironically, a replacement body part could spell a problem of the future such as the disqualification of the super athlete who could break the 3-minute mile because of his artificial heart and lungs.

ARM

The electronic arm has a microcomputerized power station tucked under an artificial elbow, and features an elbow that bends, a wrist that rotates, and a forefinger and thumb that close. The patient thinks the action, and an electrode receiving the brain signal sets off the power station to activate the arm.

BLOOD

Synthetic blood is a chemical compound composed of carbon and fluorine. Acting as a temporary replacement until a more acceptable donor is found, synthetic blood does the job of red blood cells in transporting oxygen and carbon dioxide to and from body tissues. The first Americans to receive synthetic blood were Jehovah's Witnesses who, for religious reasons, refused normal blood transfusions.

BRAIN

Brain Pacemaker The brain pacemaker consists of 3 metal electrodes, each 1 millionth of an inch in diameter, implanted on the brain's surface. The electrodes discharge tiny, painless electric currents to relieve or modify a host of neurological afflictions such as back pain or schizophrenic behavior.

BREAST

Artificial breasts are available in a variety of silicone-gel shapes and sizes to ensure the physical, social, and emotional recovery of the annual 100,000 women who lose one or both their breasts to cancer.

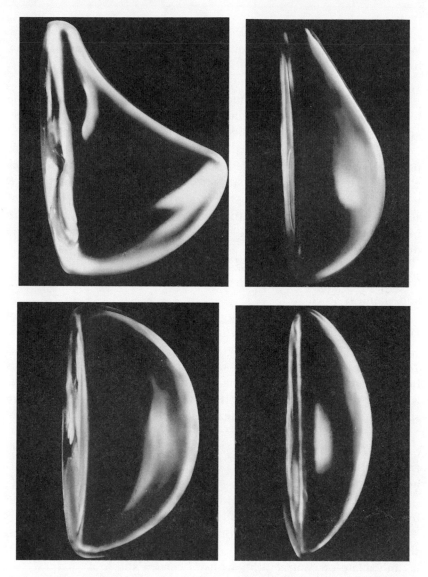

Artificial breasts are available in a variety of silicone-gel shapes and sizes for victims of breast cancer—more than 100,000 women each year. These are Silastic ® Gel-Filled Mammary Implants: Contour Design; Low Profile Contour Design; Round Design; and Low Profile Round Design. Courtesy Dow Corning Wright Corporation, Arlington, Tennessee.

While implanted mainly for cosmetic reasons, silicone chins and noses have many different center thicknesses for shaping.

EAR

Inner Ear Tympanum vent tubes do the job of real tubes that become blocked and fail to carry ear fluid away to the eustachian tube. These artificial tubes are made of silicone, stainless steel, or polyethylene.

The electronic ear is an artificially stimulated cochlea. A microprocessor implanted in a drilled cavity in the mastoid bone activates electrodes implanted on the surface of the cochlea, sending sound waves to the brain and allowing the deaf to hear speech. The quality of sound perceived by the deaf is that of a robot talking. "Walter Cronkite might sound like Donald Duck," said Dr. William Dobellein, one of the designers of the electronic ear, "but at least he'll be understandable."

Middle Ear Tiny bone implants are artificial replacements of the hammer, stirrup, and anvil. These ear bones are made out of Teflon and stainless steel.

Outer Ear The outer ear is a lightweight framework of silicone and Dacron mesh covered by a skin membrane.

ELBOW

The plastic-and-titanium elbow was first developed in 1970 and has been improved in design by replacing the upper and lower arm bones with their titanium counterparts. This allows the elbow to handle more stress, such as the lifting of a heavy object.

EYE

Acrylic Lens The acrylic lens for the eye does not cause tissue reactions, and transmits almost 100 percent light without ever degenerating.

Computerized Glass Eye The blind can see geometrical images formed by tiny, computerized points of light with this kind of artificial eye.

Cornea Inside and behind the drilled hole of an eyeball, a mushroom shaped, plastic bolt can be anchored and secured to a nut. Even though it can't dilate or contract, the artificial cornea still looks natural.

Eye Socket When the real eye socket is fractured or lost through injury, the silicone-rubber eye socket can be implanted to support the eyeball.

FINGER, TOE, AND WRIST

These bones vary with special kinds of hinges for joint rotation. A special bone preparation is required prior to inserting the implant.

HAND

When a patient thinks "open" or "close" he can open, close, or swivel the electronic hand through 360 degrees. A tiny motor that operates the lifelike hand is activated by the brain-stimulated electrodes attached to the forearm stump. This particular artificial body part works best on children.

HEART

Artificial Heart The most famous prototype, the Jarvik 7, pumped the blood of pioneer recipient Barney Clark for 112 days. Lighter-weight artificial hearts like the Utah 100 are under development. Success of the artificial heart, some people speculate, could eventually mean its failure because it would add billions of dollars to America's and other developed nation's medical bills, resulting in social rejection of a life-extending treatment for the first time in history. On the other hand, if a way is found to bring medical costs of implantation and support systems down, the second or third generation of artificial hearts will be a boon to humanity, saving millions of lives.

Assist Devices The left-ventricular assist device (LVAD), developed by the artificial heart engineering team of the University of Pennsylvania Hershey Medical Center gives temporary circulatory support to the lower 2 pumping chambers of a damaged or repaired heart that requires a rest period following surgery.

Coronary Arteries Ranging in diameters from 1/5 to 1 1/3 inches (5 to 35 millimeters), and 20 inches (508 millimeters) long unstretched, artifi-

Lighter-weight artificial hearts such as the Utah 100 are being developed and tested. Courtesy University of Utah Medical Center.

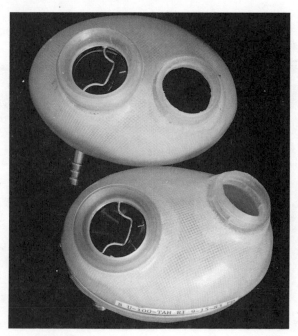

cial coronary arteries keep blood loss at a minimum when repairing real heart arteries. The knit Teflon or Dacron-fiber coronary artery resembles a flexible auto radiator hose.

Pacemakers Blessed are the pacemakers! Between 1978 and 1983, 1,250,000 patients with heart blocks (heart contractions that slow from the normal 72 beats to 30 beats per minute or lower, eventually causing death) had pacemakers installed at a cost of $6.25 billion that included materials (the electronic pacemakers) and surgeons' labor. During its typical 10-year life span the lithium pacemaker stimulates the heart to pump tens of millions of gallons of blood on only a total of 2,200 watts of power, barely enough to power an ordinary household electric iron for 2 hours.

Valves Artificial aortic, mitral, and tricuspid valves of the heart direct blood flow and are available in many versions. As of 1982, the number of pyrolytic carbon, titanium, and polyester heart valves implanted was about 300,000, or roughly the population of the state of Wyoming.

HIP

An assembly consisting of a metal ball fused to a titanium stem, the artificial hip seats and cements on the upper end of the leg bone, and couples with a plastic socket cemented to the patient's pelvis. Hip replacements are common: in the United States, 80,000 patients receive them annually.

A variety of artificial heart valves can replace the body's wornout natural ones. More than 300,000, roughly the population of Wyoming, have been implanted. Courtesy National Institutes of Health.

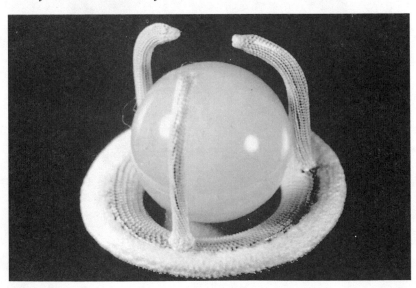

JAWBONE

HA—hydroxylapatite—is a jawbone-packing compound that fills a tooth-removed space in the jaw, preventing the jaw from deteriorating due to the tooth loss. Unlike silicone, HA is not a synthetic material: 65 percent of the jawbone and 95 percent of tooth enamel is HA, and a portion of the millions of tons of HA mined annually is used in fertilizers.

KIDNEY

WAKs are not members of the Women's Army Corps, but Wearable Artificial Kidneys—portable dialysis units that behave as motorized microfilters while disposing of the body's wastes. A far cry from the first baby-carriage-sized artificial kidneys of 4 decades ago, the WAK is compact enough to be worn externally and to fit under the seat of an airplane. The WAK replaces the dialysis machine and its cleansing fluid, medication, water softeners, tubes, clamps, and injections—necessary supplies that added up to 3 tons annually for earlier kidney patients.

KNEE

There are a variety of titanium and plastic knee systems to choose from depending on the shape, type, or rotation required, and the amount of bone and tissue loss. The artificial knee—a metal ball inside an acrylic socket—offers a bending range of 120 degrees and allows the foot to rotate 20 degrees in and out. Some 40,000 knee replacements are installed annually.

LIVER

Doctors have experimented with a few different kinds of artificial livers, none of which comes close to duplicating the highly complex natural organ. One technique uses activated charcoal and an ion-exchange resin to purify the blood of its poisons. This procedure, however, has a low success rate, but it may yield to a more sophisticated method, still on the drawing board, that uses donor cells from a liver cancer to perform many normal liver functions in a human. The donor is our fellow mammal, the rat.

LUNG

A temporary, external-support device for the patient's lungs undergoing rest or repair, the extracorporeal carbon dioxide removal (EC-CO$_2$R) technique uses a mechanical breather and a primitive artificial lung to circulate blood through a thin membrane. As of 1983, the ECCO$_2$R procedure has reversed acute respiratory failure in a half dozen patients, some of whom have stayed on the machine for almost 1 week.

MUSCLE

Pectoralis Muscles These are silicone pecs that replace surgically removed, or congenitally absent, ones; very little function exists in this type of implant other than the restoration of some lost body tone.

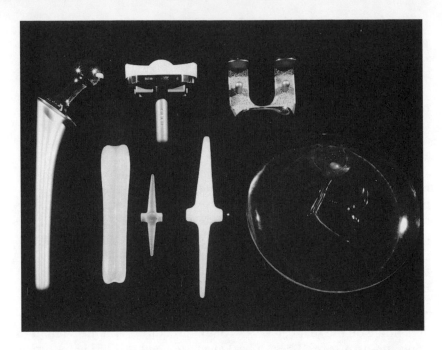

In a 5-year period, more than 4 million people have had spare body parts implanted. Here are a few of the many parts available to spare-body-parts shoppers.

Top: Whiteside OrthoLoc™ Knee Prosthesis, tibial (left) and femoral components. Bottom: Titan™ Hip Prosthesis; Silastic Penile Implant (Gerow Design); Silastic Finger Joint Implant H.P. (Swanson Design); Silastic Wrist Joint Implant H.P. (Swanson Design); and Silastic Mammary Implant. Courtesy Dow Corning Wright Corporation, Arlington, Tennessee.

Skeletal Muscles Made of a crimped, stretchable Dacron inner tube and a silicone-rubber outer tube, the artificial skeletal muscle is implanted opposite its real muscle antagonist to perform many normal muscle movements.

NERVES

As of 1983, surgeons have implanted artificial nerves in the limb muscles of a dozen quadriplegics, restoring movement in their once nerve-dead arms, hands, and fingers. Using his elbow, the patient flips a belt-worn microprocessor on electrifying the artificial nerve, activating the muscle. The nerves are stainless steel wires 1/40 of an inch thick. A hypodermic needle inserts the nerves into selected muscle sites. After the needle is withdrawn, the nerve stays in place, thanks to the nerve's barblike tip that grabs the muscle, much like a fishhook.

PANCREAS

A programmable pump that feeds a steady trickle of insulin into the bloodstream, the artificial pancreas is implanted in the diabetic's chest and is about the size and shape of a hockey puck.

PENIS AND TESTICLES

Inflatable Penis This is a totally implantable hydraulic system consisting of a pump, a reservoir for biocompatible hydraulic fluid, and fluid-carrying tubules. For $6,000 you get the artificial inflatable penis, fully installed and guaranteed to duplicate the erection of a real penis for intercourse.

Penile Sheath An implantable sheath of silicone to increase the diameter of the penis during intercourse, the penile sheath can provide the partner greater sexual satisfaction.

Solid Penile Implants These are hinged silicone-rubber rods ranging in length from 3.14 to 6.3 inches (80 to 160 millimeters) and in diameter from 0.275 to 0.55 inches (7 to 14 millimeters). In treating total physiological impotence, these penile implants are hinged to allow the penis to hang normally when not engaged in intercourse.

Sperm Reservoir A 2-inch-long (51-millimeter), silicone-rubber, semi-capsulelike implant sutured to the epididymes of the testicles to recover sperm, the artificial sperm reservoir is one answer for men who regret getting a vasectomy and want to have children again.

Testicles Made of Dacron felt and silicone gel, artificial testicles can be ordered in infant, petite, small, medium, and large sizes for patients having cause to replace their testicles. They do not generate sperm.

Totally Constructed Penis A flap of skin is surgically molded around a silicone rubber frame to resemble a penis.

Several types of penile implants are available to men with physically caused impotence. The Surgitek® Flexi-Rod® Penile Implant shown here comes in many sizes, with lengths from 3.1 to 6.3 inches (80 to 160 millimeters). They are hinged to lie flat against the leg when not in use. Courtesy Medical Engineering Corporation, Racine, Wisconsin.

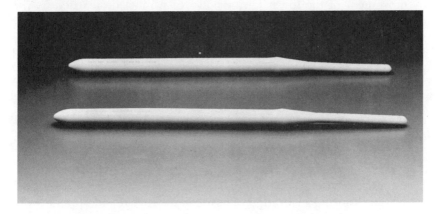

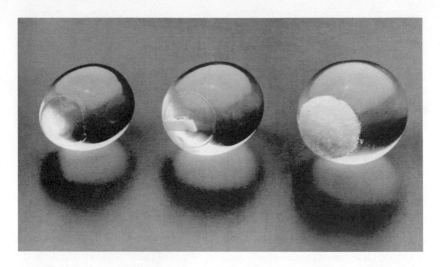

Artificial testicles such as the Surgitek Testicular Prosthesis comes in infant, petite, small, medium, and large sizes for patients who must have their testicles replaced. They do not generate sperm. Courtesy Medical Engineering Corporation.

SKIN

Custom-fitted to match the burnt skin's configuration, synthetic skin helps the damaged skin to repair itself, protecting it from infection. It does not induce rejection by the body when implanted. A strange mixture of materials make up the synthetic skin: acrylic, cowhide, and shark cartilage.

SPHINCTERS

These are J-shaped silicone tubings implanted in the ureter to control urination.

TONGUES

The silicone-rubber tongue clips on the lower teeth and is manipulated by movement of the lower jaw, a skill which must be learned by the patient. Eating with the artificial tongue can be accomplished, as long as the food is in small chunks which fall into grooves on the side of the device and go down with gravity. It is estimated that this artificial implant improves the quality of speech by 80 percent.

VAGINAS

A skin wrapped around a silicone-rubber frame 1/5 inch (5 millimeters) thick, with a retention loop for external anchoring and a central drain, the artificial vagina is available in sizes small through large.

VOICES

The mechanical voice implant is a plastic tube and valve assembly that replaces the larynx. It channels exhaled air from the windpipe into the esophagus, causing a vibration of tissue in the throat and upper esoph-

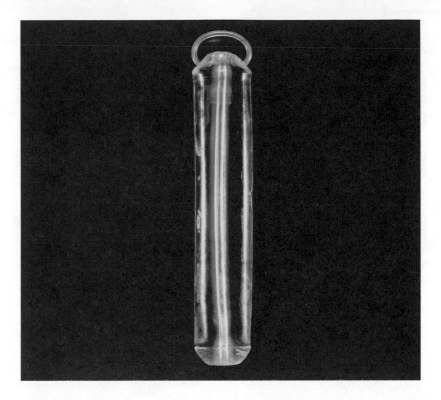

Surgitek Vaginal Stents are available for women victims of accident or disease and are available in small, medium, and large sizes. Courtesy Medical Engineering Corporation.

agus. This enables the patient to form words that are understandable but a bit on the raspy side.

MICROSURGERY

All Things Great and Small

Microsurgery requires surgeons to think and act small.

The microdimensions of blood vessels and nerves that doctors must "tie" together requires a new kind of coordination in performing the operation—some doctors describe it as working in an Alice-in-Wonderland world as they peer through a ceiling-suspended microscope.

Microsurgery has been likened to Chinese carvings on a piece of ivory no bigger than a grain of rice. When magnified, the intricate detail of the carving is amazing. The master carver acquired the skill by constantly closing his eyes and concentrating on his hands.

In the same way, microsurgeons must learn a whole new vocabulary of minute hand, muscle, and nerve movements if they want to sew together nerves the diameter of thick thread or arteries the diameter of a narrow string.

An experienced microsurgeon, Dr. William Shaw, says that he can readily spot an inexperienced surgeon performing microsurgery: "It looks like an earthquake under the microscope."

The Living Divot

Doctors perform microsurgery to sew or otherwise join severed ends of nerves, blood vessels, bones, muscle, and skin—all achieved with tiny needles several hundredths of an inch long, thread finer than human hair, and a microscope that magnifies tissues up to 40 times.

One of the more recent examples of microsurgery has been the restoration of the penis's sexual function after a small, blocked artery leading to the penis and causing impotence was bypassed by inserting another artery.

Ever since 1965, when a Japanese surgeon claimed to have performed the first kind of microsurgery anywhere by reconnecting a severed arm and its corresponding nerves and blood vessels, over 300 operations have been performed in the United States alone. Toes have replaced fingers, skin has been lifted from one area of the body and grafted onto another area, severed feet, fingers, hands, legs, and arms have been reattached, and muscle has been lifted from the leg to save an injured arm from amputation. (Without transplanted muscle, the arm would have been denied blood—and lost.) Because the muscles are so rich in blood, this type of microsurgical transplant, in which exposed bones have been covered with chunks of muscle, has been compared to a living divot. Through microsurgery, it can be used to fill in many holes.

LASERS

The Healing Light

It's quicker, cleaner, more precise, and has a better scorecard in treating a gamut of human afflictions than many presently used clinical techniques. Following its application, there is minimal scarring, little or no side effects, and effective—if not total—cure. It is the medical laser—not a military death ray, but a light scalpel for life. Its benefits for medicine are as diverse as its beams are narrow.

Consider that the laser's hair-thin beam has: eliminated permanently the cause of the pressure buildup of glaucoma in the eye; effectively remated the sheared nerve bundles of a crushed hand; been used to graft synthetic skin without rejection; vaporized brain tumors without damaging adjacent, functional tissue; and cleanly cauterized bleeding ulcers 60 times faster than conventional electric-spark treatment.

Gynecologists and urologists use lasers to destroy cancers of the cervix and penis, venereal warts, and uterine membrane inflammations. Ophthalmologists use them to perform eye surgery, and dentists to detect tooth decay. Skin specialists remove unwanted birthmarks with lasers, and heart surgeons direct a microbeam of laser light to scour the coronary arteries' inside walls of plaque (buildup of fatty deposits).

And just in case you happen to be on the lookout for safe, comfortable options to a nagging conscience over that embarrassing tattoo, check out the laser tattoo remover.

An Out-of-This-World Laser

Although the first man-made laser was not assembled until after the middle of this century, a grand-scale natural laser has been emitting its radiation for millions of years. It is the planet Mars.

The continuous light of the red planet operates on the same principle as man-made laser beams—stimulated emission of radiation.

Because the thin upper atmosphere of Mars is made up of 95 percent carbon dioxide and absorbs sunlight which "pumps" molecules to a higher energy state, and because its light is monochromatic (red, due to the planet's iron-oxide surface), Mars is a natural laser similar to the man-made CO_2 surgical laser.

However, most surgical carbon-dioxide (CO_2) lasers emit 20 watts of light and can beam down to a spot 1/66 of an inch (1/25 of a millimeter). Mars's laser continuously emits 1 million megawatts of power into the solar system—enough power to keep 1,000 hydroelectric plants running full steam.

The Cosmic Measuring Tape

The laser can emit light of one fixed wavelength. This property of light is called "monochromatic." Another property of the laser, and closely related to its being monochromatic, is its nondivergent, or coherent, beam. In the world of macrophysics, where masses of objects are large enough to be humanly observable, coherence is rarely found, because the scattering of particles in nature is random. For example, the light from an incandescent bulb is noncoherent because its beam spreads outward from the instant it leaves the burning filament.

Laser light, however, is coherent. In theory, it can travel infinitely without any diffusion.

In reality, the beam does spread out, but only at the rate of 1/2 inch per mile (1.27 centimeters per 1.6 kilometers). Mirrors set up on the moon's surface by American astronauts reflect back to earth laser light beamed from earth. In this way, the laser, as a cosmic measuring tape, calculates the fluctuating distances between moon and earth.

Each beam starts from earth a couple of millimeters wide and ends up on the moon's surface 2 miles (3.2 kilometers) wide.

By contrast, the beam from a searchlight—if one could be made powerful enough—would spread out to over 12,000 miles (19,350 kilometers) wide.

Aiming the Beam

In the early 1960s, a dermatologist named Leon Goldman "shot" his arm with a low-powered laser to see what it would do to his skin. After many experiments on himself and his patients, Goldman, along with other specialists, found that many skin disorders could be cleared up with laser light. Shortly thereafter, eye specialists took Goldman's cue and used lasers to weld detached retinas back in place. Today, the laser cauterizes, vaporizes, and analyzes tissues, blood vessels—even individual cells. Indeed, lasers promise to become the indispensable surgical tool of the twenty-first century.

Predictions of immediate commercial use, however, are hard to make. Safety regulations on using lasers have yet to be spelled out, and doctors who use them must be exceptionally well trained.

The need for pinpoint accuracy can never be overstated when talking about laser surgery. While vaporizing a brain tumor, the laser beam can wipe out or forever alter speech, sight, hearing, intellect, or personality if the powerfully intense light goes so much as half a centimeter (less than a quarter inch) awry.

Aiming the Invisible Light

Different kinds of clinical lasers emit different kinds of light. With argon-gas and ruby-crystal lasers, the beams are visible. But the light of a carbon-dioxide laser is infrared—invisible.

Visible and invisible light is a very small part of the entire spectrum of electromagnetic waves.

The length of these waves, or wavelength, is measured from one wave's crest to the next. The spectrum of light comes about because there are many different wavelengths of visible light. The light of an incandescent bulb emits many wavelengths of light at one time. But the light of a laser emits only one wavelength.

The CO_2 laser, known for its power (usually around 20 watts but flashed in microsecond pulses of light) to smite tumors and turn them into smoke, emits infrared light.

When surgeons use a CO_2 laser, they first locate the tumor with a beam from another source (this one giving off visible but harmless light) to determine the precise placement of the invisible but scorching beam. Diameters of both beams are identical—from a fraction of a millimeter to a couple of millimeters wide, depending on the size of the targeted tumor.

When the CO_2 beam is fired, it can cook the tumor like frying bacon. Heat from the laser beam turns most of the fluid-filled tumor into steam. What's left is the rim of the tumor adjacent to delicate nerves the surgeon wishes to save. The rim is then peeled off like the skin of a peach.

In this way, the surgeon performs the feat of using invisible light to remove a tumor.

Timing the Split Second

Laser light can be in the form of a steady stream of light, lasting indefinitely. But in clinical use, the time duration, or pulse of light, is very short—just a fraction of a second.

In treatment for glaucoma, each pulse of laser light focused on eye tissue is 1/10 of a second. If that sounds like a very short time span, it's actually 10,000 times longer than the pulse of light sent by CO_2 lasers to zap brain tumors.

Another type of eye disease, senile macular degeneration, requires treatment with the argon laser. The length of time this laser's beam focuses on abnormal eye blood vessels is 1 trillionth of a second, or 100 billion times shorter than our first example.

The finest example of laser's split-second timing is a recent creation at Bell Laboratories. Dubbed the "laser stopwatch," it enables the Bell people to watch activity of the atom's electrons in the early stages of their movement through integrated circuitry chips. Probably the world's fastest strobe light, this laser's smallest recorded duration of time for a pulsed beam is 30 millionths of a billionth of a second—0.000000000000030 second.

Another one of history's fleeting moments, folks.

The Beam's Drill

Ophthalmologists—eye surgeons—use the argon laser to fight glaucoma, a disease that causes blindness and afflicts 10 million people worldwide.

Inside the eye, where cornea meets sclera, is a microscopic, spongy drainage system that carries off the eye's fluids through drain channels 1 micron (1/25,000 of an inch) in diameter. This 20-layered meshwork of tissue is known as the trabecular network. When a drain loses its tautness and becomes blocked, the fluid has nowhere to go and backs up. Pressure sets in on the optic nerve. The deterioration continues—often without the patient's knowledge—until irreversible damage occurs to the optic nerve and blindness results.

If eye decay by glaucoma is detected early enough, treatment—eyedrops—can be administered in time to prevent blindness. But the patient must return again and again for the eyedrops, and even that is no guarantee against eventual blindness.

Eye surgeons have a better alternative to repetitive eyedrop treat-

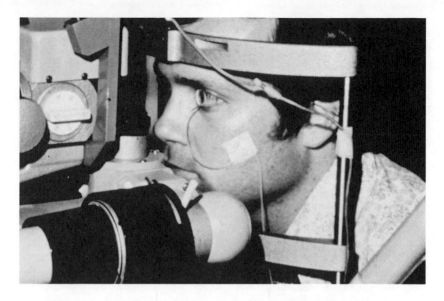

Eye surgeons use the medical laser to reverse glaucoma, a disease that afflicts 10 million people worldwide. The blue-green microbeam repeatedly flashes for 1/600 of a second to reopen drainage channels in the eye's trabecular meshwork. Courtesy National Institutes of Health.

ment if they have access to an argon laser. The procedure is done on an outpatient basis, takes 15 minutes, and is simple, safe, and painless.

The patient, having been administered anesthetic eyedrops, places his chin on a rest at the end of a horizontal binocular microscope to which an argon laser is attached.

The surgeon aims the laser at a precise location in the eye, then triggers the light beam. The blue-green light, flashed for just 1/600 of a second at 1-watt power, reflects off a mirror into the eye's drainage system, leaving a burn hole 1/20 of a millimeter (1/500 of an inch) wide. Like an old sponge that has been restored, the channels are reopened for fluid drainage and the pressure falls immediately as the surgeon repeats firing at the trabecular ring 100 times.

All the laser holes from this procedure, if placed one next to the other, would equal the width of one match flame.

The Light Scalpel

Different lasers are used for different treatments in medicine. The CO_2 laser explodes cancers and tumors because diseased body tissues contain 80 percent water—and water absorbs the CO_2 laser's beam. The

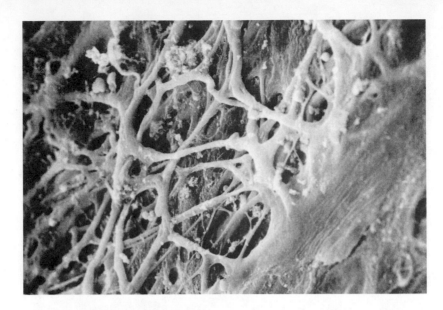

Two magnifications (1,260X and 6,000X) of the eye's trabecular meshwork. The argon medical laser burns hole about 1/500 of an inch (1/20 of a millimeter) in diameter into the tissue to allow drainage and reverse glaucoma. Courtesy Edward Y. Zavala, Sharp Cabrillo Hospital.

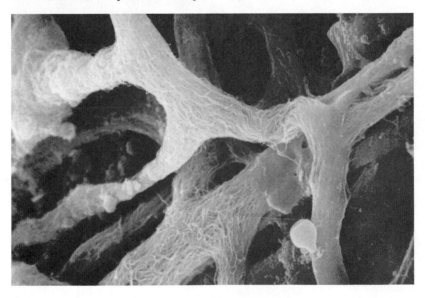

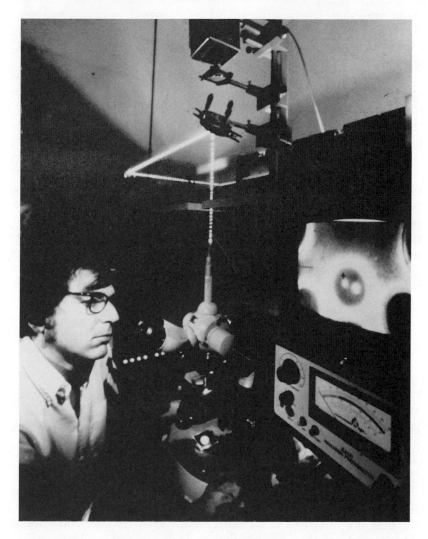

Laser use in medicine and research has expanded dramatically in the last decade. Here a researcher uses its microbeam to surgically slice chromosomes in a living cell and observe what happens at the most critical stages of cell division. The beam is reduced in size through a light microscope. Such reduction has allowed a researcher to carve his own initials on a human blood cell. Courtesy National Institutes of Health and the Resources Information Center.

argon laser is a cauterizing tool—a hot scalpel. Water does not absorb its blue-green beam; therefore, the argon laser, instead of vaporizing, burns holes through tissues and cauterizes leaky blood vessels.

The argon laser has several advantages over the CO_2 laser: It is cheaper, its beam is visible, it coagulates blood more effectively, and it has more precise aiming capacity. With the use of fiber-optic cables, the argon laser can travel into the stomach to cauterize a bleeding ulcer, and it can make life-saving journeys into the heart and other body organs as well.

What's more, its beam can be focused down to the minutest fraction of a pinhead. A classic example is the argon laser's role in the study of the mechanics of cellular reproduction. To observe exactly what happens at the most critical stages of cell division, researchers slice chromosomes, the carriers of heredity, with an argon laser. Reduced in size through a light microscope, the laser's microbeam is 400 billionths of an inch (10 billionths of a meter) in diameter—70 times smaller than the beam's own wavelength. Such a microbeam has allowed a researcher to carve his own initials on a human blood cell.

To Beam or Not to Beam

Can hospitals or clinics afford lasers in their ever-tightening budgets? Will an administrator be wary about adding them to his budget when conventional surgical techniques still produce results with acceptable rates of success?

What is "acceptable?" What is "expensive?"

The answers may be in this scenario for laser cost effectiveness.

Six thousand Americans die each year following surgery for severe stomach-intestinal bleeding. Patients who have this kind of internal bleeding are too often in a catch-22 trap: They're in no condition to survive surgery; yet, surgery's their only viable option for survival. A proven laser gastrointestinal photocoagulation system can seal off the leaky blood vessels without cutting the patient open. Its cost: $50,000.

If 10 systems were installed in hospitals around the country, the cost would come to $83 per patient.

Without them, the price becomes 6,000 American lives.

COMPUTERIZED IMAGING DEVICES

Deducing from X Rays

Wilhelm Roentgen, a German physicist, discovered the X ray in 1895, and it became one of medicine's most valuable diagnostic tools. With an X-ray machine, doctors can see internal parts of the body by looking right through the skin. A bone fracture, a lung tumor, an oversized, overworked heart—all can be seen and studied by the physician to make inferences about appropriate surgical treatment.

But despite their value to the diagnosis, conventional X-ray photographs often do not tell the whole story. As high-frequency electromagnetic waves generated in a vacuum tube, X rays are absorbed by dense tissues like bone and liver, but they pass right through less dense organs like lungs. Also, X rays produce two-dimensional photographs —pictures without depth that make it almost impossible for a doctor to gauge depth or distinguish soft tissues by looking at just one or several X rays. Add to this the fact that denser tissues like bone and heart conceal other structures behind them, and it is easy to understand why the doctor's conclusion about types of treatment—his professional opinion—is often a judgment call at best.

To Scan a CAT

Many computerized scan systems are finding their way into diagnostic and research centers to do what X rays do and much, much more.

One system that has been around since 1973—it is actually a glorified X-ray machine—is the computerized axial tomography scanner, or CAT scanner. CATs locate brain tumors and eliminate the need for exploratory surgery with computerized three-dimensional viewing. Twenty-seven percent of planned surgery is canceled because of results of CAT scans with an average saving of more than $1,000 per patient.

Like X rays, CATs are limited because the object imaged must remain still. While scanning during the course of a 360-degree rotation about the patient, the CAT takes 5 to 10 milliseconds per scan, with each scan giving 500 X-ray transmission measurements.

But, while an X ray is only one cross-sectional view, the CAT produces up to 2,000 different cross-sectional views of the organ, and each view is a 1/12-inch (2-millimeter) slice of the organ, or the thickness of a quarter.

DSR Dynamics

The Dynamic Spatial Reconstructor (DSR) also provides 3-D images of the human body, but it is state-of-the-art technology and makes the CAT scanner look antique by comparison. Only one DSR unit presently exists in the world, installed at the Mayo Clinic in the United States.

The Dynamic Spatial Reconstructor (DSR) produces 3-D images of the living human body—75,000 cross sections in just 5 seconds. Courtesy Mayo Clinic.

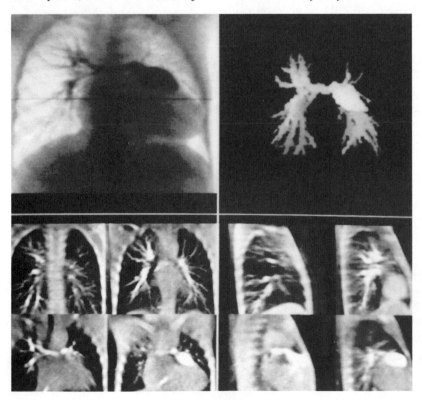

DSR's imaging scanner can produce up to 240 different sliced views of a moving organ such as a beating heart in only 1/100 of a second, and then reconstruct the data into a high-tech image of the organ from any possible perspective. In the 5 seconds that it takes an average CAT scanner to produce just one cross-sectional image of the entire body, the 15-ton DSR scanner can generate 75,000 cross sections!

Teacher's PETT

PETT—Positive Emission Transverse Tomography—allows doctors to observe chemical reactions of the brain during such actions as speaking, hearing, and thinking, or the changes in chemistry before, during, and after a stroke.

Invaluable in teaching doctors and researchers about the many types of neurological disorders, PETT works by computerized imaging and the patient's ingestion of a tiny radioactive isotope such as C^{11}-labeled carbon monoxide. To detect abnormal heart walls, the patient need only ingest a few millicuries of radiocarbon—10 billionths the amount of carbon monoxide required to generate danger symptoms in the body.

More with Less

DSA—Digital Subtraction Angiography—subtracts, via computer, unwanted background of distracting and unimportant organs to give sharp image resolution of blood vessels and related structures. DSA gets its name from the digitized fluoroscopy apparatus employed, as well as from its background subtraction techniques.

Ultrasound—Not Just for Babies

Though it has been around hospital labor rooms for years watching fetal development, even ultrasound has become computerized for 3-D imaging. In using brief pulses of ultrahigh-frequency acoustic waves (lasting 1/100 of a second) to produce sonar maps of congenital heart defects and heart-valve malfunctions, ultrasound delivers more than 30 scans per second.

Of all of the devices in the computerized imaging family (with the possible exception of nuclear magnetic resonance) ultrasound is the

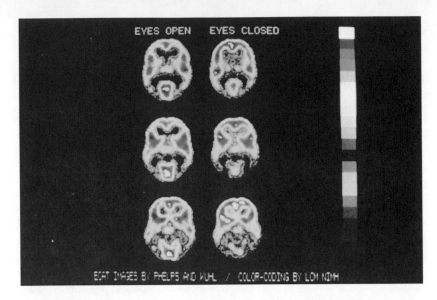

PETT (Positive Emission Transverse Tomography) scanning of the human brain allows doctors to observe chemical reactions of the living brain during such activities as speaking, hearing, and seeing. The images show differences in a brain when eyes are open and when they are closed. Courtesy National Institutes of Health.

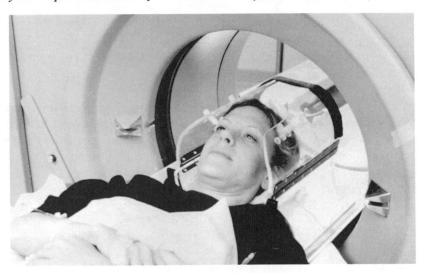

GLIMPSES FROM NOW:

least body-invasive instrument as well as the cheapest, currently arriving at the hospital for under $125,000.

NMR—Dead or Alive

NMR—nuclear magnetic resonance—is becoming the most valuable of all computerized scanning devices because it can be used to study both diseased and healthy tissues from a wide variety of morphological, functional, anatomical, and physiological viewpoints. What makes NMR stand out from computerized X-ray scanners is that most X-ray studies cannot distinguish between a living body and a cadaver, while an NMR scan "sees" the difference between life and death in great detail.

The Medical Magnet

Analysts can study both patients or chemical samples using the same nuclear magnetic resonance—NMR—machine. The procedure is the same in either case, except for adjusting the magnetic field strength.

When the patient enters the cylindrical bore of an NMR machine, he is surrounded by a 9-ton magnet. The atomic nuclei of the patient's body are then subject to the NMR's powerful magnetic field of 3,500 gauss, or 350 times that of the earth's magnetic field.

The nuclei align themselves in the magnetic field. Next, radio waves of 15 megahertz—the frequency next to the 14 megahertz frequency band for amateur radio operators—are applied against the field. The amount of energy it takes to knock the nuclei out of their field alignment is measured and used as the "signature" data, which is relayed to the computer for reconstructing the image of the body part being studied.

The strength of the magnetic field is far greater for chemical samples. When analysts want to examine chemical spectra, they will place the sample in the machine and turn up the magnetic field to 15,000 gauss, or 1,500 times the earth's magnetic field.

Monstrous Figures

Nuclear magnetic resonance might conjure up an image of a science fiction film robot, but it's actually one of the most exciting diagnostic tools in high-tech medicine. NMR comes housed in an 8-foot-wide cube with a circular opening that could make the patient entering the machine for the first time for diagnosis feel like Jonah entering the whale.

But Jonah got a free ride compared to the $700-per-half-hour patient fee. That figure sounds high until it is compared to the hospital installation fee which can cost as much as $150,000. But even that amount is only one tenth the total cost of purchase: $1.5 million.

What X Rays Don't See

Nuclear magnetic resonance can save the lives of patients suffering from abnormalities of the brain and central nervous system. NMR works on the principle that protons (subatomic particles within each atom's nucleus) of hydrogen have a particular angular momentum relative to its (hydrogen's) environment. When placed in a magnetic field, these tiny, spinning tops give off a certain energy frequency, or "signature," which is then graphically illustrated by the machine's computerized imaging system.

Since hydrogen is a component of water; since both healthy and diseased tissues are made up of about 80 percent water; and since the distribution of fluid (usually blood) is known to be altered in many diseased states, NMR can discriminate between healthy and diseased tissues with more sensitivity than conventional radiographic instruments like X rays and CAT scans. This is particularly true for persons with minute brain lesions that would ordinarily go undetected.

A Device with a Familiar Ring

Patients at high risk from radiation are welcome to the radioactive-free, diagnostic core of the nuclear magnetic resonance machine, as are those suffering from abnormalities of the heart, bladder, spinal column, discs, knees, or other body parts not receptive to current examining methods. The invitation also extends to those patients reluctant to undergo the sometimes painful dye-injection techniques of other diagnostic tools.

There is one requirement a patient undergoing NMR treatment would have to agree to, but this one is painless and amusing. A small device is attached to the sophisticated machine, but this gadget looks more apropos on a formal dining table. Its presence is owed to the high intensity of the machine's magnet. Patients use it if they need to signal the radiologist.

The device is a tiny, nonmagnetic, brass bell.

NMR and the DNA Twist

In 1952, Felix Bloch of Stanford and Edward Purcell of Harvard were awarded Nobel Prizes for their pioneering efforts in the field of nuclear magnetic resonance spectroscopy. Then, and for some time afterward, scientists were using NMR to reveal the distribution of atoms in a sample of chemical material. It was only in the 1970s that NMR began to find its way into the diagnostic rooms of medicine.

Though doctors can gather anatomical images with NMR that signal the early stages of disease, researchers are still using the machine to watch the chemistry of living systems.

At one research facility studying the behavior of chromosomes (carriers of heredity that reside in the nucleus of the cell) analysts found a contradiction to the notion that the DNA helix is a rigid structure. By

A Nuclear Magnetic Resonance (NMR) scanner can distinguish between diseased or healthy tissue in the human body with extreme sensitivity. It is one of the newest and most exciting tools in diagnostic medicine. In fact, it has even shown that the molecules of DNA bend and twist 1 billion times every second! Here biomedical engineers construct the magnetic core of an NMR machine. Courtesy National Institutes of Health.

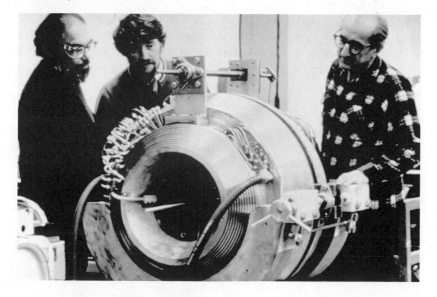

FUTURE BODY, FUTURE BRAIN

subjecting strands of DNA to the magnetic core of an NMR device, the researchers found that the molecules of DNA bend and twist 1 billion times every second.

GENE SPLICING

Out of the Lab, Onto the Assembly Line

When James Watson and Francis Crick discovered the spiral staircase-like structure—the double helix—of DNA in 1953 at Cambridge University in England, they were ushering in a new kind of industrial age—the manufacturing of new life forms and products associated with life.

Their discovery paved the way for the Brave New World of recombinant DNA. (DNA stands for deoxyribonucleic acid, a giant molecule that replicates itself and codes for the production of every living creature, be it bacteria, bird, or man.) Also referred to as "genetic engineering," "gene splicing," or "today's biotechnology," recombinant DNA is beginning to enable gene manipulators to cure cancer, forecast disease and aberrant behavior, increase the quantity and quality of food, mass-produce sorely needed antibodies and hormones, and, even more revolutionary than nuclear fission, create new life forms.

All this has led to the sprouting of about 200 genetic engineering firms around the world. And many more are on the horizon. The U.S. Patent and Trademark Office has approved more than 3,000 biotechnological patents. For not only has the genetic code been completely deciphered (by the year 2000 scientists will have chemically determined and rebuilt the human genome—the entire aggregate of about 150,000 genes of the human organism), but gene researchers have now learned the universal language genes use to communicate their own genetic "programs." They have determined how to cut apart and splice (recombine) genes. They know how to make genes (animal and human) grow inside bacteria. They can even synthesize genes in a test tube.

Such is the state of the biotech industry of the 1980s.

But the idea of such business ventures was far from the mind of Watson in 1951. At that time, just 2 years prior to his and Crick's historic discovery, Watson applied for a fellowship to study X-ray crystallography at Cambridge, a tool he needed to become acquainted with and use in solidifying his hunches about the helical structure of DNA.

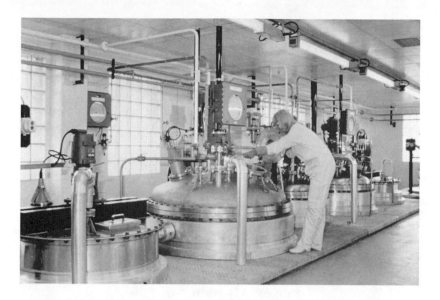

By the year 2000, biotechnology in medicine and agriculture will have grown to a $125-billion industry—all from a $3,000 stipend in 1951. These are purification tanks for man-made insulin from DNA technology. Courtesy Eli Lilly and Company.

His request for the fellowship was initially denied, and Watson was naturally disappointed. He considered the option of returning to his former specialty, cell physiology, but that would have meant abandoning hope for determining the structure of DNA. Fortunately for millions of people, and many millions more not yet born, the fellowship board reversed its decision, and awarded Watson $3,000 to pursue his studies of the alpha helix at the Cambridge lab. Watson and Crick went on to use X-ray diffraction to reveal the secret code of life.

And by the year 2000, biotechnology in medicine and agriculture will have grown from a hard-to-get $3,000 stipend to a $125-billion industry.

Unraveling DNA

The coiling of DNA inside the human body is a marvelous example of packaging at its best. If all the DNA throughout your body could be unraveled, its stranding would cover the distance between earth and the sun and back a thousand times, or enough to wrap around the earth 7 million times at the equator!

Scaling the Egg's Genes

The female egg, the ovum, is the largest cell in the human body, but even so, it is only 140 micrometers (about 1/180 of an inch) in diameter —barely visible to the naked eye.

This seems small until it is compared to the size of one of its chromosome's genes in the cell nucleus. A gene is almost 1.8 million times smaller than the egg cell, which is similar in scale to comparing a weather- or hot-air balloon (with a 24-foot, 7.3-meter, diameter) to the planet earth!

4-Letter Alphabet of Life

There are two reasons why DNA is referred to in more scientific papers than any other acronym.

First, DNA contains all the information needed to manufacture and

A scanning electron microscope image of DNA (deoxyribonucleic acid), the stuff of life that contains all the coded information necessary to maintain and reproduce a living cell. About 13 feet (4 meters) of coiled DNA occupies each body cell. Courtesy National Institutes of Health.

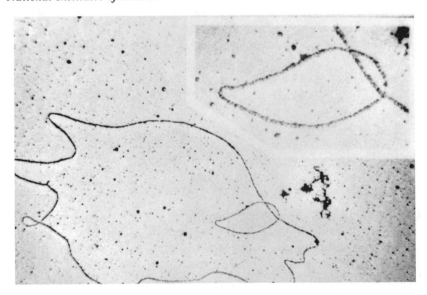

GLIMPSES FROM NOW:

maintain a living cell. This information is coded. Second, DNA reproduces itself. The result has been life when life first began, life as we know it today, and life as we will know it tomorrow.

For 3 billion years, from single-celled plants and animals to man, over 2 billion different species have owed their kind of existence to DNA, whose code contains only 4 "letters" (molecules called bases) grouped into "words" (the sequence of those bases) 3 letters long.

Pairs and Stairs

DNA manipulates and replicates cells using a coding mechanism as old as life itself. The code consists of DNA's shape of a double helix—

This model of the DNA double-helix molecule hangs in the National Library of Medicine. Some 2 billion different species over time have owed their existence to this microcosmic spiral staircase. Courtesy National Institutes of Health.

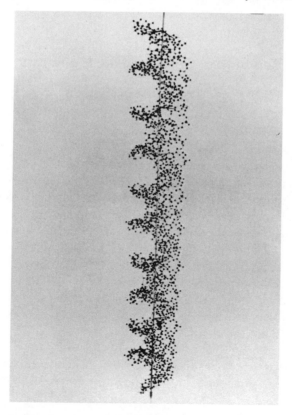

spiral staircase—and 4 chemical compounds—bases—that make up the ends of the spiral ladder's rungs. The rungs are hydrogen atoms that bond the ladder's 2 sides—sugar-phosphate backbones—together.

Each of these bases—cytosine (C), guanine (G), adenine (A), and thymine (T)—take their opposite places at each end of a rung on the molecular ladder, but their pairing is like a marital contract. Cytosine mates only with guanine, and adenine mates only with thymine. It is this fundamental law of DNA behavior that accounts for cell duplication, reproduction, and life.

The cell begins to replicate itself as DNA begins to come apart, figuratively, at the seams. Each rung—pair of bases—of the ladder splits like a zipper coming undone. Free-floating bases—nucleotides at large in the nucleus of the cell—begin converging on both halves of the unzippering ladder. Obeying the code, only a wandering base identical to that which was split off can attach itself on the half-ladder. The disassembly and reassembly continue until 2 complete DNA ladders are formed, each the same as the original. The DNA spiral-staircase molecule has duplicated itself, and life goes on.

Templates, Codons, and Humanity

Each pair of bases, held together by hydrogen bonds, forms the shape of the spiral staircase. This shape is never changed by the paired base sequence because the molecular shape of the CG pair is always identical to the AT pair.

As a cell begins to divide and reproduce, the coiled strand of DNA splits down its center. The sequence of paired bases is preserved, with CG seeking out GC and AT looking for TA. The original DNA strand is now a template for a new DNA strand.

All this business about templates for new DNA strands is very nice, but it would still add up to nonsensical information if it weren't for the fact that every 3 letters (bases) along the DNA spiral staircase form a "word," or codon. Each codon specifies 1 of the 20 amino acids. It is the particular sequence of these codons along the double helix that determines the gene, which in turn directs production of enzymes and proteins, forming the characteristics that comprise you, such as your blood type, color of your eyes and hair, and so on.

After 10,000 years, all of us still bear a close resemblance to 500 generations of human ancestors, thanks to the remarkable constancy of DNA.

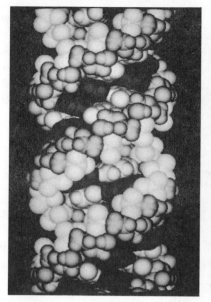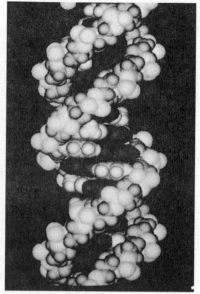

These 2 computer-image models of DNA (left) and RNA (right) show their structural differences. RNA (ribonucleic acid) is DNA with an extra oxygen atom. Both molecules synthesize proteins within the cell. Because both substances have a remarkable consistency in reproducing themselves, each of us bears a close resemblance to 500-plus generations of human ancestors. Courtesy Richard J. Feldmann, National Institutes of Health.

Treading the Basepaths

A gene is a nucleic acid, a giant double-helical molecule coiled within itself. Within this molecule are smaller molecules called bases. It is the particular sequence of these bases along the spiral ribbons of DNA that embodies the genetic code of life.

The number of different bases that may compose a gene are only 4, yet these bases may repeat themselves in varying sequences many times over the stretch of a nucleic-acid molecule. Some nucleic acids are only 100 bases long; others are hundreds of millions of bases long.

The gene-splicing industry now depends on a data bank for DNA/RNA sequencing. (RNA—ribonucleic acid—is DNA with an extra oxygen atom. The 2 molecules work together in protein synthesis within the cell.) Run by a scientific research firm, the bank stores, maintains, and distributes data to subscribers by magnetic tape and phone. Its purpose is to prevent duplication of data collection, since more than 500,000 nucleic acids are sequenced each year.

If an engineer needs the base sequencing of a particular nucleic acid, he can save himself much time and energy by referring to the gene bank. The sequencing information stored within this bank deals with molecules that are an average 750,000 bases long. (Virus nucleic acids are typically 170,000 bases long.)

The Body's Big Crapshoot

Genes design the arrangement of amino acids, which combine with each other to form proteins, the cellular workhorses that produce all the ingredients necessary for the functioning of living things. In all of nature only 22 amino acids have been found; yet, when put together in an infinite array of combinations, these amino acids become the building blocks for over 1 billion different proteins.

Genes supervise this molecular construction with incredible precision. The way the gene's "words"—molecules, or bases, along the DNA chain—line up dictates the route amino acids will take to combine with each other. One example is vasopressin, a hormone that increases blood pressure and regulates the kidneys. Over the course of vasopressin's molecular structure, enough amino acids repeat themselves so that there are 40,320 possible ways to design and build vasopressin. Yet, the body, from one generation to the next, selects only one. The gene for vasopressin sees to it that the body gets the one unique amino acid combination the body can use.

Vasopressin is simple in design when compared to insulin. There are 8 million, million, million, billion possible arrangements of insulin, made up of just 15 different amino acids. The body chooses only one.

Even the possibilities for insulin do not begin to compare with those for the structure of hemoglobin. In this blood-forming compound, 20 different amino acids are used 7 times each to form a 140-amino acid peptide (chain sequence of molecules). As far as the body is concerned, there is only one correct sequence of amino acids. Any combination other than the correct one will result in sickle-cell anemia. This blood disorder afflicts 33,000 Black Americans every year, yet the batting average of the hemoglobin gene is staggering when one considers the 135,000,000,000,000,000,000,000,000,000,000,000,000,000,000, 000,000,000,000,000,000,000,000,000,000,000,000,000,000,000, 000,000,000,000,000,000,000,000,000,000,000,000,000,000,000, 000,000,000,000,000,000,000,000 (1.35×10^{167}) possibilities for the arrangement of the amino acids of hemoglobin.

When Murphy's Law was formulated—if anything can go wrong, it probably will—it wasn't talking about our designer genes.

Genes, the Inflation Beaters

Before the end of the 1980s, scientists will have scrapped conventional methods of making interferon—the drug scientists hope will cure certain forms of cancer—in favor of the recombinant DNA method. In doing so, these genetic engineers will be beating inflation in a marvelous way.

The current technique is to sift gallons of blood for white cells, then induce those cells to produce tiny amounts of interferon. The entire yield of the precious protein after 500,000 gallons of this "broth" is just a small fraction of an ounce—1 gram. And this 1 gram of interferon carries a price tag of a whopping $50 million.

Through recombinant DNA, genetic engineers will extract the appropriate genetic material—plasmids—from a virus, inject it into bacteria, and harvest the ensuing bacterial crop to collect interferon. The method will be certainly cost effective, reducing the price of obtaining the wonder drug some 10 billion times.

Cloned Antibodies

By engineering certain mouse and human cells, geneticists are cloning antibodies—monoclonal antibodies. Monoclonal antibodies are uniform, pure, and reproducible, making them extremely versatile in researching cancer, heart disease, multiple sclerosis, viruses, immunity disorders, and many kinds of body functions. In a more active role, these man-made fighters for the immune system are being injected into patients to fight cancer and desensitize allergies.

Furthermore, valuable drugs are being made even more valuable by the purifying feats of monoclonal antibodies. By mixing interferon with its antibody, scientists have purified interferon 5,000 times in one step.

The Supergene, Outstanding in Its Field

In the human body, an average of 3,000 genes—giant molecules that code for the production and maintenance of living cells—occupy the length of a single chromosome, the rod-shaped carrier of heredity. Most of these genes individually code for a different body characteristic or function; some act in concert to do the same; while others apparently have no function at all, perhaps having been carried over for millions of years as an evolutionary microvestige, no longer useful in the human scheme of things.

All genes and their functions (or nonfunctions) occupy their respective places on chromosomes and can therefore be "mapped." An example of genetic mapping is the gene that causes color blindness and hemophilia. This gene is normally found on the chromosome commonly recognized and referred to by scientists as the "X" chromosome —one of the chromosomes involved in sexual determination. To date, scientists have mapped well over 100 genes.

One complex DNA cluster that stands out among the mapped genes is the Supergene. It is found on the scientifically designated sixth chromosome and represents about one thousandth of the total amount of DNA in the cell.

The Supergene does the job of 50 genes. It figures decisively in the acceptance or rejection of organ transplants; determines to a great extent the body's immune system; influences our vulnerability to certain cancers; helps determine the rate at which people age; influences chemical communication and mating behavior between members of a species, and more.

So distinctive is its makeup that, in one case, the Supergene was used to prove that fraternal twins actually had 2 different fathers.

Thoughts to Make You Recoil

An "antiaging" drug is emerging from biotechnology as scientists observe the coiling idiosyncracies of DNA.

The body is made up of tens of trillions of cells. Each normal body cell contains a nucleus and each nucleus houses 46 chromosomes, each of which in turn contains some 3,000 genes.

About 13 feet (4 meters) of DNA occupy each cell. To do this inside a space of only 20 microns (1/1,250 of an inch) requires a highly sophisticated form of packing—coiling. Coiling forms a double helix, which in turn wraps itself around beads of protein to form a "super helix." This super helix coils itself into a "super-super helix," which is also coiled.

Laser studies show that such coiling induces stress along the DNA double helix. Further evidence by laser microbeams shows that damage to the helix may result from this stress; but, to a certain extent, the body can repair this damage.

Scientists now believe that aging sets in when the body fails to repair the supercoiling damage. This also leads to a decrease in DNA supercoiling.

Tests are being devised to identify drugs that promote DNA supercoiling, or the repair of supercoiling damage. In time, you may be able to purchase a drug that may indeed recharge your batteries by recoiling your genes.

FUTURE BODY, FUTURE MIND

Computer Doc

If medicine is any indication of how computers are taking over society, then future societies may see silicon doctors instead of human doctors.

Computers in medicine provide three-dimensional viewing for imaging devices like CAT and NMR, are storage and retrieval systems

High-tech medicine is dependent on the computer revolution for its progress. This machine, the SMAC-20 (Sequential Multiple Analysis Computer), can rapidly analyze 20 different substance levels in a blood sample at one time. Courtesy National Institutes of Health.

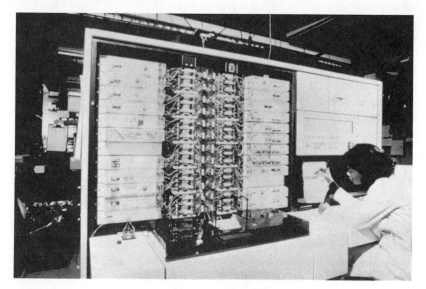

for medical research, automate clinical laboratories, analyze 20 different chemical compounds of the blood at once, simulate the heart, assist the pharmacist with patient drug histories, provide simulation of giant molecules like DNA, are surgical tools, act as microprocessors for artificial limbs and organs, and even give dentists three-dimensional images of teeth from as few as 8 differently angled X rays. But the following application perhaps gives the best example of the computer's role in medicine today and tomorrow.

A patient in discomfort will call a computerized doctor's office, dialing a specific code number for identification in addition to the doctor's phone number. The computer will answer the phone, at the same time retrieving the patient's file using the ID number. The computer will ask the patient to describe his particular affliction; then, based on that information plus the patient's medical history, the computer will recommend the appropriate treatment and transmit a prescription to a computerized data-linked pharmacy.

The dialogue between computer and patient will be so realistic that the latter will be unaware that the voice on the other end is not that of a human, but that of a computer.

Low-Invasive Scouring and Vacuuming

Doctors must often remove tissues from the body for examination—biopsy—in order to know the extent of organ damage. This form of invasive diagnosis could be drastically reduced over the next 25 years, with the use of computerized imaging devices like NMR and PETT that provide doctors with computerized pictures of the potentially diseased organ without conducting a biopsy.

Another form of highly invasive medical treatment, open-heart bypass surgery, could be performed by the less invasive technique of using a laserscope. The laserscope, still in the testing stages, beams light through one channel of a dual-channel catheter to scour plaque from the inside walls of the coronary artery, while the catheter's other channel vacuums up the vapor and debris.

Brain Mending

Scientists may someday transplant healthy brain tissue into brains of humans with damaged tissue. The transplant could substitute good, functional neurons for neurons whose failure to secrete hormones causes disease.

There are several possible sources for brain-tissue transplants. One is neuroblastomas—tumors made up of primitive nerve cells in children. Since these nerve cells can be cultured or frozen alive for a long time, scientists may be able to make them grow into mature nerve cells, making them a good source of transplant material.

Another donor source could be, depending on the disorder, the patient himself. In Sweden, one man who had Parkinson's disease donated one of his adrenal glands to himself. Surgeons removed the gland, extracted the cells that can also produce dopamine, and reimplanted them in the brain.

Brain transplants using tiny portions of tissue from monkey brains will probably raise many ethical questions. But this form of transplant is more feasible than it might sound at first because hormones and proteins like vasopressin and hemoglobin that are secreted by monkey neurons are identical in molecular structure to those of humans. And because the brain is immunologically tolerant—the donor can be unrelated to the recipient and the transplanted tissue will still take—doctors are confident they can transplant brain tissue from monkeys into brains of humans without bad reactions. Allowing monkeys to help man could correct such disorders as diabetes insipidus, Alzheimer's and Parkinson's diseases, epilepsy, paralyses following strokes, even loss of certain senses due to brain damage.

It would mean that man could borrow tissue from his evolutionary past of 30 million years ago to help make his future body.

Will You Need an Artificial Body Part?

The artificial body parts business is big, and it will get bigger as people live longer and infant mortality continues to decline. As of 1980, 3 million metal, ceramic, and plastic body parts have been installed to patch up some of the United States' 14 million amputees and victims of cerebral palsy, spinal deformities, muscular dystrophy, multiple sclerosis, Parkinson's disease, and disabling arthritis.

Based on the present trend, your chance of wearing an artificial body part somewhere, sometime in the next 20 years is about 1 in 12.

Drugs that Self-Destruct

Early in the twenty-first century, drugs housed in plastic and released via magnetic command will be implanted in patients for timed release into their bodies. After a period of time, these time-release implants will gradually erode—self-destruct—with the housing being absorbed and expelled by the body, eliminating surgical excision. While they will increase the physician's ability to deliver drugs to the patient in the most effective way, implantable self-destruct drugs may turn syringes, pills, and capsules into museum pieces.

Out-of-This-World Drugs

America's space shuttle missions promise to lower the high healthcare costs for diabetics. Experiments in zero gravity performed on the shuttle *Challenger* while it orbited the earth in the summer of 1983 were successful in separating and purifying the highly coveted pancreatic islet cells—those that make insulin—from the exocrine cells.

The reason is the absence of gravitational influence on the cell-purification process. Without gravity, the cells won't settle when they are suspended in the separating medium; purification is therefore more efficient and less expensive, yielding 400 times more product in space than on earth.

In addition to purifying the insulin-producing cells of the pancreas, other substances like the pituitary gland's growth hormone, used to treat skin burns, will also be extracted in space-orbiting labs. The potential for highly efficient commercial manufacturing of drugs and hormones in the next 10 years will be "far out."

Brainy Orgasms

The pleasure centers of the brain can be electronically stimulated when electrical current-carrying electrodes are attached to these sites with accuracy. In a few decades, this fact may allow people to buy bunches of orgasms simply by pressing a button on a control box. The sex machine Woody Allen envisioned in his film *Sleeper* could become a reality.

A Big Step for Paralytics

Good news is on the horizon for paraplegics from scientists at Stanford University and Chicago's Illinois Institute of Technology.

Stanford scientists may be on the verge of using certain nerve-regenerating proteins from skin and muscles to regenerate damaged

---

342

brain and spinal-cord nerves. When nerve cells are damaged, Schwann cells—cells that form a sheath around nerves of skin and muscle—manufacture nerve-regenerating proteins. These Schwann cells are absent in brain and spinal-cord nerves; but doctors believe that providing the Schwann-cell-produced proteins to damaged central nerves could stimulate their regrowth.

Chicago bioengineers, relying on their knowledge that walking involves a complicated interaction of gait and swing in the torso and upper limbs, have connected upper-back-attached electrodes to a microprocessor, which in turn was hooked up to electric stimulators on the patient's legs. When the patient moves his upper body, the electrodes capture signals measuring 1 millivolt each. The microprocessor amplifies this tiny signal to 80 to 100 volts. Only $1/3,333$ of a second long, each pulse occurs 10 to 30 times a second, and goes unnoticed in the patient. But the current is enough to turn on the previously paralyzed muscles to walk and make that big first step toward freedom from wheelchair confinement.

In the next decade, about 2,000 paraplegics could be walking again, thanks to giant leaps in nerve research and bioengineering.

The Complete Human Genome Catalog

Gene researchers are currently feeding a central computerized data base with a cataloging of genes for their specific location in the human body cell's 46 chromosomes as well as for their chemical makeup and particular sequences of nucleotides. If the average rate of 4 genes per month continues, scientists will have the gene sequences of all the human chromosomes—the complete human genome—determined before the end of the twentieth century.

Genetic Preventive Maintenance

Although genetic engineers are presently involved in splicing genes to produce disease fighters like interferon, insulin, and human growth hormone, they will someday be capable, in tandem with doctors, of practicing genetic preventive maintenance so that future generations will not inherit diseases like Down's syndrome, sickle-cell anemia, and certain types of cancer, all of which presently affect some tens of millions of people worldwide. This might be accomplished by scientists first referring to a central data base, then altering the sex cells of the parent—carrier of the disorder—by substituting a good gene for a

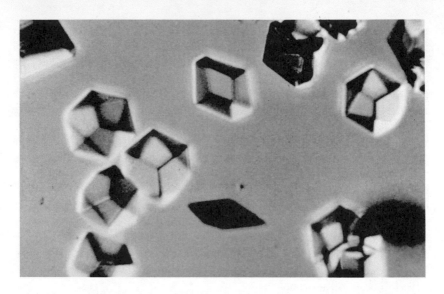

Magnification of the first human insulin crystals created by recombinant DNA technology. Humulin®, the man-made insulin produced by Eli Lilly and Company, was the first commercial product for human health care created by high-tech DNA. Courtesy Eli Lilly and Company.

harmful gene. Alteration of unwanted DNA could also be done to ovum and sperm cells of the test-tube baby during its early embryonic stages.

This kind of DNA manipulation could be more desirable than cloning. (Cloning is the duplication of a biological organism such as a human being by replacing the nucleus of an egg cell with one from the organism being duplicated.) Using the gene-splicing technology for genetic preventive maintenance, man could control the evolution of his own gene pool for the first time in history, eventually elevating his physical self to higher biological states of perfection.

By producing clones instead, man would only be carbon-copying his imperfect self.

Genetic Predestination

Around the turn of the next century, in addition to being able to clone bodies and practice genetic preventive maintenance, genetic engineers could attempt to produce the ideal body and mind. A market of genetically manipulated body cells could exist for people desiring their offspring to be such social paragons as accomplished artists, revered

GLIMPSES FROM NOW:

politicians, or sports idols—all brought to fruition by test-tube fertilization and surrogate mothering. If society allows this practice of ectogenesis to spread, a type of oversight group—a committee of creation—could be established to determine if the fetus is genetically suitable for inclusion in the human race.

Complex ethical and social considerations make such a practice extremely unlikely to be accepted by society. Who of us would have wanted such a committee deciding on whether we were to be or not to be?

Vestigial Man, Developed Man

Just what might man look and sound like 14 million years from now?

Experts speculate that our eyes and ears could be twice their present size due to the ever-increasing amounts of information those sense organs are required to absorb. Our noses, however, will diminish in size because the hairs of our nostrils will lose their function in not having to scent prey and warm incoming currents of cool air while we live in an atmosphere of constant air conditioning. Our jaws and teeth could get smaller because we won't have to grasp and tear soft food. But our palate, larynx, and tongue could get bigger to accommodate our speed in conversing to exchange huge blocks of information—a zany dialogue similar to revving up the tape recorder by switching it to the next highest speed setting.

Future Fatheads?

Experts disagree on what our cranial size will be in the far future.

Some say that man will develop a much bigger head than he presently has so he can retain much more information than now. Others insist, however, that the human hat size will stay about the same as long as women continue to deliver their newborn at the pelvis; a greatly increased skull size would make childbirth as we know it impossible.

Besides, experts say, why worry about needing a bigger housing for the brain when, after all these 14 million years of human evolution, our brains are still working at only 10 percent capacity!

Our Height Advantage Has Its Limits

If it took 12 million years for man to double his height from that of Ramapithecus—one of the earliest known human predecessors of Homo sapiens—does it mean that at the end of another 12 million years his height will be 13 feet?

Assuming man's body proportions stay the same, then 13 feet will not be a height advantage, since his weight would have increased 10 times while the cross-sectional area of a support member like the thigh would have increased only 4½ times. This would make man a rather unwieldy creature, reverting him to the former status of walking on all fours—a definite negative evolutionary trait contrary to previously positive developments in the line of evolution.

The more accepted view by experts is that man will reach his optimum height—7, or possibly 8, feet—in 2 million years, thereby preserving the present rules of basketball for another 2,000 millennia.

Society's Future Brains

Both kinds of brains—human and electronic computer—have passed through stages of evolution. The human brain's evolution from that of Homo erectus (containing basic survival instructions on thirst, flight from danger, hunger, reproduction, and parental caring) to Homo sapiens (where the old brain is still active but is now covered by the cerebral cortex—seat of memory, learning, and abstract thinking) took 400 million years. And because it has remained essentially unchanged for the last 100,000 years, the evolution of the human brain as we know it is, in all probability, finished.

The modern computer, on the other hand, has only evolved in the last 25 years—from the silicon-chip IBM 360 computer of 1960 to the microchip computers of today.

Now, scientists speculate that, by implanting in the brain electrodes carrying microvoltages of electricity, the day is not far off when man could hook his own brain up with a computer. Such a silicon-carbon computer hybrid could lead to an eventual transfer of the mind to the metallic lattices of the computer, paving the way for New Immortal Man, able to roam the galaxies for a million years without the constraints of his present biological housing.

GLIMPSES FROM NOW:

End of an Era

For the last 100,000 years, the human brain has been weighing in at 3 pounds, taking up 1/10 of a cubic foot in volume, and consuming the electrical energy output of a 25-watt light bulb. With these modest packaging dimensions, the human brain is still able to contain from 10 billion to 100 billion items of information.

In the last 30 years, the size, weight, and electronic brain capacity of the artificial computer brain have changed radically.

The model computer of the early-generation computers was the IBM 360. It occupied hundreds of cubic feet, used 100,000 watts of electrical energy, and had a memory of a few million items of information. If the IBM 360 computer in 1960 were to equal the human brain in terms of information capacity, it would have occupied most of the space of the Empire State Building, cost some $500 million, and consumed 1 billion watts of electrical energy. Such was the crudeness of artificial intelligence in 1960, achieved, by the way, with tiny silicon chips, which had replaced the 2 previous generations of bulky computer hardware made up of transistors and vacuum tubes.

Since then, the speed of computers has been doubling every 2 years. Today's supercomputers can do up to 160 million calculations per second and be housed in the space of a small bookshelf. Using the technique called massive parallelism, each of the computer's processing elements connects to 2 others below it in a binary treelike fashion until 1 million elements are wired together after only 19 levels of branching.

By 1995, in line with their past history of evolution, computers will catch up to the human brain in terms of electronic brain capacity. Using 20 watts of power, these artificial forms of intelligence will house 10 billion facts in a box the size of a briefcase, possibly marking the start of a new era of silicon-based life—and ending the era dominated by carbon-chemistry life as we know it.

A Biochip Revolution?

The brain of Homo sapiens is the result of 400 million years of evolving nerve tissue, neuron layer by neuron layer, through the trial and error of natural selection. Now, in less than 2 decades, the artificial intelligence of computers has evolved to its number-crunching state by quadrupling its computing power on a single silicon chip every 3 to 4 years.

In another decade, the computer could evolve from silicon electronics to organic, living electronics if a recent technology known as the biochip proves successful. Growing and thriving as an implant in human brain tissue (providing that metal electrodes can be made compatible with tissue), the biochip could mean sight for the blind, sound for the deaf, and feeling and use of limbs for the paralyzed. In the far future the biochip could begin a new evolutionary spiral for the human brain in terms of the brain's own capacity to accumulate and manipulate information.

The biochip results from the latest efforts of scientists who are constantly striving for new breakthroughs in computer technology—not that the computer's evolution up until now is anything less than remarkable. For 18 years the number of transistors in the computer's integrated circuit doubled from 1 in 1959 to 262,144 (2^{18}) in 1977. Then, in the late 1970s, the trend slowed down until 1981, when Hewlett-Packard announced a chip with more than 600,000 "on-off" binary elements.

Even with that amazing number, the computer's electronic technology still pales in comparison with nature's modus operandi. Just a single green plant leaf has 10 million more electronic elements at the atomic level per square millimeter than the best current silicon chip.

In a biochip, metal and silicon are replaced with protein molecules, using a combination of microminiaturization and the mechanism of DNA. This technology of molecular electronics may prove to be man's answer to nature's green-leaf circuitry. The making of a biochip starts with strategic protein synthesis. Genetically engineered DNA is inserted into *E. coli* or other bacteria which in turn make the right protein for the biochip. A single protein layer is placed on a glass slide and covered with a very thin plastic called a resist, which is then bombarded with electron beams that dig grooves 1/7,100 of an inch (3.5 microns, about half the diameter of a red blood cell) wide in its surface. The protein sandwich is finally dipped in silver, coating the grooves which become the microscopic wires for the biochip's organic circuitry. It amounts to laying down slivers of silver on protein, resulting in protein-sized conductors.

The protein molecules have the same switching, oscillatory, and storage behavior as the silicon transistors of a chip, but hydrogen atoms from the protein's amino-acid group are used to spur free electrons through the protein's latticework, the biochip's molecular mainframe. The electron's rate of movement constitutes electrical current, and information is passed on in a way similar to an electron's motion along the micropathways of a silicon chip's integrated circuit. Scientists estimate that the biochip will be able to compute 1 million times faster than today's best chip.

Future Brain

The biochip could be ideal for brain implantation to help the handicapped. The brain-implanted molecular computer could stimulate, for example, the brain's visual-cortex cells of a blind person. Scientists have already placed platinum electrodes on the visual cortex of a blind person, enabling him to see the faintest outline of shapes. But the electrodes are too big to affect single nerve cells. A type of biochip now on the drawing board will offer 10,000 microelectrodes that would enmesh with individual nerve cells. The microelectrodes would then hook up to a tiny video camera mounted on the blind person's glasses to send digitized signals back to the nerve cells, a setup that could make artificial sight a thousand times more accurate than today's crude platinum electrodes.

If and when the organic computer known as the biochip reaches this stage of brain-implantation development, the revolution will have begun. Working to help the brain calculate faster and react sooner, the biochip could troubleshoot and prevent body breakdowns such as heart attacks, strokes, and the spread of cancer. Its microsize would enable man to store 1 million billion elements per cubic centimeter, meaning that all the memory elements of every computer made up to now could be had in a cube 1 centimeter on a side.

Present-day biochips have conductive velocities 1 million times faster than that of human nerve cells, and circuit switches 100 million times faster than those of human nerve junctions. This is only a beginning. It is estimated that before the millennium runs out, a biochip called a soliton, 1 billionth of a meter wide, could compute in less than 1 trillionth of a second. Scientists envision a day when such a computer would be implanted in the brain to infiltrate the brain tissue, living with it and learning from it. Such a brain-fused biochip "computer" possessing three-dimensional circuits, increased speed, less energy consumption, and microdimensions, could be the consciousness jewel of humankind, the new brain, containing the collective knowledge of planet earth.

Selected Bibliography

BOOKS

Asimov, Isaac. *The Genetic Code.* New York: Orion Press, 1971.

———. *The Human Body: Its Structure and Operation.* New York: New American Library, 1963.

———. *The Human Brain: Its Capacities and Functions.* New York: New American Library, 1965.

Berkow, Robert, ed. *The Merck Manual of Diagnosis and Therapy.* 14th ed. Rahway, New Jersey: Merck and Company, Inc., 1982.

Bernstein, Ellen, ed. *1983 Medical and Health Annual.* Chicago: Encyclopaedia Britannica, Inc., 1982.

———. *1984 Medical and Health Annual.* Chicago: Encyclopaedia Britannica, Inc., 1983.

Blakeslee, Thomas R. *The Right Brain.* Garden City, New York: Anchor Press/ Doubleday, 1980.

Bush, Patricia J. *Drugs, Alcohol, and Sex.* New York: Richard Marek Publishers, 1980.

Calvin, William H., and George A. Ojemann. *Inside The Brain.* New York: New American Library, 1980.

Davis, Goode P., Jr., and Edwards Park. *The Heart: The Living Pump.* Washington, D.C.: U.S. News Books, 1981.

The Diagram Group. *Man's Body: An Owner's Manual.* New York: Bantam Books, Inc., 1976.

———. *Sex: A User's Manual.* New York: G. P. Putnam's Sons, 1981.

Editors of Time-Life Books. *A Commonsense Guide to Sex, Birth & Babies.* Alexandria, Virginia: Time-Life Books, 1981.

Fishbein's Illustrated Medical and Health Encyclopedia (24 Volumes). Westport, Connecticut: H. S. Stuttman, Inc., 1981.

Fisher, Arthur. *The Healthy Heart.* Alexandria, Virginia: Time-Life Books, 1981.

Guiness Book of World Records-1982 Edition. New York: Bantam Books, Inc., 1982.

Guyton, Arthur C. *Textbook of Medical Physiology.* 6th ed. Philadelphia: W. B. Saunders Company, 1981.

Hafez, E. S. E., ed. *Scanning Electron Microscopy of Human Reproduction.* Ann Arbor, Michigan: Ann Arbor Science, 1978.

Hecht, Jeff, and Dick Teresi. *Laser: Supertool of the 1980s.* New Haven, Connecticut: Ticknor & Fields, 1982.

Hopson, Janet L. *Scent Signals.* New York: William Morrow & Co., 1979.

Jastrow, Robert. *The Enchanted Loom: Mind in the Universe.* New York: Simon & Schuster, 1981.

Jensen, Karen. *Reproduction: The Cycle of Life.* Washington, D.C.: U.S. News Books, 1981.

Kessel, Richard G., and Randy H. Kardon. *Tissues and Organs.* San Francisco: W. H. Freeman and Company, 1979.

Le Vay, David. *Human Anatomy and Physiology.* Sevenoaks, Kent, England: Hodder and Stoughton, 1981.

Ludwig, H., and H. Metzger. *The Human Female Reproductive Tract.* Berlin, Germany: Springer-Verlag Berlin Heidelberg New York, 1976.

Lygre, David G. *Life Manipulation.* New York: Walker & Company, 1979.

Lynch, Wilfred. *Implants: Reconstructing the Human Body.* New York: Van Nostrand Reinhold Company, Inc., 1982.

Madison, Arnold. *Transplanted and Artificial Body Organs.* New York: Beaufort Books, Inc., 1981.

McCary, James Leslie. *Human Sexuality.* New York: D. Van Nostrand Company, 1973.

Merkin, Gabe, and Marshall Hoffman. *The Sportsmedicine Book.* Boston: Little, Brown & Company, 1978.

Miller, Jonathan. *The Body in Question.* Boston: Little, Brown & Company, 1982.

Montagu, Ashley. *Touching: The Human Significance of Skin.* 2nd ed. New York: Harper & Row, 1978.

Moore, Francis. *Transplant: The Give and Take of Tissue Transplantation.* New York: Simon & Schuster, 1972.

Morgan, Chris. *Future Man?* New York: Irvington, 1980.

Murphy, Wendy. *Touch, Taste, Smell, Sight and Hearing.* Alexandria, Virginia: Time-Life Books, 1981.

NIA. *Changes . . . research on aging and the aged.* Bethesda, Maryland: National Institute on Aging, Department of Health and Human Services, 1980. NIH 81-85.

———. *Special Report on Aging 1982.* Bethesda, Maryland: Department of Health and Human Services, 1982.

Nicogossian, Arnaud E., and James F. Parker, Jr. *Space Physiology and Medicine.* Washington, D.C.: National Aeronautics and Space Administration, Scientific and Technical Information Branch, 1982. NASA SP-447.

Nilsson, Lennart. *Behold Man.* Boston: Little, Brown & Company, 1974.

———. *A Child Is Born.* New York: Delacorte Press/Seymour Lawrence, 1980.

Nourse, Alan E. *The Body.* Alexandria, Virginia: Time-Life Books, 1980.

Page, Jake. *Blood: The River of Life.* Washington, D.C.: U.S. News Books, 1981.

Panati, Charles. *Breakthroughs.* New York: Berkley Books, 1981.

Pask, Gordon, and Susan Curran. *Micro Man.* New York: MacMillan, 1982.

Pines, Maya. *Medicines and You.* Bethesda, Maryland: National Institute of General Medical Sciences, Department of Health and Human Services, 1981. NIH 81-2140.

Podolsky, Doug M. *Skin: The Human Fabric.* Washington, D.C.: U.S. News Books, 1981.

Ratcliff, J. D. *"I Am Joe's Body."* New York: Berkley Books, 1980.

Rayner, Claire. *Everything Your Doctor Would Tell You If He Had The Time.* New York: G. P. Putnam's Sons, 1980.

Restak, Richard M. *The Brain: The Last Frontier.* Garden City, New York: Double-day & Company, Inc., 1979.

Rothenberg, Robert E. *The New American Medical Dictionary and Health Manual.* New York: New American Library, 1975.

Steen, Edwin B., and Ashley Montagu. *Anatomy and Physiology* (Vols. 1 and 2). New York: Barnes & Noble Books, 1959.

Thomas, Clayton L., ed. 14th ed. *Taber's Cyclopedic Medical Dictionary.* Philadel-phia: F. A. Davis Company, 1981.

Thomson, William A. R. *Black's Medical Dictionary.* 32nd ed. New York: Harper & Row, 1979.

The United States Pharmacopeial Convention, Inc. 1983 USP DI, Vol. I: *Drug Information for the Health Care Provider.* Rockville, Maryland, 1982.

————. 1983 USP DI, Vol. II: *Advice for the Patient.* Rockville, 1982.

Wagman, Richard J., ed. *The New Complete Medical and Health Encyclopedia* (4 Volumes). Chicago: J. G. Ferguson Publishing Company, 1977.

Watson, James D. *The Double Helix.* New York: New American Library, 1969.

Wertenbaker, Lael. *The Eye: Window to the World.* Washington, D.C.: U.S. News Books, 1981.

Wilentz, Joan. *The Senses of Man.* New York: T. Y. Crowell, 1968.

Wingate, Peter. *The Penguin Medical Encyclopedia.* Harmondsworth, Middlesex, England: Penguin Books, 1979.

The World Almanac and Book of Facts 1983. New York: Newspaper Enterprise Association, Inc., 1982.

The World Book Illustrated Home Medical Encyclopedia (4 Volumes). Chicago: World Book-Childcraft International, Inc., 1980.

PERIODICALS

The following magazines and newsletters were often consulted.

American Health: Fitness of Body and Mind. American Health Partners, New York, N.Y.

America's Health. World Wide Medical Press, Inc., New York, N.Y.

Bulletin of Bureau of Pharmaceutical Services. School of Pharmacy, University of Mississippi, University, Mississippi.

Digestive Diseases Clearinghouse Fact Sheet. Centers for Disease Control, Depart-ment of Health and Human Services, Atlanta, Georgia.

FDA Consumer. Food and Drug Administration, Washington, D.C.

The Harvard Medical School Health Letter. Department of Continuing Education, Harvard Medical School, Cambridge, Mass.

Health. Family Media, Inc., New York, N.Y.

JAMA, Journal of the American Medical Association, Chicago, Ill.

Medical Hotline. Medical News Associates, New York, N.Y.

Medical World News. HEI Publishing, Inc., New York, N.Y.

Morbidity and Mortality Weekly Report. Centers for Disease Control, Department of Health and Human Services, Atlanta, Georgia.

News & Features from NIH. National Institutes of Health, Bethesda, Md.

The NIH Record. Division of Public Information, The National Institutes of Health, Bethesda, Md.

OMNI. Omni Publications International Ltd., New York, N.Y.

Research Resources Reporter. Division of Research Resources, National Institutes of Health, Bethesda, Md.

Science Digest. The Hearst Corporation, New York, N.Y.

Science News. Science Service, Inc., Washington, D.C.

Science Times. Section of *The New York Times.* New York, N.Y.

Yale-New Haven Hospital Health News Service. New Haven, Connecticut.

Index

Italicized page numbers indicate references to illustrations

Accidents and shift work, 295
Acetylcholine, 19–20
Acupuncture, 95
"Adam's apple," 180
  See also Larynx
Adaptation of pain receptors, 59
Adenoids, 171, 180–81
Adrenal gland, 16, 17
Afterimages, 39, 41
Aging, 278–85
  and bladder control, 199
  and bone loss, 118–19
  and breathing rate, 161
  and diabetes, 194
  and DNA coiling, 338–39
  and drug pharmacokinetics, 284–85
  and dryness of mouth, 177
  and hearing loss, 53
  and intelligence, 14–15, 279–80
  and lung capacity, 174
  and muscle strength, 111–12
  premature, 280–81
  and sleep requirements, 280
  and surgery, 283
  and taste loss, 61
  and testosterone production, 213
  and tremors, 93
  and weight gain, 276
Air pollutants and breathing, 167–70
Albumin, 142–43
Alcohol consumption
  and cold stress, 287
  and dreaming, 27–28
  and drug interactions, 265
  and jaundice, 192
  and sex, 215
  and urine production, 199
  and vitamin deficiencies, 265
Alimentary canal. *See* Digestive system
Allergies, 171, 216, 286
Alveoli, *162,* 163, 165, *255*
Ambergris, 72
  See also Musk
Ammonia in urine, 200

Amnion, 242
Amniotic fluid, 242–43
Amotivational syndrome and marijuana
  use, 268
Amputation and phantom limb
  sensation, 93
Amyand, Claudius, 202
Anabolic steroids, 268, 270
  See also Testosterone
Anemia, 146, 165, 177
Anesthetics, 90
Anger and heart disease, 125–26
Angina, 128, 140
Angioplasty, 127–30, *132,* 146
Antacids, 275
Antagonism of drugs, 263
Antibiotics, 260, 275
Antibodies, 148, 286, 336
Antigens, 147, 286, 301
Anus, 186, *187*
  hemorrhoids of, 203–4
Anxiety and pain, 92
Aorta, 153, *154*
Apnea, 173, 280
Apollo moon program and heart
  disease, 126
Appendix, *187,* 202
Aqueous humor, 35, 38
Arm
  electronic, 304
  nerves of, 79
Arteries, replacements for, 302, 307–8
Arteriosclerosis, 157–58, 220
Arthroscope, 114
Artificial body parts, 304–13, *310,* 341
Artificial flavors, 65
Artificial insemination, 236–37
Artificial respiration, 160
Aspirin and heart disease, 140–41
Asthma and biofeedback, 87
Athletes
  "bonking," 293
  and heat exhaustion, 290
  "hitting the wall," 292–93

leg pain and breathing pattern, 163–64

motor nerve performance, 87–89

salt consumption, 276–77

Auditory nerve, 47, *48*

Auscultation, 163

Autonomous nervous system, 84, 86, 87–88, 93

Axons, 8–9, 11–13, 81

Baby Fae, 303

Back pain, 90–92

Bacteria, 104

Bad breath, 176

Balance

disorders of, 49, 50–51

mechanisms of, 51–52

Balloon heart surgery. *See* Angioplasty

Bedwetting, 199

"Bends," the, 165

Beta-blockers, 139–40

See also Heart, drugs for

Beta cells of pancreas, 193–94

Bile, 186, 190, 191–92

Biochip, 347–49

See also Computer technology

Biofeedback, 86–87

Biopsy, 340

Birth control devices

vaginal ring, 227

vaginal sponge, 228

Birth control pills, 224–27, *225*

and jaundice, 192

for men, 228–30

and pheromone production, 70

risk with smoking, 266

Bitterness, 62

Bladder, 199–200

Bloch, Felix, 329

Blood, 141–53

color and oxygenation, 164

composition of, 142

plasma, 142–43, 165

synthetic, 144–46, 304

Blood-brain barrier, 15

Blood cells

platelets, 145, *151*, 151–53, *152*

production of, 115, 147

red, *142*, 143–44, *145*, 165

white, *145*, 146–50

Blood clots, *151, 152*

Blood pressure, 125, 220

Blood sugar

and fructose, 278

liver control of, 190–91

and pancreatic function, 193

"Blue bloods," 164

Body odor, 69, 74

Body temperature and sleep, 26

Bone, 112–19

composition of, 112

growth and anabolic steroids, 270

marrow. *See* Marrow

Bones

hyoid, 113

sesamoid, 113–14

Brain, 1–24

chemistry, 18–23

computer images, *36*, 325, *326*

electrical energy in, 9–10

electrode recording of, 3, *5*

electronic link with computer, 18

fluid retention affecting, 219

future evolution of, 7, 345

nerve-cell connections, 8–9, *9*. *See also* Axons; Dendrites; Neurons

pacemaker for, 304

prenatal development, 1–2

reaction time in vision, 37

size and age, 14–15

structures, *4, 6*

surgery, prenatal, 248, *249*

tissue transplants, 2–3, *16*, 16–17, 340–41

Brain stem, 8

Breast, artificial, 304, *305, 310*

Breathing

description, 159–61

styles of, 171–72

voluntary and involuntary, 166–67

See also Lungs

Bronchioles, 163

Brown, Louise, 232

Bruxism, 175–76

Burns

and artificial skin, 103–4

and kidney damage, 197

Caffeine

as diuretic, 198

and hearing, 53

and intoxication, 271

Calcium

in bones, 112, 118

in kidney stones, 201

Calcium blockers, 140

See also Heart, drugs for

Cancer, 225, *262*

Capillaries, 40, 155–56

Carbon dioxide, 165, 166

Carbon monoxide poisoning, 146

Carr, Elizabeth Jordan, 231

Carrel, Alexis, 300

Cartilage, 112

CAT scanner, 323–24

Central nervous system (CNS) disorders, 15–16

Cerebral cortex, *4*, 4–5

Chest, nerves of, 79

Chin, artificial, 306

Heart disease
  aspirin for, 140–41
  risk factors, 125–26
  and sleep apnea, 280
Heart-lung machine, *130, 131*
Heat, sensation of, 60
  See also Touch
Heat exhaustion, 277, 290
Heatstroke, 289–90
Hemispheres, brain, 4–7, 26–27
Hemoglobin, 144, 336
Hemorrhoids, 203–4
Hepatitis, 192
Hiccuping, 93, 178–79
Hip, artificial, 308, *310*
Hippocampus, *4,* 23
Hormonal implants, 227
Hormones
  in birth control pills, 225, 226
  and brain structures, 4–5
  and fluid retention, 219
  human growth hormone (hGH), 285–86
  and impotence, 219–20
  and menopause, 282–83
  and premenstrual syndrome (PMS), 217
  and prostate enlargement, 203
  taste and smell, effect on, 70
  See also Estrogen; Testosterone
Hot flashes, 282
Human growth hormone (hGH), 285–86
Hyalin membrane disease. *See*
  Respiratory distress syndrome
Hydrocephalus, 248
Hydroxylapatite (HA), 309
Hyoid bone, 113
Hyperventilation, 173
Hypnosis in pregnancy and labor, 251–52
Hypothalamus, 8, 28
Hypothermia, 287–88

Immune system, 286
Immunoglobulins, 286
Immunosuppressant drugs, 303
Impotence, 215–16, 219–20, 221–23
Impotence testing device, 221, *221*
Indigestion, 188–89
Infants
  brain development, 115
  breathing, 170–71
  heart rates, 122
  taste sensitivity, 61
  touch requirements, 57–58
Infections
  of ears, 48–49
  of respiratory tract, 180–81
  of urinary tract, 197
Infertility. *See* Fertility research

Insomnia, 24
Insulin, 192, 193, *331,* 336, *344*
Insulin pumps, 194, 261
Intelligence and aging, 14–15, 279–80
Interferon, 337
Internal clocks, 294–95
Intestinal gas, 188
Intestine, large, 186
Intestine, small, 186, *187,* 192
Intoxication, 271, 290
  See also Alcohol consumption
Inversion therapy, 295–96
In vitro fertilization (IVF), 230–33, *231*
Ion balance in brain, 9
Iris, 32, *33,* 38, 41
Irritable bowel syndrome (IBS), 189
Itching, 58–59, 92–93
  See also Touch

Japan, heart disease in, 125–26
Jarvik, Robert K., 131, 133, 134
Jarvik 7 artificial heart, 131, 133–34, *136, 137, 138*
Jaundice, 192
Jawbone, 115
  artificial, 309
Jet lag, 294
Joints, artificial, 306–9, *310*
Jones, Georgeanna, 231
Jones, Howard, 231

Kegel, Arnold, 209
Kidneys, 194–99, *195,* 260, 276
  artificial, 197–98, 300, 309
Kidney stones, 201–2
Kidney transplants, 300
Klinefelter's syndrome, 244
Knee, artificial, 309, *310*
Kneecap, 113–14
Knee surgery, 114
Kolff, Willem J., 134

Lactose intolerance, 189, 277–78
Larynx, 177, 178, 180, 181, *182*
  artificial, 185, 312–13
  surgery to remove, 184–85
Laser
  research, *321*
  surgery using, 129–30, 315–19, 322, 340
  types of, 319–22
Lashley, Karl, 22
Learning behavior and brain chemistry, 21, 22
Legs
  nerves of, 79. *See also* Sciatic nerves
  pain and breathing pattern, 163–64
Lens, 35–36
Life span, 281
  See also Aging

Neurotransmitters, 18–20, *19, 20,* 97,
     98, 110
Neutrophils, 148–49
     See also Phagocytes
Nicotine
     and hearing, 53
     and heart disease, 125
     lungs, effects on, 169–70
     and urination, 198
     and vitamin deficiencies, 266
Nitroglycerin, 137–38, 261
Nitrous oxide, 90
Nocturnal emissions. *See* Wet dreams
Nocturnal jerk, 24
Nodes of Ranvier, 11
Nose, 74, 306
Nosebleeds, 75
"Nose brain." *See* Limbic system
Nose kiss, 74
Novocain, 90
Nuclear Magnetic Resonance (NMR),
     327–30, *329*
Nutrient absorption, 264
     See also Vitamins

Odors, 67
     See also Smell
"Old mammalian brain." *See* Limbic
     system
Optic nerve, 36–37
Oral contraceptives. *See* Birth control
     pills
Organ transplants. *See* Transplants
Orgasm, 206, 207, 342
Osborne, Charles, 179
Osteoporosis, 118–19, 282–83
Otitis media, 48–49
Oxygen, blood levels of, 173–74

Pacemakers
     in brain, 304
     controlling erection, 94–95
     heart, 135–37, 308
Pain
     as protective function, 89
     receptors, 59
     reduction, 90
     referred, 92
     sensation of, 58–59. *See also* Touch
     types of, 59–60
Palate, 178, *182*
Pancreas, 186, *187,* 192–94
     artificial, 310. *See also* Insulin pump
Parathyroid glands, 112, 118
Parkinson's disease, *16,* 16–17, 93, 341
Patella. *See* Kneecap
Pelvic inflammatory disease (PID), 224
Penile prosthesis, 222–23, *223, 310, 311*
Penis, 212–13, 220
     artificial, 311. *See also* Penile prosthesis

Peptides, 18, 21, 22
Peritonitis, 202
Pert, Candace, 17
PETT scan, *36,* 325, *326*
Phagocytes, 144, 147, 148–49
Phantom limb sensation, 93
Pharmacokinetics, 260, 284–85
Pheromones, 68–69, 73, 214–15
Phosphorus, bone content of, 112
Pituitary gland, 8, 195, 199, 270, 285
Placebos, 259
Plasma, 142–43, 148, 152, 165
Platelets, 145, *151,* 151–53, *152*
Pleura, 172
PMS. *See* Premenstrual syndrome
Poisons, 62, 191, 192
Positive Emission Transverse
     Tomography. *See* PETT
Potentiation of drugs, 262–63
Pregnancy, 251–53
     and caffeine, 271–72
     and nicotine, 271–72
     and urination, 198, 199
     and varicose veins, 157
Premature births, 253–56
Premenstrual syndrome (PMS), 216–19
Prenatal development, 242
     of heart, 124, 243
     of lungs, 254, *255,* 256
     of sex organs, 243–45
     of touch, 53
Prenatal imaging, 245–48
Prenatal surgery, 246–50, *249*
Primrose-oil, 218
Progeria, 280, 281
Prosopagnosia, 23–24
Prostaglandins, 218
Prostate gland, 202–3, 270
     surgery, 94, 222
Puberty, 282
Pubococcygeal (PC) muscle, 208–9
Pulmonary blood vessels, 153
Pulmonary system, 161
     See also Breathing; Lungs
Pupil, 38
Purcell, Edward, 329

Rabies, 303
Radiation sickness, 293–94
Rapid-eye-movement sleep. *See* REM
     sleep
Rectum, 186, *187*
Reflexes, 85
REM sleep
     and bruxism, 176
     and dreaming, 27
     and sexual response, 28-29
     and sleeptalking, 26
Reptilian brain. *See* Brain stem
Respiration. *See* Breathing; Lungs

Respiratory distress syndrome (RDS), 254, 256
"Restaurant coronary," 179
Retina, 33, 34
  surgery to reattach, 31–32, 316
Rhodopsin, 34
Ribonucleic acid. *See* RNA
RNA, 335, *335*
Robinson, James, 203–4
Robotics, 86, 111
Rod cells, 34–35, 38
Roentgen, Wilhelm, 323

Sacher, George, 279
Sacromeres, 124
Salazar, Alberto, 159
Saliva, 63–64, 177, 185
Salt, 64, 276–77
Saltiness, 62
Scabs, 152
  See also Blood clots
Schaie, K. Warner, 279
Schwann cells, 343
Sciatic nerves, 79, 80–81, 82, 85, 87
Sclerotherapy, 157
Scotophobin, 21
Scratching, 92–93
  See also Itching
Semen
  allergy to, 216
  composition of, 239. *See also* Sperm cells
Semicircular canals, 49, 51
Senses, comparison of, 54
Sensory information, screening of, 75
Serotonin, 26, 152
Sex
  and autonomous nervous system, 84
  and blood pressure, 125
  and hypothalamus gland, 8
  nerves controlling, 94
  as remedy for insomnia, 24
Sex differences
  in bladder training, 199–200
  in blood weight, 143
  in bone loss, 118
  in brain structures, 4–5
  in breathing rate, 161
  in larynx size, 180
  in muscle strength, 112
  in muscle weight, 107–8
  in sense of smell, 70
  in sexual response, 94
  in underarm scents, 69
  in vocal cords, 182–83
Sex organs
  muscles of, 111
  prenatal development, 243–45
  See also Penis; Vagina
Sexual cycles, 212
Sexual intercourse, 205–6, 215
Sexual scents. *See* Pheromones

Shaw, William, 314
Shepard, Alan, 50–51
Shunammitism, 73
Sickle-cell anemia, 336
Sight. *See* Color vision; Eyes; Vision
Skin, 100–6
  artificial, 103–4, 312
  laboratory culture of, 104
  sensitivity of, 53–54, 55–56
  shedding of, *102,* 102–3
  thickness of, 103
Skull. *See* Cranium
Sleep, 24–29
  and aging, 280
  body temperature effecting, 26
  death from lack of, 24
Sleeptalking, 25–26
Smell, 66–75
  loss of sensation, 291–92
  memory of, 66, 71
  receptor cells for, 67–68
Smoking. *See* Nicotine
Sneezing, 179–80
Snoring, 178, 280
Sourness, 62
Space adaptation syndrome (SAS), 296–97
Space missions and medical research, 342
Space technology, 37, 158
Sperm banks, 236
Sperm cells, *238,* 238–41, *240*
Spermicide, 228
Sphincters, artificial, 312
Spinal column, 115–17
  and back pain, 90–91, *91*
  parts of, *91*
Spinal cord, 77–79, *78, 79*
  anesthetics of, 90
  damage to, 96–97
Spinal nerves, *80*
Stapedectomy, 49–50
Steptoe, Patrick, 231, 232, 233
Stomach, 186, *187*
Stress, 86–87, 126
Stroke, 87, 146
Stuttering, 181–82
Sulzman, Frank, 294
Surgery
  on elderly patients, 283
  prenatal, 246–50, *249*
Swallowing, 48, 178
Sweat glands, 104–6, *105*
Sweetness, 61–62
Synapses, 12–13, 81–82
Synaptic vesicles, 11

Taste, 60–66
  loss of sensation, 61, 63, 292
Taste buds, 61–63
Taste preference
  changes in, 64

About the Author

NEIL McALEER was born in 1942, in Richmond, Virginia, and now lives in New Cumberland, Pennsylvania. He holds a bachelor's degree from the University of New Mexico and a master's degree in English literature from Southern Illinois University, where he studied under John Gardner, the novelist, and Harry T. Moore.

From 1974 to 1979 he was editorial director of a Pennsylvania publishing house, where he created a successful list of science books, including the best-selling *Colonies in Space,* and established other new publishing directions with such books as *The Beatles Forever.*

His own work includes both fiction and nonfiction. *Earthlove,* a fantasy novel, was his first published book, followed by *The Cosmic Mind-Boggling Book,* a popular science book. Several magazine articles and poems have also been published. *The Body Almanac,* his second nonfiction work, is his third published book, and he is currently working on his fourth book project.